# INTENSITY MODULATED RADIATION THERAPY FOR HEAD AND NECK CANCER

# INTENSITY MODULATED RADIATION THERAPY FOR HEAD AND NECK CANCER

*Editor*

**K.S. CLIFFORD CHAO**

*Associate Professor of Radiation Oncology*
*Washington University School of Medicine*
*St. Louis, Missouri*

*Current affiliation:*
*Associate Professor of Radiation Oncology*
*The University of Texas*
*M.D. Anderson Cancer Center*
*Houston, Texas*

*Assistant Editor*

**GOKHAN OZYIGIT**

*Fellow, Department of Radiation Oncology*
*Washington University School of Medicine*
*St. Louis, Missouri*

*Current affiliation:*
*Research Fellow, Department of Radiation Oncology*
*The University of Texas*
*M.D. Anderson Cancer Center*
*Houston, Texas*

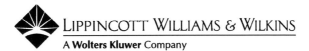

Philadelphia • Baltimore • New York • London
Buenos Aires • Hong Kong • Sydney • Tokyo

*Acquisitions Editor: Jonathan Pine*
*Developmental Editor: Lisa Consoli*
*Production Editor: Robin E. Cook*
*Manufacturing Manager: Colin Warnock*
*Cover Designer: Mark Lerner*
*Compositor: TechBooks*
*Printer: Walsworth*

© 2003 by LIPPINCOTT WILLIAMS & WILKINS
530 Walnut St.
Philadelphia, PA 19106 USA
www.LWW.com

All rights reserved. This book is protected by copyright. No part of this book may be reproduced in any form or by any means, including photocopying, or utilized by any information storage and retrieval system without written permission from the copyright owner, except for brief quotations embodied in critical articles and reviews. Materials appearing in this book prepared by individuals as part of their official duties as U.S. government employees are not covered by the above-mentioned copyright.

Printed in the USA

**Library of Congress Cataloging-in-Publication Data**

Intensity modulated radiation therapy for head and neck cancer / editor, K.S. Clifford Chao ; assistant editor, Gokhan Ozyigit.
    p.  cm.
   Includes bibliographical references and index.
   ISBN 0-7817-4104-1
   1. Head—Cancer—Radiotherapy.   2. Neck—Cancer—Radiotherapy.   I. Chao,
K.S. Clifford.   II. Ozyigit, Gokhan.
   RC280.H4 I46   2002
   616.99′4910642—dc21                           2002028650

Care has been taken to confirm the accuracy of the information presented and to describe generally accepted practices. However, the authors, editors, and publisher are not responsible for errors or omissions or for any consequences from application of the information in this book and make no warranty, expressed or implied, with respect to the currency, completeness, or accuracy of the contents of the publication. Application of this information in a particular situation remains the professional responsibility of the practitioner.

The authors, editors, and publisher have exerted every effort to ensure that drug selection and dosage set forth in this text are in accordance with current recommendations and practice at the time of publication. However, in view of ongoing research, changes in government regulations, and the constant flow of information relating to drug therapy and drug reactions, the reader is urged to check the package insert for each drug for any change in indications and dosage and for added warnings and precautions. This is particularly important when the recommended agent is a new or infrequently employed drug.

Some drugs and medical devices presented in this publication have Food and Drug Administration (FDA) clearance for limited use in restricted research settings. It is the responsibility of the health care provider to ascertain the FDA status of each drug or device planned for use in their clinical practice.

10 9 8 7 6 5 4 3 2 1

*To our patients from whom we have learned to excel.*

*To Helen, David, and Nick whose support has make this project possible.*

# CONTENTS

*Contributing Authors  viii*
*Foreword  ix*
*Preface  xi*
*Acknowledgments  xiii*

**1**  Physics of Intensity Modulated Radiation Therapy for Head
and Neck Cancer  1
*Daniel A. Low*

**2**  CT and MR Imaging of Head and Neck Cancer  18
*Franz J. Wippold II*

**3**  Positron-Emitting Tomography (PET) Imaging in Head and Neck Cancer  30
*Wade L. Thorstad and K.S. Clifford Chao*

**4**  Dose Prescription and Target Delineation for Nodal Volumes  38
*K.S. Clifford Chao*

**5**  Paranasal Sinuses and Nasal Cavity  50
*Gokhan Ozyigit and K.S. Clifford Chao*

**6**  Nasopharynx  68
*K.S. Clifford Chao and Gokhan Ozyigit*

**7**  Oral Cavity  85
*Gokhan Ozyigit and K.S. Clifford Chao*

**8**  Tonsillar Fossa and Faucial Arch  100
*K.S. Clifford Chao and Gokhan Ozyigit*

**9**  Base of the Tongue  114
*K.S. Clifford Chao and Gokhan Ozyigit*

**10**  Hypopharynx  127
*Gokhan Ozyigit and K.S. Clifford Chao*

**11**  Larynx  139
*Gokhan Ozyigit and K.S. Clifford Chao*

**12**  Neck Node Metastasis of Unknown Primary  155
*Gokhan Ozyigit and K.S. Clifford Chao*

**13**  Management of Acute and Late Effects of Radiation Therapy in
Head and Neck Cancers  160
*Gokhan Ozyigit*

*Index  169*

# CONTRIBUTING AUTHORS

**K.S. Clifford Chao, M.D.**
Associate Professor of Radiation Oncology
Washington University School of Medicine
St. Louis, Missouri

*Current affiliation:*
Associate Professor of Radiation Oncology
The University of Texas
M.D. Anderson Cancer Center
Houston, Texas

**Daniel A. Low, Ph.D.**
Associate Professor
Division of Medical Physics
Department of Radiation Oncology
Washington University School of Medicine
St. Louis, Missouri

**Gokhan Ozyigit, M.D.**
Fellow, Department of Radiation Oncology
Washington University School of Medicine
St. Louis, Missouri

*Current affiliation:*
Research Fellow, Department of Radiation Oncology
The University of Texas
M.D. Anderson Cancer Center
Houston, Texas

**Wade L. Thorstad, M.D.**
Instructor
Chief of Head and Neck Science
Department of Radiation Oncology
Washington University School of Medicine
St. Louis, Missouri

**Franz J. Wippold II, M.D., F.A.C.R.**
Associate Professor of Radiology
Chief of Neuroradiology
Mallinckrodt Institute of Radiology
Washington University Medical Center
St. Louis, Missouri

# FOREWORD

Several advances in technology have combined to move radiation oncology into a new era, which I refer to as the three-dimensional (3-D) radiation therapy era. Modern imaging technologies, including x-ray computed tomography (CT) and magnetic resonance imaging (MRI), provide a fully 3-D model of the cancer patient's anatomy that allows radiation oncologists to more accurately identify tumor volumes and their relationship with other critical normal organs. Powerful CT-simulation and three-dimensional radiation therapy treatment planning (3DRTP) systems have been commercially available for over a decade and are rapidly replacing the conventional radiation therapy x-ray simulator and two-dimensional dose planning process as the standard of practice. In addition, the latest generation medical linear accelerators have sophisticated computer-controlled multi-leaf collimators (MLCs) systems that provide beam-intensity modulation features capable of precise shaping of dose distributions.

These technological advances have spurred the implementation of external beam radiation therapy techniques, in which the high-dose region can be conformed much more closely to the target volume than previously possible, thus reducing the volume of normal tissues receiving a high dose. This form of external beam irradiation is referred to as three-dimensional conformal radiation therapy (3DCRT). It generally uses an increased number of radiation beams that are shaped using beams-eye-view planning to conform to the projection of the target volume. The radiation beams normally have a uniform intensity across the field, or, where appropriate, have the intensity modified by simple beam fluence modifying devices like wedges or compensating filters. This form of 3DCRT must now be referred to as "traditional 3DCRT" because a more advanced form of conformal therapy, called intensity modulated radiation therapy (IMRT) has evolved, and appears to be ideally suited for the radiation treatment of head and neck cancer. IMRT can achieve even greater conformity than traditional 3DCRT techniques as a result of the optimization of the radiation beam fluence incident on the patient. Although the technology of IMRT planning and delivery shows great promise, clinical expertise in its use is lagging behind, particularly in the head and neck area, due to the complexity of the target volume(s) shape and the normal tissue anatomy.

It should be understood that IMRT is not just an add-on to the conventional radiation therapy process, or even the traditional 3DCRT process. Rather, it represents a significant change in practice, particularly for the radiation oncologist. The 2-D treatment planning approach emphasizes the use of a conventional x-ray simulator for designing beam portals based on standardized beam arrangement techniques and bony landmarks visualized on planar radiographs. In contrast, IMRT planning emphasizes an image-based virtual simulation approach in defining tumor and critical structure volumes, and requires a detailed specification of the dose prescription including dose and/or dose-volume constraints for the all targets and critical structures for the individual patient, in order to determine the optimized beam fluences.

A critical question is (and always has been) how well the target volume(s) and critical structure volumes can be defined for the cancer patient. For IMRT treatments, the question is even more important, as it is now recognized that IMRT is more sensitive to clinical and geometric uncertainties than conventional radiation therapy because of the sharper dose gradients that were created around target volumes and critical structures. Thus, the IMRT planning process puts new demands on the radiation oncologist to critically specify target volumes and critical structure volumes with far greater accuracy and precision. Moreover, IMRT places new demands on the radiation oncology physicist to insure adequate quality assurance measures are in place, e.g., the need for new precision in tumor imaging, patient set-up reproducibility, organ motion assessment, and treatment delivery verification.

This textbook provides the reader a strong foundation regarding the current state of IMRT in the treatment of head and neck cancer. Beginning with a basic background in IMRT treatment planning and quality assurance and modern imaging modalities, the text continues with pertinent overview of the natural course, lymph node spread, diagnostic criteria, and therapeutic options for each head and neck cancer subsite. Most importantly, practical guidelines on target determination and delineation based on the patterns of primary tumor extension and lymph node spreading are presented.

In summary, it is imperative that the treating physician and physicist fully appreciate the need to account for the clinical target definition and spatial uncertainties in the planning and delivery of a cancer patient's IMRT treatment. The publication of this comprehensive text on the use of IMRT in the treatment of head and neck cancer is especially timely to address these important issues.

*James A. Purdy, Ph.D.*

# PREFACE

Intensity modulated radiation therapy (IMRT) provides an excellent opportunity to improve tumor control and spare normal tissue. It is especially true for head and neck cancers, due to the close proximity of the tumor to the spinal cord, brain stem, parotid glands, and optic pathway structures. While traditional therapies are frequently inadequate in tumor target coverage and normal tissue sparing, IMRT optimizes both. With appropriate clinical input and precise computer algorithms that consider not only target and normal tissue dimensions but also dose-volume constraints, IMRT delivers a better target coverage with steep dose gradient once it reaches surrounding normal tissues. This cutting edge technology is now used not only in academic centers but also in community clinics.

Although technical development of IMRT hardware has advanced, clinical knowhow is lagging behind, especially in the head and neck area, due to the complexity in anatomy and versatility in tumor extension and spreading nature. In this book, we provide practical guidance for clinical evaluation, decision making, and technical proficiency in the application of IMRT for the management of patients with head and neck cancers. We first give a practical overview of IMRT physics and quality assurance in Chapter 1. Because successful implementation of IMRT depends on proficient understanding in anatomical imaging (computed tomography or magnetic resonance imaging), essential information to update readers on this topic is provided in Chapter 2. Integrating functional imaging to assist in a better target delineation or for dose escalation may soon be a clinical reality. In Chapter 3, we share our experience in implement functional imaging fusion in IMRT planning. In the remaining chapters, we provide concise, pertinent overviews of the natural course, lymph node spread, diagnostic criteria, and therapeutic options for each head and neck cancer subsite. We emphasize the importance of understanding basic anatomy and the corresponding imaging sections that are being used for target and normal tissue delineation. The guidelines on target determination based on the patterns of primary tumor extension and lymph node spreading are provided. More than 250 full-color, detailed illustrations to clarify each step in clinical implementations of head and neck IMRT. Clinical outcomes for patients treated with IMRT and with conventional techniques are also included. We believe this timely book will assist residents, fellows, and clinicians of radiation oncology in learning or practicing head and neck IMRT. The intention was to provide a foundation that enables different clinics and institutions to exchange clinical experiences. The information presented in this book will be refined as clinical and physical research advances.

# ACKNOWLEDGMENTS

The editor is indebted to Edna Major for her assistance in preparing the manuscript. Special thanks to the Assistant Editor, Dr. Gokhan Ozyigit, whose expertise in imaging processing has provided high quality figures for readers to apprehend the image-based anatomy and target delineation.

# 1

# PHYSICS OF INTENSITY MODULATED RADIATION THERAPY FOR HEAD AND NECK CANCER

## DANIEL A. LOW

## 1. DIFFERENCES BETWEEN IMRT AND 3DCRT

### 1.1. Dose Distribution Conformality

- Both intensity modulated radiation therapy (IMRT) and 3D conformal radiation therapy (3DCRT) dose distributions can be very conformal.[1-11] Typically, the radiation field edges extend to the edge of the projected target volumes. However, with IMRT, the fluence intensity at the target edges can be enhanced to partly compensate for the beam penumbra (reduced scattered radiation and distributed source distribution), whereas for 3DCRT, the portal boundary must be extended beyond the target volume to increase the dose near the target periphery.

- The prescription isodose surfaces of 3DCRT dose distributions are generally convex because all beams contribute to the prescription dose level. For IMRT, assuming a sufficient number of beams are used, the prescription isodose surface can have concavities, allowing greater conformation than possible with 3DCRT.

- Lower isodose surfaces (values that are intended to avoid critical structures) may wrap around critical structures due to converging radiation beam paths. However, the convexity of 3DCRT dose distributions is strongly dependent on the beam directions. While the beam directions are still important with IMRT, more flexible critical structure avoidance is usually possible.

- This greater conformality has important clinical consequences. Improved patient immobilization may be required to take full advantage of the conformal dose distribution shapes. Target volume margins should be applied using the same process as that for 3DCRT. Larger target volume margins associated with poor immobilization will limit the advantage obtained when using IMRT.

- Some treatment planning systems use more rudimentary dose calculation algorithms when optimizing fluence than when doing the final dose distribution calculation for display and analysis. If the algorithm used during optimization does not have a penumbra model, the fluence near the target volume edges may be insufficient to counteract the lateral scatter loss and the subsequent lack of coverage near the target surface. To counteract this, a target volume with a "block margin" may be used for prescription to ensure that the clinical target volume is adequately covered.

- The dose distribution can be highly complex in all three dimensions, with multiple concavities that are often not easily appreciated using only transverse views. A thorough inspection of the full dose distribution is necessary to determine if the concavities are appropriately positioned relative to critical structures. Most treatment planning systems have the capability of providing a margin for critical structures to allow the treatment planner to position steep dose gradients a safe distance from the critical structures.

### 1.2. Multiple Simultaneous Prescription Dose

- Typical 3DCRT treatment courses involve treatments to multiple target volumes, each with different prescription doses. The treatment courses are delivered sequentially, with the larger, lower-dose target volumes being treated first and then boost fields used to complete the dose distribution delivery to the smaller, higher-dose targets. Therefore, two or more sets of treatment fields are required during the course of therapy. The dose per fraction is often the same for all subplans.

- A similar situation exists with critical structures, where the beam geometry is altered during the course of therapy to block the critical structure at the tolerance dose. The tolerance dose is often reached using a relatively high dose per fraction and subsequently a very low dose per fraction (scatter dose).

- Because of limitations on the early commercial IMRT treatment planning systems, IMRT treatment plans were delivered with a single set of beams.[6,8,12] To prescribe different target doses required prescribing to different doses per fraction. The radiobiologic consequences of this require that a change be made to the total target prescription doses relative to the sequential dose prescriptions. Either the dose per fraction of the higher-dose target must be increased or the dose per fraction of the lower-dose target must be decreased, or a combination of the two, relative to the standard of practice. Either method requires consideration of the radiobiologic effects of the change in dose per fraction relative to the standards of practice.

- Although some treatment planning systems allow the planning of sequential subplans, with the doses to earlier subplans used in the consideration of target and critical structure dose limits, the process of assigning critical structure limits between the successive treatment plans is sufficiently complex that most users still optimize to a single treatment course with multiple target doses per fraction.

## 1.3. Temporal Delivery

- The IMRT treatment plan is optimized by a computer adjustment of a set of rectangular voxels for each beam direction.[13,14] The voxel intensities correspond to beam fluence intensities. For most cases, the modulated fluence distribution is delivered using a temporal sequence of complex radiation portals.[11,15–18] The specific sequence of portals is dictated by the treatment planning system (TPS) model of the linear accelerator and MLC. Often the dose distribution calculation utilizes only the idealized fluence distribution, not the delivery sequence used by the linear accelerator. The relatively complex geometry of the multileaf collimators (MLCs) causes dosimetric artifacts that are not computed in the treatment plan. Although these are often not considered clinically significant, they will yield differences between measurement and calculation that makes quantitative evaluation of the delivered dose more difficult.[19]
- The delivery sequence is delivered using complex, often small, portals that, under other conditions, would be considered difficult to model accurately. In IMRT, hundreds of such portals may be used for a single treatment. The treatment planning system considers the delivered dose to be a superposition of the individual portal doses. Unmodeled patient motion will yield differences between the planned and delivered dose.[20] Because of the complex nature of the interaction between patient motion and the delivered dose, very few studies have been conducted to quantify the effects of motion on the delivered dose.

## 1.4. Small Complex Fields

- The small complex fields typically used in IMRT cause challenges in the modeling of the dose per monitor unit (MU), the depth dose, and the surface dose. The field can be as small as $0.5 \times 1.0$ cm$^2$. Larger fields often have complex shapes, with the distance between all points in the field within 1 to 2 cm from the field edges. Modeling of the dose to these fields is difficult due to the lack of lateral electronic equilibrium and the complex partial blocking of the source distribution. Typically, the smallest field size used in commissioning 3DTPS is 3 to 4 cm$^2$; the dose distribution of the smallest bixel used for the IMRT field should be well characterized by the treatment planning system.[21]

- Validation of the dosimetry of these fields is similar to validation of stereotactic treatment planning systems. Dosimeters capable of accurately measuring dose distributions in small field are necessary for the characterization and validation of the small fields used in IMRT.[22–25]

- The dosimetry of small complex fields becomes more difficult in the presence of heterogeneities.[26] Electron transport distributions are strongly affected by heterogeneous media. For unmodulated fields, neighboring regions largely compensate for the change in secondary electron path lengths in one portion of the field. However, this compensation does not exist when heterogeneous fluences are used. Dose calculation algorithms that do not correctly account for secondary electron transport effects will incorrectly compute the dose to IMRT fields in heterogeneous media. For the head and neck, these regions include the trachea, nasal passages, and bones.

## 2. TYPES OF IMRT

- Most of IMRT is delivered using four approaches, two that use conventional MLCs and one that uses a dedicated IMRT MLC, and physical modulators (compensators). The sequence of portals is determined by a sequencing algorithm provided by the TPS.

## 2.1. Static Multileaf Collimation

- Static multileaf collimation (SMLC) uses conventional MLCs installed on linear accelerators. The nonuniform fluence distribution is delivered using a sequence of fixed irregular fields. Each field is delivered using MUs determined by the IMRT treatment planning system. Every linear accelerator manufacturer supports SMLC. The capabilities and performance of the SMLC delivery varies with the manufacturer and model of linear accelerator. The principal differentiator of SMLC is that the leaves do not move while the linear accelerator beam is on.

- Because the fluence distribution is delivered by fixed portals, the boundary between bixels is relatively sharp. Position errors (either patient or linear accelerator) that causes a shift in the fluence distribution yields dose errors that are narrow (<3 mm) but can be of large magnitude (13% mm$^{-1}$).[27]

## 2.2. Dynamic Multileaf Collimation

- DMLC also uses conventional MLCs installed on linear accelerators. The principal difference between DMLC and

SMLC is that the leaves move during irradiation.[17,28–34] Because the leaves are moving, a fluence gradient is produced by the passing of the leaves. Shallow and steep fluence gradients are produced by fast and slow leaf velocities, respectively.

- Unlike SMLC, if a minimal fluence is desired in the center of a field, the leaves are required to close during passage over that area. Some MLC manufacturers use leaves that travel in a straight line (as opposed to a radial arc) and correspondingly use rounded leaf ends to maintain a constant penumbra as a function of off-axis distance. This means that the leaves cannot fully block the radiation at the abutment and that the net leakage between the closed leaves is significant. Some leaf-sequencing algorithms use hybrid sequencing algorithms that employ dynamic sequencing until a minimal fluence is required for a bixel. The beam is turned off and the leaves are moved across the bixel with the beam off. The sequence is restarted after passage and delivery is restarted.

## 2.3. Tomotherapy

- Tomotherapy is a form of dynamic IMRT that uses a narrow multileaf collimator while the linear accelerator is rotated during beam-on.[6,21,35–38] Typically, the dose and rotation rates are kept constant during delivery. The treatment planning system optimizes the fluence from each beam direction. The dose calculation model is similar to that used in conventional arc irradiation, where the smooth rotation is modeled as a series of equally spaced fixed fields. In tomotherapy, the fluence distribution is optimized from each direction and the leaf sequence is programmed to produce the optimized nonuniform fluence.
- The leaves operate in a binary fashion and are typically opened and closed pneumatically, stopping at manual stops. The leaf transit times are rapid (<100 ms). A bixel is modulated by opening the leaf the fraction of gantry angle corresponding to the relative fraction of fluence required from the specific direction.

### 2.3.1. Nomos Peacock

- The first commercial IMRT delivery system (MIMiC) used the tomotherapy process.[6,21,39–45] The NOMOS Peacock system was designed to be attached at the collimator of a conventional linear accelerator. The MIMiC acted as a tertiary multileaf collimator with the secondary collimators set to a fixed rectangular field.
- The collimator consisted of two opposed banks of 20 leaves that operated independently. The leaves typically subtended $0.84 \times 1.0$ cm$^2$ (projected to isocenter) or $1.7 \times 1.0$ cm$^2$ bixels (depending on mechanical stop settings) to deliver the dose to two abutting cylindrical regions of 0.84 cm thickness each.
- Because the dose was delivered to a relatively narrow region (1.68 cm in the direction parallel to the gantry

rotation axis), most tumors required delivery of more than one abutting arc (termed *index*). The beam penumbra for this tertiary collimator was very sharp. For 6-MV beams, the penumbra in the index direction was measured to be 20% mm$^{-1}$.[38,46,47] Therefore, very accurate movement of the patient was required to obtain an accurate dose in the abutment region. The manufacturer provided a device (CRANE) that rigidly attached to the treatment couch. The CRANE had a manually operated rack and pinion system with a digital readout that provided couch motion accuracy of 0.2 mm.

- The radiation fields abutted to better than 5% along the linear accelerator central axis. However, the abutment between indexes was not perfect. The small divergence at the field edges caused some abutment dose heterogeneities. The value of the heterogeneity was a function of the off-axis distance and position, total gantry angle rotation of the arc, and field size (0.84 cm or 1.70 cm leaf setting). These abutments were evaluated by Low et al. for target volumes, but they have not been evaluated for critical structures.[38]

### 2.3.2. Tomotherapy, Inc.

- A dedicated tomotherapy unit, built by Tomotherapy, Inc., has been developed and is in clinical use.[48–55] The unit uses a 6-MV linear accelerator mounted in a commercial CT gantry. A single bank of leaves dynamically collimates the beam as the gantry rotates. Unlike the Peacock system, the couch moves continuously during irradiation, yielding a helical delivery. This reduces the effects of abutment positioning errors in the delivered dose. Additionally, the tomotherapy unit has a bank of radiation detectors opposite the dynamic MLC to capture the transmitted fluence. This will be used to provide a reconstructed megavoltage CT of the patient during the treatment.

## 2.4. Physical Modulators

- The tool required to deliver IMRT has the capability of generating customized nonuniform fluence distributions. This can also be accomplished by using physical filters, or modulators, that are custom designed and fabricated. There are some specific advantages and disadvantages of using physical modulators.[56,57]
- The use of physical modulators does not preclude the use of a separate portal aperture-defining device. The modulator material can be a machined metal or alloy, or it can be a metal mixture that fills a machined tray (e.g., out of Styrofoam). Physical modulators can be made thick enough to attenuate approximately 30% of the fluence relative to the maximum fluence transmission (the thinnest portion of the modulator). Because portal attenuators typically reduce the fluence to less than 3%, the filters are unable to provide this function. Therefore, they are used

in conjunction with custom fabricated metal apertures or MLCs.

- The minimum transmitted fluence provided by filters is greater than the minimum available using MLCs. Theoretically, this means that filters should be less capable of providing optimal fluences than MLCs. However, a reduction in treatment plan quality has not been proven in clinical cases.
- The filters require replacement for each portal, necessitating entry into the linear accelerator vault, even when MLCs are used to define the portal outline.
- The presence of filters has some important effects on the radiation beam. The beam spectrum is hardened as it passes through the filter, and the hardening is a function of the filter thickness, and therefore a function of the position within the beam aperture. The filter also scatters the beam, providing a background of scattered photons in the patient that extend outside the portal boundary.
- Elements of the quality assurance of filters are more straightforward than those for MLC-based IMRT. The filter can be physically examined, and the thickness distribution can be used to check alignment relative to the beam. As with MLC-based IMRT, quantitative evaluation of the filter thickness requires fluence or dose measurements.

## 3. IMRT DOSIMETRY

The practice of IMRT requires the use of quantitative dosimetric techniques that are more complex than those used for traditional radiation therapy treatments. The dynamic delivery and small complex portals make quantitative verification more difficult than before. At the same time, the modeling of the delivered dose is more challenging, leading to an increased need for good dosimetry techniques.

## 3.1. Dosimeter Requirements

- Ideally, the quality assurance (QA) of IMRT would be done with dosimeters that have the following properties:
  - □ A three-dimensional measurement of sufficient size to encompass the high-dose regions and neighboring critical structures
  - □ Tissue or water equivalence (energy dependence)
  - □ No dose rate dependence
  - □ High spatial resolution ($\leq 1$ mm$^3$)
  - □ Relatively low expense
  - □ A permanent record of the delivered dose
  - □ Integrated dose for use with time-dependent dose delivery.

Unfortunately, no dosimeters have all the listed properties, so compromises are required. The following are the most common dosimeters used in the measurement of IMRT dose distributions.

## 3.2. Ionization Chamber

- The ionization chamber is the most commonly used dosimeter in radiation therapy. When matched with a high-quality electrometer, it is highly linear and has virtually no dose rate dependence. All radiation therapy physicists are familiar with the operation of ionization chambers.
- Ionization chambers measure ionization in air, not dose directly, so protocols have been developed to determine the absorbed dose to water or tissue as a function of measured ionization.[58-61] These protocols include calibrations by accredited laboratories that have standards traceable to the National Institute of Standards and Technology (NIST). Because a clinic's calibrated ionization chambers may not have properties that are suitable for IMRT measurements (e.g., cross-sectional size), clinical IMRT measurements are often conducted using uncalibrated ionization chambers. The sensitivity of these chambers are determined by calibrating the dose per MU for a photon beam using a calibrated chamber and transferring that calibration to the working chamber.
- They are typically used to measure integral dose by allowing the electrometer to integrate charge during irradiation. Some users integrate the charge separately for each beam or couch index, recording the charge and summing the results. This allows for recovery in the event that one of the beams is incorrectly delivered, and allows an independent determination of the dose contribution from each beam or index.
- Cylindrical ionization chambers have the advantage of providing the same cross-sectional area, and, consequently, the same sensitivity as a function of incident beam angle if the ionization chamber is placed with its axis parallel to the rotational axis of the linear accelerator. This limits measurement artifacts caused by changes in dose sensitivity as a function of incident beam angle.
- Ionization chambers measure dose at a single point and require the entire IMRT dose distribution to be delivered to measure the dose at that point. This is very inefficient, especially considering that the complex nature of IMRT dose distributions requires that dose measurements be conducted at numerous locations, so ionization chamber measurements are not sufficient. Further, the size of ionization chambers causes them to sample the dose distribution over a volume, rather than at a true point.[62] This causes the measurement to be the average (volume average) of the dose distribution throughout the ionization chamber volume. If the dose distribution is relatively uniform throughout the volume encompassed by the chamber, the measurement will be accurate. If steep dose gradients pass through the chamber, the volume averaging will provide a result that is difficult to interpret. The calculated dose that is compared against measurement should be the mean dose throughout the chamber volume.

- Because of volume averaging, the measurement by ionization chambers of beam penumbras (often used by IMRT treatment planning systems) is not recommended. The resulting penumbra gradient will be shallower than the physical gradient, so the resulting penumbra model will be inaccurate, causing inaccurate dose distribution calculations.[62]
- Linear arrays of ionization chambers are available for specialized applications. These were initially designed to measure the dose distributions of dynamic wedges, where the dose gradient lies in a straight line. They have been used to some extent for IMRT, but their geometry makes them impractical for most IMRT measurements.
- While volume averaging is a concern when steep dose gradients pass through the ionization chamber, conducting measurements in homogeneous regions that are nearby steep dose gradients also has ramifications for measurement accuracy. The inaccurate positioning of the ionization chamber relative to the dose distribution or the possibility of inaccurate dose distribution delivery or modeling can place the ionization chamber within the steep dose gradient region. The resulting measured dose will differ from the expected dose, and interpretation of the difference may be difficult. Taking account not only of the calculated dose at the point of measurement but also of the doses nearby is important when interpreting such results. More important, the data acquired at such points are not as valuable as those acquired at points far from steep dose gradients.

## 3.3. Radiographic Film

- Radiographic film is the most common multidimensional detector available to the medical physicist. If used correctly, it can provide an accurate, inexpensive, high-resolution measurement of dose in a plane. The use of radiographic film requires careful attention to detail.[63-68]
- Processed radiographic film has a smooth relationship between the optical density (OD) and the absorbed dose. At zero dose, the OD is termed the *base and fog,* to describe the optical attenuation from the inactive film base and converted silver halide from radiation exposure prior to the experiment and chemical processes. The exposed film has a greater OD, such that the difference in OD between the irradiated and unirradiated film is termed the *net OD.* The shape of the calibration curve has a nearly linear response at low OD, and the slope of OD versus dose decreases with increasing dose. The sensitivity (change in OD with respect to change in dose) therefore decreases with increasing dose.
- Quantitative measurements of the OD distribution on the film require a densitometer.[69,70] Because OD has a logarithmic relationship to transmitted light, many commercial densitometers have a logarithmic response, in that

the sensitivity of the densitometer is constant as a linear function of OD. Typically, densitometers with a logarithmic response provide more accurate measurements of larger ODs (OD > 2) than densitometers with linear responses. Quantitative film measurements require that the densitometers have the following characteristics:

1. *High spatial resolution and linearity.* The densitometer should accurately determine the position of each measurement point and have a spatial resolution of at least $1 \times 1$ mm$^2$ to ensure limited averaging across steep dose gradient regions.
2. *Sufficient dynamic range for ODs of interest.* The detector and digitization system should provide an adequate signal to digitize the greatest OD of interest. Most commercial densitometers have the capability of measuring radiographic films with OD of more than 3, which is adequate for clinical use.
3. *Stability.* After a suitable warmup period, the densitometer should not change sensitivity. This allows the user to separately scan the calibration and measurement films without a change in the densitometer sensitivity.
4. *Light scatter artifacts.* The densitometer should be free of significant light scatter artifacts (see later).

- The relationship between film OD and dose is different for each film batch, and a strong function of the state of the film processor chemicals and their temperature. The same dose can yield very different net optical densities, even from the same batch, when the processor conditions change. Not only does the net OD change at a specific dose, but the shape of the sensitometric curve changes such that a simple normalization of a previously measured curve by a film measured to a single dose does not yield an accurate curve.
- The sensitometric curve is typically obtained by irradiating a set of films to a series of doses, from 0 (to determine the base and fog) to just over the maximum dose expected in the measurement films (to avoid the need for extrapolation). The calibration films are scanned using the same device as the measurement film. A polynomial fit is usually required to fit the relationship between dose and OD. As long as the calibration is consistent with the measurement, either net or raw OD can be used. Examples are shown in Fig. 1.1.

## 3.4. Thermoluminescent Dosimeters

- Thermoluminescent dosimeters (TLDs) are commonly used in IMRT dose verification measurements.[42,71,72] Although they are not as convenient as ionization chambers, by placing multiple TLDs in a phantom, one can simultaneously acquire measurements at numerous points. Like radiographic film, the quantitative use of TLDs requires care. Because the sensitivity of TLDs changes as they age,

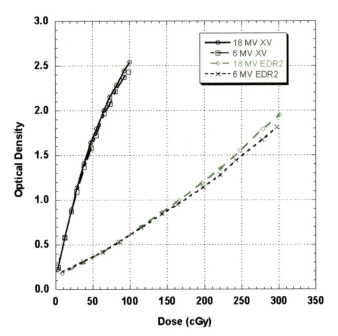

**FIGURE 1-1.** Examples of radiographic sensitometric curves for two commonly used radiographic films. Note that one of the films (EDR 2) has a response that allows it to be used with typical single fraction doses. This removes the requirement of scaling monitor units for the quality assurance procedure.

individual TLDs cannot be calibrated. However, their sensitivity relative to a batch of TLDs can be very stable, as long as the batch thermal history is consistent. The relative sensitivity of the chips can be determined by irradiating the batch to a common dose (e.g., 200 cGy) and reading their responses to determine the sensitivity of each chip relative to the group average. The individual chips are separately identified and a relative calibration factor is assigned to each. (The sensitivity measurement is often made a few times to determine the stability of the response and to reduce the individual measurement uncertainty.) At each experiment, a few chips are irradiated separately to a known dose, and after applying their sensitivity corrections, used to determine the sensitivity of the measurement chips. After their readings have been corrected, the sensitivity is used to determine the measurement doses.

- The sensitivity should be monitored periodically to determine which chips, if any, have been damaged enough to change their sensitivity significantly.

### 3.5. Phantoms

- Phantoms can be classified into two general categories: anthropomorphic and geometrically regular. Anthropomorphic phantoms are characterized by their humanlike shape. This can be either external, with a homogeneous internal structure, or heterogeneous, with internal air and bony anatomic structures. Regular geometric phantoms are characterized by their geometric shapes. They are made in cubic, circular, and elliptical cylindrical shapes. There are tradeoffs with the use of each type.[73]
- Anthropomorphic phantoms mimic specific clinical sites. To this extent, they are generally the correct size and shape with respect to the site being studied. This means that the physical beam characteristics (depth dose and scatter properties) are the same as those for the patients. The internal heterogeneous construction tests the dose calculation algorithm and the user's implementation in a manner that is more realistic than that for homogeneous phantoms. However, the interpretation of differences between calculated and measured doses will include the question of whether the discrepancy is due to errors in the effects of the heterogeneities. This can make identification of the source of discrepancies more difficult.
- Setup and alignment of anthropomorphic phantoms can be difficult. The surface of anthropomorphic phantoms is usually rounded. Stable positioning of the phantom on the treatment couch is difficult and often requires the preparation of the same immobilization devices used to treat patients. Although this at first seems like a test of the immobilization system, the dosimetric consequences of using these systems can be easily verified independently. The available locations for dosimeters and the types of dosimeters are often limited. This is especially true for the use of radiographic film, which requires compression to remove air gaps that can cause dosimetric artifacts. The shape of the phantom requires careful (and time-consuming) trimming of the film, and careful marking of the film to determine, after processing, its orientation in the phantom.
- Although geometrically regular phantoms do not mimic patient shapes, they have some desirable characteristics. Figure 1.2 shows an example of geometric phantoms used for IMRT dose-quality-assurance procedures. The phantoms can be machined to close dimensional tolerances, allowing for precise positioning of dosimeters. The phantoms can be made so that preparing film is straightforward. Some use whole sheets in ready-pack form, negating the need for a darkroom to prepare the phantom for irradiation. Others use rectangular films that require only cutting using a paper cutter or equivalent. These phantoms are typically easier to align than anthropomorphic phantoms because they have flat surfaces and alignment marks can be placed in precise relationships to the dosimeter positions. Hybrid phantoms, those that have the external appearance of anthropomorphic phantoms but precise internal construction (Fig. 1-3), may provide an excellent compromise between the two types.

### 3.6. Dose Distribution Evaluation

- Quantitative dose distribution comparisons are very important in the quality assurance process.[74,75] Although the comparisons are made ideally using digital versions of the

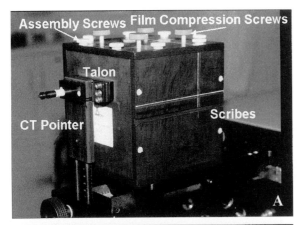
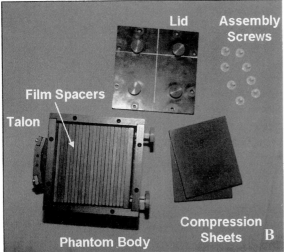
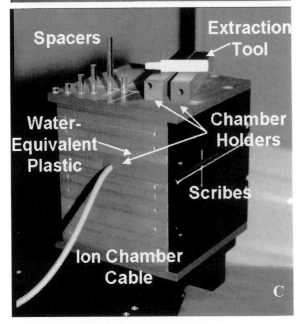

**FIGURE 1-2.** Phantom used for IMRT dosimetry measurements. **A:** Film phantom. **B:** Internal construction of film phantom, showing compression plates. **C:** Ionization chamber phantom. (These figures from Low DA, Gerber RL, Mutic S, et al. Phantoms for IMRT dose distribution measurement and treatment verification. *Int J Radiat Oncol Biol Phys* 1998;40:1231–1235, by permission.)

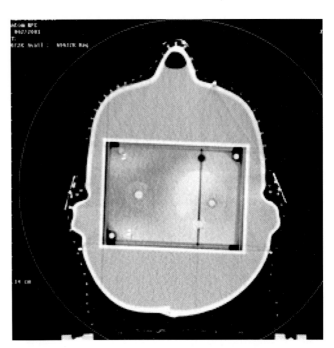

**FIGURE 1-3.** Cross-sectional computed tomographic scan through a hybrid anthropomorphic phantom developed by the Radiological Physics Center for the quality assurance of IMRT dose distributions. Note that while the external construction is shaped like the human head, the internal cavities are geometrically shaped to allow precise positioning.

dose distributions, comparisons are possible using hardcopy printouts of isodose distributions. Printouts are prepared using common distance scales and isodose curves, and are overlaid on a light box. The comparison is limited to the doses corresponding to the isodose levels, and evaluations of position or shape differences in shallow gradient regions is difficult, because small dose differences correspond to large position shifts. In this discussion, the two compared distributions will be referred to as measured and calculated, although they also apply to calculated dose distribution comparisons.

- In any comparison, one of the most important considerations is the independent determination of the measurement and calculation coordinate systems. The steep gradients formed by IMRT must be placed in the correct location relative to the predicted position. If the position is incorrect, the sparing of critical structures may be compromised. The only way to ensure that the steep gradients are in the correct position is to accurately determine the positions of the dose measurements and independently determine the positions of the calculated dose points. The measured dose positions are usually determined by understanding the geometry of phantoms and dosimeters or by marking the dosimeter relative to the phantom. Once the position of the phantom relative to the linear accelerator has been determined, the positions of the dose measurement points relative to the linear accelerator are known. The calculated positions are determined using the treatment planning system itself, either by having the co-ordinates downloaded with the dose distribution export, by obtaining the positions from the treatment planning system using one of the dose examination tools, or by querying the internal data files to identify the calculated dose positions.

- The most straightforward dose comparison tool involves taking the numerical difference between the calculation and measurement. Of course, if the measurement was conducted using a scaled set of MUs to accommodate the dosimeter's dynamic range, the measured dose will be appropriately scaled before the comparison. Van Dyk determined that this comparison is overly sensitive to spatial shifts between the dose distributions in steep dose gradient regions.[76] Even if the two dose distributions are identical, but are shifted relative to one another, the numerical difference will be large in steep dose gradient regions.

- Figure 1.4A shows a calculated IMRT dose distribution (to be used as the reference distribution). For evaluation of the dose comparison tests, a second (the evaluated) distribution was simulated by copying the calculated distribution, scaling the $x$ position of the dose distribution so that the positions differed by 4 mm and 2 mm at the left and right edges of the high-dose regions, respectively. The modified distribution is shown in Fig. 1-4B. For this analysis, we assume that an acceptable dose difference criterion is 3%.

- The corresponding dose difference is shown in Fig. 1-4C. The differences are as large as 20%, even though the same dose distributions were used. The large differences are caused by the spatial shifts in steep dose gradient regions.

- Because of the relative sensitivity of the dose difference test in steep gradient regions, a second test was designed to identify the distance between isodose lines.[74] This test, called the *distance-to-agreement* (DTA) *test,* measured the distance from a point in the measured distribution to the nearest point in the calculated distribution with the same dose. This does an excellent job of determining the spatial offset of two dose distributions in steep gradient regions but is overly sensitive in low-dose gradient regions. For this reason, the DTA test is typically limited to 1.0-cm distances and distances beyond that are truncated to 1.0 cm. Figure 1.4D shows the DTA for the doses shown in Figs. 1.4A and 1.4B. Because the modified dose distribution was created by scaling the unmodified distribution, the DTA follows a somewhat predictable pattern, with roughly 4- and 2-mm values in the left and right sides of the figure, respectively. Even with the relatively straightforward method used to create the modified distribution, the DTA is difficult to interpret, because large DTAs typically extend over wide regions where the dose difference is relatively small and distract from the regions where the DTA is important.

- Typically, dose-difference and DTA tests are desired in shallow and steep dose gradient regions, respectively. If acceptability tolerances are selected for each test (e.g., 3% and 3 mm), the points that fail both tests (the composite test) can be identified. These are the regions of greatest concern. Figure 1.4E shows an example of the composite test results from the dose distributions of Figs. 1.4A and 1.4B. Because the test is binary, the regions of failure are identified by homogeneously colored areas.

- One of the difficulties with the composite test is that it provides a binary result. The use is not provided a continuous scale of values with which to determine how badly the comparisons failed the criteria. Low et al. developed a modification of the composite test.[75] They renormalized the measured and calculated distributions (both dose and distance axes) to the acceptance criteria, thereby providing comparisons of only unitless quantities. The distance between each point in the measured distribution is computed for all points in the calculated distribution. The minimum distance is termed $\gamma$. In regions of shallow dose gradients, the value of $\gamma$ is the same as the dose difference divided by the dose-difference criterion. Therefore, in these regions a value of $\gamma = 1$ indicates the dose difference is the same value as the dose-difference criterion (e.g., 3%). Conversely, in regions of steep dose gradients, the value of $\gamma$ is the same as the DTA divided by the DTA criterion. This test automatically switches as a function of the local dose gradient. In addition, because $\gamma$ is a continuous variable, it can be plotted or histogrammed, and the magnitude of $\gamma$ can be used to determine by how much the comparison passes or fails the test. Figure 1.4F shows an example of the $\gamma$ distribution for the examples of Figs. 1.4A and 1.4B. The regions that fail the $\gamma$ test are very similar to the composite evaluation, but the magnitude of failure is clearly identified in the example.

## 3.7. Response to Discrepancies

- One of the most important reasons to conduct quantitative dose measurement validation is to provide information for adjustment of the user's linear accelerator model parameters to better model the accelerator's performance in the treatment planning system. Unfortunately, discrepancy analysis can be difficult because of the complexity of the planning and delivery process. The following is a partial list of the possible sources of discrepancies between film measurement and calculation:
  1. Treatment planning system
     1.1. Input data inaccurate (e.g., depth doses, output factors, beam penumbra, leaf offsets)
     1.2. TPS accelerator model inaccurate
     1.3. Dose calculation algorithm limitation
     1.4. Leaf-sequencing algorithm
  2. Experiment (the dose measurement)
     2.1. MLC leaf sequence data transfer from TPS to accelerator

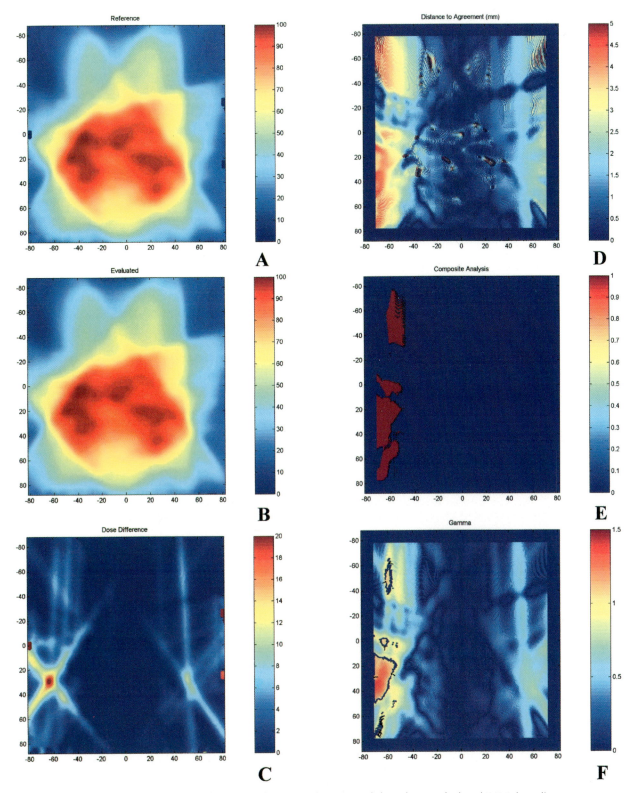

**FIGURE 1-4.** Examples of dose distribution evaluation tools based on a calculated IMRT dose distribution and the same distribution modified by rescaling the horizontal axis such that the left and right edges of the steep dose gradients were 4 and 2 mm different from the unmodified distribution. **A:** The unmodified distribution (labeled reference). **B:** The modified distribution (labeled evaluated). **C:** Dose difference (in percent: of the dose distributions in **A** and **B**). **D:** Distance-to-agreement (in mm). **E:** Composite evaluation (1 = fail, 0 = pass) using 3% and 3-mm criteria. Note that because the modified distribution was created by scaling the unmodified distribution by only 2 mm on the right side, the DTA was not greater than 2 mm where the dose difference was greater than 3%, so the composite evaluation passes on the right side. **F:** $\gamma$ analysis (3% and 3-mm criteria). An additional contour is added at $\gamma = 1$ to aid in the determination of the regions that fail both criteria. The scale shows the magnitude of $\gamma$.

2.2. Experimental setup
  2.2.1. Geometry (error in position/orientation of phantom)
  2.2.2. Irradiation error (e.g., wrong MUs, collimator settings, angles)
  2.2.3. Bad film calibration curve
  2.2.4. Inconsistent processor
2.3. Delivery
  2.3.1. Incorrect MLC leaf calibration
  2.3.2. Incorrect linear accelerator operation (e.g., leafs sticking)
3. Data analysis
  3.1. Film scanning and readout
    3.1.1. Densitometer artifacts
    3.1.2. User-input data (e.g., film position relative to calculated dose distribution)
    3.1.3. Incorrect registration of calculation and measurement

- Although this list is very long, techniques are being developed to isolate some of the causes of error using straightforward test procedures. For example, the MLC calibrations have tests that are easily conducted, and if the system passes, the calculated and measured dose discrepancies are unlikely to be due to that cause.

## 4. LINEAR ACCELERATOR QA

The concepts of linear accelerator QA have been well established for conventional and conformal therapy. The integration of IMRT adds some significant additional constraints to the accelerator operation; therefore, additional QA processes are required.[77] Typically, IMRT dose distributions are delivered using conventional MLCs that have been modified to automatically deliver a preprogrammed sequence of portals. These portals provide the fluence distribution that was optimized by the treatment planning system. Of course, if the sequence is not accurately delivered, the dose will not be accurately delivered. One of the most important immediate tasks of the physics community is to quantify the dosimetric errors caused by miscalibrations and to suggest a suite of tests to detect these errors.

## 4.1. MLC Leaf Calibration

- MLC leaf calibration refers to the relationship between the set field size (the digital position values determined by the treatment planning system and sent to the accelerator) and the delivered radiation fields.[31,78−80] With fully divergent secondary jaws, the relationship has typically been that the set position is intended to correspond to the 50% isodose at the field edge. The light field is typically calibrated to agree with this position. Ideally, the same would be done for MLCs, but many MLCs have rounded

leaf ends. This causes the 50% isodose line to lie nearly a millimeter inside the projected leaf end. The light field is therefore not collocated with the 50% isodose line, so the secondary collimator technique cannot be used for these MLCs.

- The calibration method suggested by LoSasso and others is to utilize the radiation distribution directly to determine the leaf setting.[31] They developed a technique that measures the light-radiation field offset. When the MLCs are calibrated against the light field, the offset value is typically required as input to the treatment planning system.

- For 3DCRT, the results of an error in MLC leaf calibration are that the portal boundary is not accurately defined. The tolerance on this boundary has typically been 2 mm, which when combined with planning and block margins would result in a negligible error in the portal shape. For IMRT the portals define the dose throughout the tumor, so an error in the field size results in an error of delivered dose. The change in delivered dose with respect to changes in field sizes is a function of the number and size of portals, but the errors can exceed 10% mm$^{-1}$ of leaf calibration error.[31] A consequence of this is that the maintenance personnel have to be informed that whenever the MLC is recalibrated, physics should be consulted as they would for an ionization chamber repair.

## 4.2. SMLC Operation

- Segmental multileaf collimation (SMLC) describes the technique where the MLC leaves are stationary when the beam is on, and the beam is off when the leaves are moving.[11] This yields a sequence of radiation portals that are delivered in a method that appears to be similar to the common process used in 3DCRT. All linear accelerator manufacturers support SMLC delivery, so it has become the most common method of delivering IMRT.

- As previously stated, the field edges extend within the tumor projection, and miscalibrations or misoperation of the MLCs will alter the dose within the tumor. The QA of SMLC delivery concentrates on leaf-positioning accuracy, and the most common test involves the irradiation of radiographic film with a sequence of narrow (2 cm) and long portals defined by the MLCs. Individual leaf errors of 0.5 mm can easily be detected. One difficulty with this technique is that it requires many separate irradiations to cover the entire $40 \times 40$ cm$^2$ field size, so some institutions place the film closer to the radiation source to increase the field subtended by the film.

- The SMLC delivery sequence couples MUs to be delivered with the portal outlines. There has been some discussion regarding the methods used by the accelerator manufacturers regarding the distribution of MUs to the portals. Because the delivery occurs in real time, the monitoring of delivered MUs is closely coupled with the motion of the leaves, and over- and undershooting have been reported.

## 4.3. DMLC Operation

- Dynamic multileaf collimation (DMLC) describes the technique where the MLC leaves are moving when the beam is on.[11] Currently, only Varian supports DMLC delivery. Although the issue of MLC leaf calibration is important to DMLC, the consequences of miscalibration are different from those for SMLC. Leaf calibration errors in DMLC delivery will cause the delivered fluence to differ from the desired fluence throughout the target, rather than along the internal portal boundaries. LoSasso published the idealized relationship between leaf calibration error and dose delivery errors, and showed that a reciprocal relationship exists between dose error and dynamically scanning field size, so that as the field size decreases, a given leaf calibration error causes an increasing dose delivery error.[31] As an example, a 1-mm total field size error (0.5 mm from each leaf) will cause 10% and 5% dose errors in 1-cm- and 2-cm-wide windows, respectively.
- The same tool used to test SMLC leaf calibration accuracy can be used to test calibration accuracy for DMLC. However, it does not validate the calibration under truly dynamic conditions. LoSasso suggested that a technique similar to the daily output test be used.[31,80] They use a scanning DMLC leaf pattern that ideally has a constant width and scan it across the central axis. An ionization chamber, used for the daily photon output measurement, measures the ratio of DMLC to open field readings. (More MUs are used for the DMLC field.) The benchmark ratio is determined when the MLC leaves are calibrated, and subsequent readings are compared. The greatest limitation to this test is that it checks only the MLC leaves that subtend the ionization chamber.

## 5. COMMISSIONING OF IMRT TPS

Because IMRT is a subset of 3DCRT, many of the commissioning tests will be in common with those used to validate traditional 3DCRT planning systems. Most of these tests have been described by Fraass et al. and will not be discussed here.[81] The major issues of concern are related to the differences between IMRT and 3DCRT, namely, the small field dose distribution and the leaf sequences. The following tests are based on recommendations from the literature.[72]

### 5.1. Open-Field Dosimetry

- The IMRT treatment planning system should adequately model open-field dose distributions and the dose per MU along the central axis. If the planning system can produce distributions based on homogeneous fluences, the calculations can easily be compared against clinical beam data and measurements (for the smaller field sizes). A representative set of SSDs should also be checked.

## 5.2. Single Modulated Fields

- Single modulated fields incident on a flat, homogeneous, water-equivalent phantom should be checked. No standard set of fluence distributions has been recommended, but simple distributions, such as a step wedge, pyramid, inverse pyramid, and narrow rectangular fields were used.
- The dose distributions should be measured using radiographic film with verification point dose measurements conducted using either ionization chamber or TLDs.

## 5.3. Complete Treatment Plans: Phantoms

- Single field measurements do not confirm that the spatial relationship between portals is correctly modeled. Therefore, verification measurements are required using full multibeam IMRT treatment plans. These should be conducted in a phantom that is roughly the same size as the treatment site being verified, and the dosimeters should be accurately and independently registered relative to the accelerator.
- The treatment plans require the definition of target volumes and critical structures, as well as their dose constraints. There are no generally accepted phantom target volumes, but most users have elected to mimic typical IMRT target and critical structure geometries and dose constraints. For example, a sphere can be used to mimic the prostate, with a second sphere and cylinder for the bladder and rectum, respectively.

## 5.4. Heterogeneity Corrections

- One of the most controversial aspects of IMRT is the necessity for using heterogeneity corrections. Many 3DCRT treatment plans can be accurately conducted without heterogeneity corrections (e.g., pelvis), but treatment plans of the head and neck may be compromised by assuming a water-equivalent patient. The problem is more complex with IMRT, because the dose delivered by the small, complex portals is significantly altered by the change in electron transport. There are no suggested guidelines for when to use heterogeneity corrections and which algorithms yield accurate results. The user is cautioned to conduct experimental validations in patientlike geometries before incorporating heterogeneity algorithms into IMRT software.

## 6. PATIENT IMMOBILIZATION AND LOCALIZATION

IMRT dose distributions, with their highly conformal shapes, will only be efficacious if the patient is in the correct location relative to the linear accelerator. This point is often overlooked in 3DCRT because a relatively straightforward verification of the dose is possible by examining portal films or images. In many cases, the portal film can identify if the correct portion of the patient is being treated. With IMRT the connection between portal films and dose is lost, so greater emphasis needs to be made concerning patient localization and immobilization. *Immobilization* is defined here as the process that keeps a patient immobile from the time the therapist completes the setup to the completion of beam delivery. This is contrasted with localization, which is the process of placing the target and critical structures in the same locations (relative to the accelerator) as the treatment plan. Although they are closely linked (poor immobilization will lead to poor localization), there are important differences. These differences will be explained later.

### 6.1. Immobilization Techniques

- Immobilization is accomplished using positioning tools that range from a simple flat couch (discouraging rotational motion) to elaborate thermoplastic masks, to highly invasive techniques employed by stereotactic radiosurgery. For head and neck cancer treatments, target volumes are not so small and precisely positioned as to justify invasive immobilization. However, the anatomy of the head and neck planning allows excellent immobilization using inexpensive and easily tolerated systems. In our clinic, we use a reinforced thermoplastic mask system (Fig. 1-5) for tomotherapy treatments.[6] The bar at the top of the head helps keep patients from moving in the craniocaudal direction, which is the direction most sensitive to dose delivery errors in tomotherapy.
- The system was shown to provide 1-mm immobilization accuracy when tested using portal films taken before and after irradiation.
- One concern of immobilization systems is their continued operation during the course of radiation therapy. Patients may swell at the beginning of treatment or lose weight during the course of therapy, causing the mask to not fit correctly. With sufficient swelling, the patients may complain or the therapists notice that the mask is difficult to secure and call the physicists for consultation. With weight loss, neither the therapist nor the patient may notice that the mask is no longer capable of immobilizing the patient.

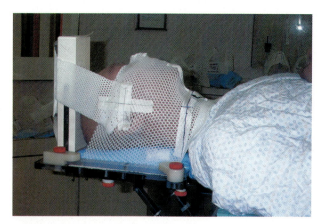

**FIGURE 1-5.** Thermoplastic mask system used at the Mallinckrodt Institute of Radiology for the treatment of head and neck cancers using tomotherapy delivery. The vertical post aids in the craniocaudal immobilization of the patient, which is critical in the treatment of serial tomotherapy.

### 6.2. Localization

- Accurate localization requires good immobilization, but good immobilization does not guarantee accurate localization because the patient can be immobilized in the wrong position or orientation. Therefore, an immobilization system must also be able to identify when the patient is not in the correct position. For the head and neck, noninvasive systems can be effective in repositioning the patient on a daily basis because of the numerous bony anatomic features.
- Inaccurate localization can cause severe dose errors by moving the low-dose region from critical structures. To illustrate this, a treatment plan for a head-and-neck patient was recomputed with simulated shifted beams (0, 5, 10, and 15 mm). For each case, the target volume, parotid glands, and spinal cord dose distributions were computed. Figures 1.6A and 1.6B show the unshifted and 10-mm shifted distributions, respectively. Figure 1.6C shows the target volume dose-volume histogram (DVH) for the four cases, showing that the shifts have minimal effect on the target volume dose (because of the adequate margin placed on the volume). Figures 1.6D and 1.6E show the DVHs for the left parotid gland and spinal cord, respectively, showing the increased doses due to the shifts. Clearly, small systematic shifts can lead to large, clinically relevant dose delivery errors.
- An important consideration of the example is that there are no portal films that identify the relationship between the dose distribution and the critical structures (specifically, the spinal cord). Unlike 3DCRT, where a portal film shows an off-cord block and its relationship to the spine, the correct positioning of this patient relative to the intended position depends entirely on the treatment planning, setup, and verification processes in the clinic. There are no direct portal films to validate that the high-dose region is avoided.

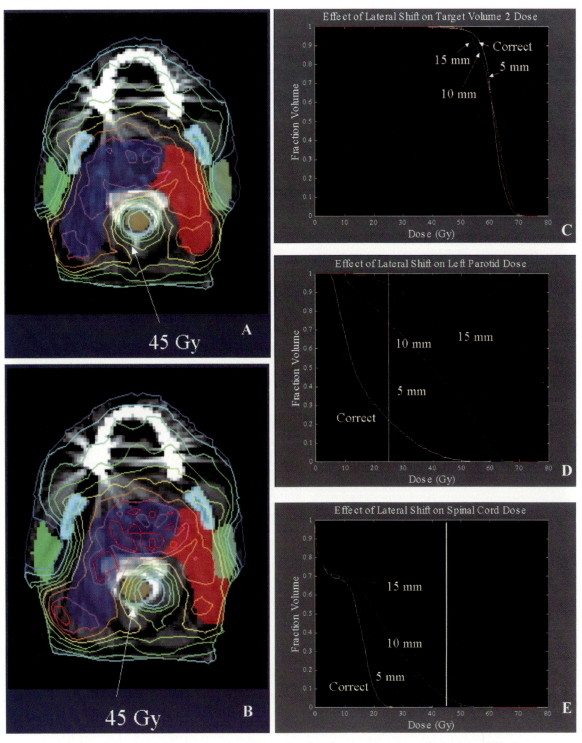

**FIGURE 1-6. A:** Unshifted isodose distribution for a head and neck patient. The isodoses differ by 10% and the 45 Gy isodose line is highlighted. **B:** Isodose distribution of patient shown in **A** with the isocenter shifted by 10 mm to the patient's right. The mismatch of the spinal cord and cold spot is clearly shown. **C:** Integral dose-volume histogram (DVH) of the target volume for the unshifted and shifted isodose distributions. **D:** Integral DVH of the left parotid gland (a line is placed at 20 Gy for reference) showing the marked increase in dose due to the patient misalignment. **E:** Integral DVH of the spinal cord (a line is placed at 45 Gy for reference) showing the marked increase in dose due to the patient misalignment.

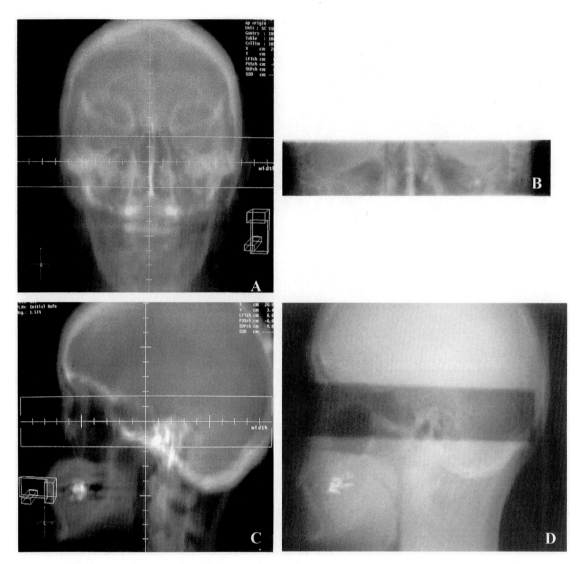

**FIGURE 1-7.** Digitally reconstructed radiographs (DRRs) and portal films for serial tomotherapy positioning validation. **A:** Anteroposterior DRR, showing the intended portal-film boundary. Note that this boundary indicates only the portal film used for positioning validation, not for dose delivery. **B:** Anteroposterior portal film corresponding to the DRR in **A**). **C:** Lateral DRR. **D:** Lateral double-exposure portal film acquired by irradiating the MLC-defined portal and then removing the MLC from the linear accelerator and opening the jaws to image the patient's head. This allows a more thorough evaluation of the head orientation.

## 7. PATIENT-SPECIFIC QA

The quality assurance of 3D conformal treatment consists of one or more checks of the treatment plan, monitor units using an independent calculation, record and verify parameters, independent monitor unit, *in vivo* dose (e.g., using diodes), patient setup parameters (e.g., central axis SSDs), and patient positioning using portal films or images. Many of these checks can be modified for use in IMRT, such as the patient setup parameters and patient positioning verification. However, the complex fluence distributions and time-dependent dose delivery sequences make other checks, such as the *in vivo* dose measurements, difficult or impossible.

## 7.1. Localization QA

- The concept of using the treatment portals for localization verification is impractical with IMRT due to the nonuniform fluences. Rather, use of independent orthogonal localization portals is effective in determining the patient orientation and position relative to the position in the treatment plan. Portal films or portal images provide the position of the patient during treatment. Figure 1.7 shows an example of digitally reconstructed radiographs and portal films for tomotherapy verification of head and neck treatments. Because of the relatively narrow maximum portal ($3.7 \times 20$ cm$^2$) and the consequences of misalignment shown in Fig. 1-6, care must be taken to check the portal films quantitatively.

## 7.2. Treatment Plan QA

- One of the most important tasks of the physicist is to check the treatment plan to determine if it is appropriate for the intended treatment. The process of conducting this review is made more difficult with IMRT, because the dose distributions are not intuitive relative to the beam orientations, and the physicist does not necessarily know if the treatment plan is the best that could be produced, given the selected beam directions and energies.
- Review of the treatment plan should include careful inspection of the normalization isodose (equivalent to reviewing the hot spot). In all cases, the dose per fraction should be considered, especially when reviewing the hot spots. Because IMRT treatment planning yields heterogeneous dose distributions, adequate tumor coverage may require the delivery of significant hot spots. Coverage of all the tumor volume may not be practical, because modern optimization algorithms allow for significant cold spots in the target as a competing objective to avoiding critical structures. It is possible to place additional margins surrounding planning target volume (PTVs) as a workaround, so that the planning system places the low-dose region outside the PTV. Of course, this will compromise critical structure avoidance.
- The dose-volume histograms should also be carefully examined, because the optimization may not have adequately spared one or more critical structures or may have inadequately treated the target.
- The spatial accuracy of the treatment plan, including patient setup reproducibility and position of isocenter relative to the patient alignment, is one of the most critical components of the review. The physicist has to be confident that the position of the beams and consequential dose distribution as shown in the treatment plan will be accurately placed with respect to the patient. Shifts from the initial setup marks to the final beam isocenter are particularly prone to error, as in many cases, the shifts are computed during treatment planning and manually executed on the treatment couch or simulator. Numerical errors, transcription errors, or misinterpretation of motion direction can easily lead to the incorrect placement of patients.

## 7.3. Dose Distribution Verification

- The process of checking the treatment plan is similar to that of checking a traditional 3D treatment plan, in that the radiation dose distribution, dose-volume histograms, and coordinate transformation information (patient shifts) are essentially identical. The complex nature of IMRT dose calculations makes the process of an independent MU check more difficult than it is for traditional 3D treatment planning. The large number and complex shapes of IMRT portals makes manual techniques impractical. While some institutions have developed their own software, direct measurements remain the most practical method of MU verification.
- Measurements are conducted using a water-equivalent phantom. Because the shape of the phantom is different from that of the patient, direct dosimetric comparisons between the treatment plan and measurement would be meaningless. Most treatment planning systems offer a feature that recalculates a patient's treatment onto the phantom geometry. Therefore, direct comparison between measurement and calculation is meaningful.[82]
- Dosimeter selection is very important for patient QA. The physicist needs to both provide a quantitative comparison and ensure that the complex dose distribution shape is accurately delivered. As stated earlier, the commonly available dosimeters do not meet both criteria, so a compromise must be made. Many use ionization chamber measurements to quantitatively validate the dose at one or two points, while also employing radiographic film (with a custom-measured sensitometric curve) for two-dimensional measurements. The ionization chamber points are selected to lie in high-dose, low-dose gradient regions, with additional points selected within the positions corresponding to critical structures.
- Depending on the complexity of the treatment plan and on the number and location of the critical structures, multiple films in different orientations may be required. For the head and neck, the dose distribution through the spinal cord and parotid glands can be validated by one or more transverse films. If the film dosimetry technique is quantitative and critical structure doses have been thoroughly validated during commissioning or by previous QA, then a separate quantitative measurement of these regions (e.g., using ionization chambers) may be unnecessary. The validation of the steep dose gradient locations may be sufficient.
- The QA does not catch all mistakes or errors. For example, if there is a contouring error such as inappropriately contouring the CT couch as part of the patient, the software will correctly recompute the dose to the phantom, and the measured and calculated doses will agree, even though the patient dose is correct. Therefore, much of the QA relies on the QA of the process used in delineating the patient, as well as patient setup.

## REFERENCES

1. Sultanem K, Shu HK, Xia P, et al. Three-dimensional intensity-modulated radiotherapy in the treatment of nasopharyngeal carcinoma: the University of California–San Francisco experience. *Int J Radiat Oncol Biol Phys* 2000:48:711–722.
2. Teh BS, Woo SY, Butler EB. Intensity modulated radiation therapy (IMRT): a new promising technology in radiation oncology. *Oncologist* 1999;4:433–442.

3. Butler EB, Teh BS, Grant WH, et al. Smart (simultaneous modulated accelerated radiation therapy) boost: a new accelerated fractionation schedule for the treatment of head and neck cancer with intensity modulated radiotherapy. *Int J Radiat Oncol Biol Phys* 1999;45:21–32.

4. Fraass BA, Kessler ML, McShan DL, et al. Optimization and clinical use of multisegment intensity-modulated radiation therapy for high-dose conformal therapy. *Semin Radiat Oncol* 1999;9:60–77.

5. Boyer AL, Geis P, Grant W, et al. Modulated beam conformal therapy for head and neck tumors. *Int J Radiat Oncol Biol Phys* 1997;39:227–236.

6. Chao KSC, Low DA, Perez CA, et al. Intensity-modulated radiation therapy in head and neck cancers: the Mallinckrodt experience. *Int J Cancer* 2000;90:92–103.

7. Chao KSC, Deasy JO, Markman J, et al. A prospective study of salivary function sparing in patients with head-and-neck cancers receiving intensity-modulated or three-dimensional radiation therapy: initial results. *Int J Radiat Oncol Biol Phys* 2001;49:907–916.

8. Zelefsky MJ, Fuks Z, Hunt M, et al. High dose radiation delivered by intensity modulated conformal radiotherapy improves the outcome of localized prostate cancer. *J Urol* 2001;166:876–881.

9. Nutting CM, Convery DJ, Cosgrove VP, et al. Reduction of small and large bowel irradiation using an optimized intensity-modulated pelvic radiotherapy technique in patients with prostate cancer. *Int J Radiat Oncol Biol Phys* 2000;48:649–656.

10. Nutting C, Dearnaley DP, Webb S. Intensity modulated radiation therapy: a clinical review. *Br J Radiol* 2000;73:459–469.

11. Intensity Modulated Radiation Therapy Collaborative Working Group. Intensity-modulated radiotherapy: current status and issues of interest. *Int J Radiat Oncol Biol Phys* 2001;51:880–914.

12. Teh BS, Mai WY, Uhl BM, et al. Intensity-modulated radiation therapy (IMRT) for prostate cancer with the use of a rectal balloon for prostate immobilization: acute toxicity and dose-volume analysis. *Int J Radiat Oncol Biol Phys* 2001;49:705–712.

13. Webb S. Optimizing the planning of intensity-modulated radiotherapy. *Phys Med Biol* 1994;39:2229–2246.

14. Webb S. A simple method to control aspects of fluence modulation in IMRT planning. *Phys Med Biol* 2001;46:N187–N195.

15. Convery DJ, Rosenbloom M. Treatment delivery accuracy in intensity-modulated conformal radiotherapy. *Phys Med Biol* 1995;40:979–999.

16. Bortfeld TR, Kahler DL, Waldron TJ, et al. X-ray field compensation with multileaf collimators. *Int J Radiat Oncol Biol Phys* 1994;28:723–730.

17. Spirou SV, Chui CS. Generation of arbitrary intensity profiles by dynamic jaws or multileaf collimators. *Med Phys* 1994;21:1031–1041.

18. Dirkx ML, Heijmen BJ, van Santvoort JP. Leaf trajectory calculation for dynamic multileaf collimation to realize optimized fluence profiles. *Phys Med Biol* 1998;43:1171–1184.

19. Siebers JV, Tong S, Lauterbach M, et al. Acceleration of dose calculations for intensity-modulated radiotherapy. *Med Phys* 2001;28:903–910.

20. Yu CX, Jaffray DA, Wong JW. The effects of intra-fraction organ motion on the delivery of dynamic intensity modulation. *Phys Med Biol* 1998;43:91–104.

21. Low DA, Chao KSC, Mutic S, et al. Quality assurance of serial tomotherapy for head and neck patient treatments. *Int J Radiat Oncol Biol Phys* 1998;42:681–692.

22. Robar JL, Clark BG. A practical technique for verification of three-dimensional conformal dose distributions in stereotactic radiosurgery. *Med Phys* 2000;27:978–987.

23. Robar JL, Clark BG. The use of radiographic film for linear accelerator stereotactic radiosurgical dosimetry. *Med Phys* 1999;26:2144–2150.

24. Somigliana A, Cattaneo GM, Fiorino C, et al. Dosimetry of gamma knife and linac-based radiosurgery using radiochromic and diode detectors. *Phys Med Biol* 1999;44:887–897.

25. Duggan DM, Coffey CW. Use of a micro-ionization chamber and an anthropomorphic head phantom in a quality assurance program for stereotactic radiosurgery. *Med Phys* 1996;23:513–516.

26. Klein EE, Morrison A, Purdy JA, et al. A volumetric study of measurements and calculations of lung density corrections for 6 and 18 MV photons. *Int J Radiat Oncol Biol Phys* 1997;37:1163–1170.

27. Low DA, Sohn JW, Klein EE, et al. Characterization of a commercial multileaf collimator used for intensity modulated radiation therapy. *Med Phys* 2001;28:752–756.

28. Convery DJ, Rosenbloom ME. The generation of intensity-modulated fields for conformal radiotherapy by dynamic collimation. *Phys Med Biol* 1992;37:1359–1374.

29. Gustafsson A, Lind BK, Svensson R, et al. Simultaneous optimization of dynamic multileaf collimation and scanning patterns or compensating filters using a generalized pencil beam algorithm. *Med Phys* 1995;22:1141–1156.

30. Källman P, Lind B, Eklof A, et al. Shaping of arbitrary dose distributions by dynamic multileaf collimation. *Phys Med Biol* 1998;33:1291–1300.

31. LoSasso T, Chui CS, Ling CC. Physical and dosimetric aspects of a multileaf collimation system used in the dynamic mode for implementing intensity modulated radiotherapy. *Med Phys* 1998;25:1919–1927.

32. Sandvoort JPC, Heijmen BJM. Dynamic multileaf collimation without "tongue-and-groove" underdosage effects. *Phys Med Biol* 1996;41:2091–2105.

33. Svensson R, Källman P, Brahme A. An analytical solution for the dynamic control of multileaf collimators. *Phys Med Biol* 1994;39:37–61.

34. Yu CX, Wong JW. Dynamic photon beam intensity modulation, presented at the XIth International Conference on the Use of Computers in Radiation Therapy, Manchester, UK, 1994 (unpublished).

35. Mackie TR, Holmes T, Swerdloff S, et al. Tomotherapy: a new concept for the delivery of dynamic conformal radiotherapy. *Med Phys* 1993;20:1709–1719.

36. Mackie TR, Aldridge S, Angelos L, et al. Tomotherapy: rethinking the process of radiotherapy, presented at the Twelfth International Conference on the Use of Computers in Radiation Therapy, Salt Lake City, 1997 (unpublished).

37. Yang JN, Mackie TR, Reckwerdt P, et al. An investigation of tomotherapy beam delivery. *Med Phys* 1997;24:425–436.

38. Low DA, Mutic S, Dempsey JF, et al. Abutment region dosimetry for serial tomotherapy. *Int J Radiat Oncol Biol Phys* 1999;45:193–203.

39. Peacock CM. A system for planning and rotational delivery of intensity-modulated fields. *Int J Imag Sys Technol* 1995;6:56–61.

40. Carol MP, Grant WH, Pavord D, et al. Initial clinical experience with the Peacock intensity modulation of a 3-D conformal radiation therapy system. *Stereotact Funct Neurosurg* 1996;66:30–34.

41. Low DA, Mutic S. A commercial IMRT treatment-planning dose-calculation algorithm. *Int J Radiat Oncol Biol Phys* 1998;41:933–937.

42. Low DA, Mutic S, Dempsey JF, et al. Quantitative dosimetric verification of an IMRT planning and delivery system. *Radiother Oncol* 1998;49:305–316.

43. Saw CB, Ayyangar KM, Zhen W, et al. Quality assurance procedures for the Peacock system. *Med Dosim* 2001;26:83–90.
44. Saw CB, Ayyangar KM, Thompson RB, et al. Commissioning of Peacock system for intensity-modulated radiation therapy. *Med Dosim* 2001;26:55–64.
45. Wu A, Johnson M, Chen ASJ, et al. Evaluation of dose calculation algorithm of the Peacock system for multileaf intensity modulation collimator. *Int J Radiat Oncol Biol Phys* 1996;36:1225–1231.
46. Carol M, Grant WH, Blier AR, et al. The field-matching problem as it applies to the Peacock three-dimensional conformal system for intensity modulation. *Int J Radiat Oncol Biol Phys* 1996;34:183–187.
47. Low DA, Mutic S, Dempsey JF, et al. Abutment dosimetry for serial tomotherapy. *Med Dosim* 2001;26:79–82.
48. Kapatoes JM, Olivera GH, Ruchala KJ, et al. A feasible method for clinical delivery verification and dose reconstruction in tomotherapy. *Med Phys* 2001;28:528–542.
49. Kapatoes JM, Olivera GH, Balog JP, et al. On the accuracy and effectiveness of dose reconstruction for tomotherapy. *Phys Med Biol* 2001;46:943–966.
50. Ruchala KJ, Olivera GH, Kapatoes JM, et al. Megavoltage CT image reconstruction during tomotherapy treatments. *Phys Med Biol* 2000;45:3545–3562.
51. Ruchala KJ, Olivera GH, Schloesser EA, et al. Megavoltage CT on a tomotherapy system. *Phys Med Biol* 1999;44:2597–2621.
52. Kapatoes JM, Olivera GH, Reckwerdt PJ, et al. Delivery verification in sequential and helical tomotherapy. *Phys Med Biol* 1999;44:1815–1841.
53. Balog JP, Mackie TR, Wenman DL, et al. Multileaf collimator interleaf transmission. *Med Phys* 1999;26:176–186.
54. Mackie TR, Balog J, Ruchala K, et al. Tomotherapy. *Semin Radiat Oncol* 1999;9:108–117.
55. Balog JP, Mackie TR, Reckwerdt P, et al. Characterization of the output for helical delivery of intensity modulated slit beams. *Med Phys* 1999;26:55–64.
56. Thompson H, Evans MD, Fallone BG. Accuracy of numerically produced compensators. *Med Dosim* 1999;24:49–52.
57. Webb S, Convery DJ, Evans PM. Inverse planning with constraints to generate smoothed intensity-modulated beams. *Phys Med Biol* 1998;43:2785–2794.
58. Saiful HM, Andreo P. Reference dosimetry in clinical high-energy photon beams: comparison of the AAPM TG-51 and AAPM TG-21 dosimetry protocols. *Med Phys* 2001;28:46–54.
59. Almond PR, Biggs PJ, Coursey BM, et al. AAPM's TG-51 protocol for clinical reference dosimetry of high-energy photon and electron beams. *Med Phys* 1999;26:1847–1870.
60. Hazle JD, Kirby TH, Gastorf RJ, et al. Results of photon absorbed-dose measurements using the AAPM TG-21 protocol for accelerating potentials up to 26 MV. *Med Phys* 1991;18:1234–1236.
61. Gastorf RJ, Hanson WF, Shalek RJ, et al. The implementation of the AAPM Task Group 21 protocol by the Radiological Physics Center and its implications. *Med Phys* 1984;11:547–551.
62. Martens C, De Wagter C, De Neve W. The value of the PinPoint ion chamber for characterization of small field segments used in intensity-modulated radiotherapy. *Phys Med Biol* 2000;45:2519–2530.

63. Van Battum LJ, Heijmen BJ. Film dosimetry in water in a 23 MV therapeutic photon beam. *Radiother Oncol* 1995;34:152–159.
64. Williamson JF, Khan FM, Sharma SC. Film dosimetry of megavoltage photon beams: a practical method of isodensity-to-isodose curve conversion. *Med Phys* 1981;8:94–98.
65. Robar JL, Clark BG. The use of radiographic film for linear accelerator stereotactic radiosurgical dosimetry. *Med Phys* 1999;26:2144–2150.
66. Hale JI, Kerr AT, Shragge PC. Calibration of film for accurate megavoltage photon dosimetry. *Med Dosim* 1994;19:43–46.
67. Evans MD, Schreiner LJ. A simple technique for film dosimetry. *Radiother Oncol* 1992;23:265–267.
68. Danciu C, Proimos BS, Rosenwald JC, et al. Variation of sensitometric curves of radiographic films in high energy photon beams. *Med Phys* 2001;28:966–974.
69. Dempsey JF, Low DA, Kirov AS, et al. Quantitative optical densitometry with scanning-laser film digitizers. *Med Phys* 1999;26:1721–1731.
70. Dempsey JF, Low DA, Mutic S, et al. Validation of a precision radiochromic film dosimetry system for quantitative two-dimensional imaging of acute exposure dose distributions. *Med Phys* 2000;27:2462–2475.
71. Tsai JS, Wazer DE, Ling MN, et al. Dosimetric verification of the dynamic intensity-modulated radiation therapy of 92 patients. *Int J Radiat Oncol Biol Phys* 1998;40:1213–1230.
72. Arnfield MR, Wu Q, Tong S, et al. Dosimetric validation for multileaf collimator-based intensity-modulated radiotherapy: a review. *Med Dosim* 2001;26:179–188.
73. Low DA, Gerber RL, Mutic S, et al. Phantoms for IMRT dose distribution measurement and treatment verification. *Int J Radiat Oncol Biol Phys* 1998;40:1231–1235.
74. Harms WB, Low DA, Wong JW, et al. A software tool for the quantitative evaluation of 3D dose calculation algorithms. *Med Phys* 1998;25:1830–1836.
75. Low DA, Harms WB, Mutic S, et al. A technique for the quantitative evaluation of dose distributions. *Med Phys* 1998;25:656–661.
76. Van Dyk J, Barnett RB, Cygler JE, et al. Commissioning and quality assurance of treatment planning computers. *Int J Radiat Oncol Biol Phys* 1993;26:261–273.
77. Xia P, Verhey LJ. Delivery systems of intensity-modulated radiotherapy using conventional multileaf collimators. *Med Dosim* 2001;26:169–177.
78. Boyer AL, Li S. Geometric analysis of light-field position of a multileaf collimator with curved ends. *Med Phys* 1997;24:757–762.
79. Boyer A, Biggs P, Galvin J, et al. AAPM Report 72, Basic application of MLC, 2001.
80. LoSasso T, Chui CS, Ling C. Comprehensive quality assurance for the delivery of intensity modulated radiotherapy with a multileaf collimator used in the dynamic mode. *Med Phys* 2001;28:2209–2219.
81. Fraass B, Doppke K, Hunt M, et al. American Association of Physicists in Medicine Radiation Therapy Committee Task Group 53: quality assurance for clinical radiotherapy treatment planning. *Med Phys* 1998;25:1773–1829.
82. Ting JY, Davis LW. Dose verification for patients undergoing IMRT. *Med Dosim* 2001;26:205–213.

# 2

# CT AND MR IMAGING OF HEAD AND NECK CANCER

### FRANZ J. WIPPOLD II

## 1. BASICS OF CROSS-SECTIONAL IMAGING

- Cross-sectional imaging has become an indispensable tool in the characterization and staging of neck pathology. Noninvasive imaging of the neck is currently performed with high-resolution rapid computed tomography (CT) and magnetic resonance (MR) imaging.
- Both of these modalities provide essential information about the deep extension of clinically detected masses, delineate additional clinically unsuspected lesions, assist in definitive therapy planning, and provide a method of surveillance following therapy.[1,2]

### 1.1. CT Imaging

- CT uses x-rays and digital computer analysis of x-ray data to create cross-sectional images of the neck and skull base.
- CT scanning of the neck should begin with a general neck survey examination before more detailed and focused protocols.
- Scanning should cover the region from the base of the skull to the clavicles. A digital lateral scout radiograph may assist in planning.
- Spiral (helical) CT scanning permits rapid scanning of large volumes of tissues during quiet respiration.[3] Volumetric helical data permit optimal multiplanar and three-dimensional reconstructions.[4,5]
- Intravenous contrast administered with a power injector through a venous catheter is essential.
- Advanced CT techniques, such as three-dimensional (3D) CT, may be useful for radiotherapy planning. Using special computer software, traces of selected anatomic structures are reformatted into a 3D-wire diagram that can then be manipulated to reveal the most optimal radiation port. This technique limits extraneous collateral radiation to other organs such as the salivary glands.[6]

### 1.2. MR Imaging

- MR imaging uses magnetic fields and radio frequency to create cross-sectional images of the neck and skull base.

- MR scanning limited to the suprahyoid neck region and base of skull can be performed with a head coil. Examinations that include the infrahyoid region require a neck coil.
- T1-weighted images display anatomic relationships and detect lesions such as lymph nodes embedded within fat. T1-weighted coronal images define the false cords, true cords, laryngeal ventricle, and floor of mouth.[7] T1-weighted sagittal images are useful for evaluating the preepiglottic space, paraglottic spaces, and nasopharynx.
- T2-weighted transaxial images characterize tissue, detect tumor within muscle, demonstrate cysts, and assist differentiation of posttherapy fibrosis from recurrent tumor.[8]
- Gadolinium-enhanced T1-weighted images improve delineation of margins in many tumors,[9] although lesions embedded in fat may be obscured unless fat-saturation techniques are used (Fig. 2-1).[10] Enhanced normal aerodigestive mucosa may also obscure small mucosal tumors. Gadolinium-enhanced, fat-suppressed T1-weighted images are especially useful in staging nodal disease.
- Magnetization transfer (MT) technique uses the transfer of magnetization between restricted protons associated with macromolecules and free water protons to improve the contrast between lesions and background tissue.[11] MT may be useful in differentiating enhancing lesions from background tissue and in defining unenhanced lesions.
- MR spectroscopy (MRS) uses MR data to quantify tissue metabolites. Although this technique is now widely employed in brain imaging, technical hurdles have impeded its application in neck pathology.
- New open-bore MR units are being used for MR guidance of biopsies.[12]

### 1.3. Comparison of CT and MR Imaging

- CT and MR imaging have different and often complementary roles. Although both CT and MR provide comparable anatomic information on the neck in most cases, CT is preferred as a screening modality.

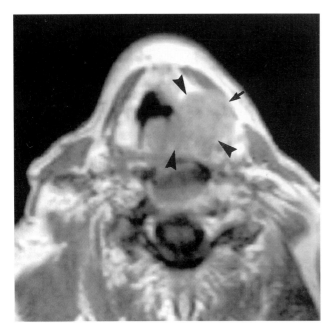

**FIGURE 2-1.** Transglottic carcinoma. Enhanced axial T1-weighted MR image demonstrating a supraglottic soft-tissue mass (*arrowheads*) invading the left paraglottic space, the left thyroid cartilage, and paraglottic muscles (*arrow*). The hyperintense fat on T1-weighted images provides excellent natural soft-tissue contrast for detecting the less hyperintense tumor. (Wippold FJ II. Neck. In: Lee JKT, Sagel SS, Stanley RJ, Heiken JP, eds. *Computed body tomography with MRI correlation,* 3rd ed. Philadelphia: Lippincott-Raven, 1998:107–182, by permission.)

- An advantage of CT includes the fast scanning speed, especially with spiral technique, that enables rapid assessment of the patient who may be dyspneic from a comorbidity of chronic airway obstruction. Spatial resolution of anatomy is superb with modern scanners. Calcifications are also well-depicted (Fig. 2-2).

- Disadvantages of CT include limitation of scanning to the transverse plane, although spiral-imaging technique has markedly improved coronal and sagittal reformation capabilities. Dental amalgam, metal instrumentation, and large shoulders may create annoying scan artifacts. Intravenous iodinated contrast agents used in CT carry a definite risk of anaphylaxis and of further compromise of impaired renal function in selected patients. The newer nonionic contrast agents may be safer than older agents for patients with previous contrast reactions or compromised renal function.[13]

- Advantages of MR include its superb soft-tissue contrast, multiplanar display, and minimal artifacts from shoulders, dental amalgam, and densely calcified or ossified cartilages. Noniodinated gadolinium MR imaging enhancement compounds are generally well tolerated by individuals with impaired kidneys.[14] MR imaging is ideally suited for evaluation of masticator, parapharyngeal, and parotid spaces, skull base, and floor of the mouth.[15]

- Disadvantages of MR imaging include degradation of images due to motion artifacts from breathing, carotid artery pulsations, swallowing, and often lengthy examinations.

- Contraindications for MR imaging include patients with cerebral aneurysm clips, cardiac pacemakers, or a history of intraorbital iron filings.

## 1.4. Fundamentals of Interpretation

- Interpretation of cross-sectional imaging requires a thorough knowledge of normal neck anatomy and an appreciation of the changes that occur with surgery and radiation.

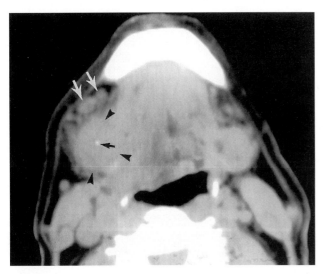

**FIGURE 2-2.** Submandibular nodes in a patient with sialadenitis. CT images showing multiple submandibular lymph nodes (*white arrows*) adjacent to an inflamed submandibular salivary gland (*arrowheads*). Note the calculus within the gland (*black arrow*).

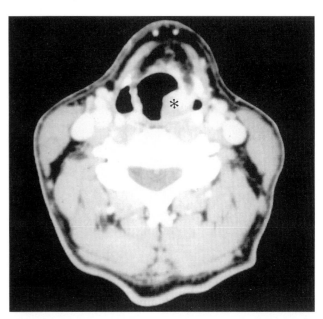

**FIGURE 2-3.** Carcinoma of the aryepiglottic fold. CT scan revealing asymmetric thickening of the left aryepiglottic fold (*asterisk*) due to a supraglottic carcinoma of the larynx. Soft-tissue asymmetry provides a helpful clue for identifying pathology. On CT images, tumors typically appear as dense soft-tissue masses.

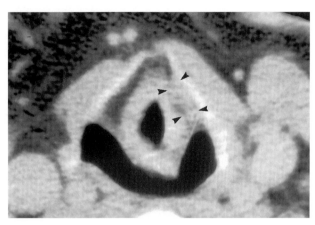

**FIGURE 2-4.** Supraglottic carcinoma. Axial CT scan reveals soft-tissue density (*arrowheads*) within the fat of the paraglottic space. High-resolution CT imaging often reveals subtleties of pathologic anatomy not readily appreciated with conventional CT imaging. Soft-tissue asymmetry is a helpful clue for detecting pathology. (Wippold FJ II. Neck. In: Lee JKT, Sagel SS, Stanley RJ, Heiken JP, eds. *Computed body tomography with MRI correlation*, 3rd ed. Philadelphia: Lippincott-Raven, 1998:107–182, by permission.)

- Asymmetric soft-tissue masses should always be viewed with suspicion for tumor unless an alternative explanation such as atrophy or an anatomic normal variant applies (Figs. 2-3 and 2-4).
- On CT images tumors usually appear as dense, enhancing soft-tissue abnormalities.
- On MR images tumors usually appear as hypointense to isointense on T1-weighted images, hyperintense on T2-weighted images, and enhancing on gadolinium-enhanced T1-weighted images (Fig. 2-1).
- Subtle soft-tissue changes and anatomic variants may be misinterpreted by the untrained eye (Fig. 2-5). This issue is especially important in the cancer patient in whom multiple sites of disease may coexist or in whom successful therapy has virtually eliminated the original pathology. For difficult cases, reliance on a trained head and neck diagnostic radiologist is crucial.

## 2. IMAGING APPROACH TO NECK ANATOMY AND PATHOLOGY

### 2.1. Spaces of the Neck

- The deep cervical fascia of the neck consists of three layers: a superficial investing layer, a middle visceral layer, and a deep, prevertebral layer.[16,17] The neck can be divided into spaces or compartments based on the deep cervical fascial planes.[17–21] This method of compartmentalization is ideal for analysis of cross-sectional images (Figs. 2-6 and 2-7).

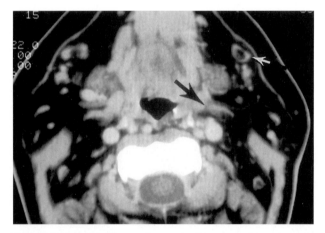

**FIGURE 2-5.** Axial CT scan demonstrating normal lymph nodes (*arrows*) with hypodense fat within the hila. These findings should not be confused with necrosis. (Wippold FJ II. Neck. In: Lee JKT, Sagel SS, Stanley RJ, Heiken JP, eds. *Computed body tomography with MRI correlation*, 3rd ed. Philadelphia: Lippincott-Raven, 1998:107–182, by permission.)

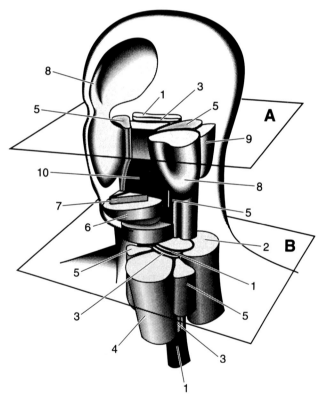

**FIGURE 2-6.** Diagram of the spaces of the neck defined by the deep cervical fascia. Axial slices through the suprahyoid (**A**) and infrahyoid (**B**) levels illustrating cross-sectional relationships of the spaces. Perivertebral space, anterior compartment (1), perivertebral space, posterior compartment (2), retropharyngeal space (3), visceral space (4), prestyloid parapharyngeal space and poststyloid parapharyngeal space (carotid space) (5), submandibular space (6), sublingual space (7), masticator space (8), parotid space (9), and pharyngeal mucosal space (10). (Smoker WRK. Normal anatomy of the neck. In: Som PM, Curtin HD, eds. *Head and neck imaging*, 3rd ed. St. Louis: Mosby Year Book, 1996:711–771. Wippold FJ II. Neck. In: Lee JKT, Sagel SS, Stanley RJ, Heiken JP, eds. *Computed body tomography with MRI correlation*, 3rd ed. Philadelphia: Lippincott-Raven, 1998:107–182, by permission.)

## 2.2. Normal Anatomy

- The cervical spaces of the suprahyoid and infrahyoid neck include the sublingual, submandibular, buccal, parotid, parapharyngeal, carotid, masticator, pharyngeal mucosal, visceral, the retropharyngeal, the posterior cervical, and the prevertebral spaces (Table 2-1, Figs. 2-6 and 2-7).

## 2.3. Pathology

- Of the spaces of the neck, the epithelial lined suprahyoid pharyngeal mucosal space and the infrahyoid visceral space are especially important sites of primary carcinoma.
- The surrounding spaces, such as the parapharyngeal, masticator and retropharyngeal spaces, are important sites of secondary tumor invasion.
- The pharyngeal mucosal space includes the mucosal surfaces and immediate submucosa of the nasopharynx and oropharynx. The oral cavity and the suprahyoid portion of the hypopharynx can also be conveniently included in this discussion.
- Imaging signs of nasopharyngeal cancer, a common pharyngeal mucosal space lesion, include blunting of the fossa of Rosenmuller, displacement of the parapharyngeal fat, and thickening of the retropharyngeal and prevertebral spaces.[22] The sphenoid and ethmoid sinuses, eustachian tube, pterygoid canal, skull base, and intracranial cavity may be invaded. MR imaging is especially useful in establishing soft-tissue and dural invasion, although CT is useful in depicting bone invasion at the base of the skull. Oral cavity and oropharyngeal cancers may spread to involve the mandible.
- The midline visceral space extends from the hyoid bone to the mediastinum. This space is important because it contains the larynx and hypopharynx, thyroid and parathyroid glands, trachea and esophagus, paratracheal lymph nodes, and recurrent laryngeal nerves, and is the site for many primary carcinomas.[21,23]
- Axial and sagittal T1-weighted MR images best demonstrate preepiglottic space and paraglottic space tumor infiltration (Fig. 2-1). In large tumors MR imaging is superior in demonstrating cartilage involvement and bone marrow infiltration. Circumferential attachment of tumor 270° or greater of the carotid diameter implies carotid involvement with a sensitivity approaching 100%.[21]

## 2.4. Lymph Nodes of the Neck

### 2.4.1. Normal Anatomy

- Ten major groups of cervical lymph nodes are recognized[17,21,24]: occipital, mastoid, parotid, submandibular, facial, submental, sublingual, retropharyngeal, and the paired anterior and lateral cervical chains (Figs. 2-2 and 2-8 to 2-13). Of these groups, the submental, submandibular, retropharyngeal, and lateral cervical chains play especially important roles in the spread of head and neck disease.

- The American Joint Committee on Cancer (AJCC) and the American Academy of Otolaryngology–Head and Neck Surgery have established guidelines using a terminology that divides the lymph node groups into a series of levels that have prognostic importance (Fig. 2-14).[25] Recently, some modifications based on imaging have also been proposed.[26]
- Level I consists of the sublingual, submental, and submandibular nodes (Figs. 2-2, 2-10, and 2-11). These nodes lie above the hyoid bone, below the mylohyoid muscle, and anterior to the posterior margin of the submandibular gland. Level IA contains the sublingual and submental nodes and Level IB includes the submandibular nodes.
- Level II includes the internal jugular chain nodes extending from the base of the skull to the carotid bifurcation (hyoid bone) (Fig. 2-13). They lie posterior to the submandibular gland and anterior to the posterior margin of the sternocleidomastoid muscle. Level IIA nodes are anterior, medial, or lateral to the internal jugular vein. If posterior to the vein, the nodes are inseparable from the vein. Level IIB nodes are posterior to the internal jugular vein with a fat plane separating the vein from the nodes.
- Level III corresponds to the internal jugular nodes from the carotid bifurcation to the omohyoid muscle (cricoid cartilage). They lie anterior to the posterior margin of the sternocleidomastoid muscle.
- Level IV refers to all nodes in the internal jugular group from the omohyoid muscle to the clavicle. They lie anterior to the posterior margin of the sternocleidomastoid muscle and lateral to the carotid arteries.
- Level V consists of spinal accessory and transverse cervical nodes that occupy the posterior cervical triangle. They lie posterior to the posterior margin of the sternocleidomastoid muscle. Level VA extends from the skull base to the inferior margin of the cricoid arch, and level VB extends from the cricoid arch to the clavicle.
- Level VI contains the pretracheal, prelaryngeal, and paratracheal nodes. These nodes lie between the carotid arteries from the hyoid bone to the manubrium.
- Level VII includes the nodes in the tracheoesophageal groove and upper mediastinum. They lie between the carotid arteries below the manubrium and above the innominate vein.[26]

### 2.4.2. Pathology

- Imaging criteria for lymphadenopathy are based on nodal size, internal heterogeneity, presence of clusters, shape, and associated findings.[25,27,28]
- The maximum transaxial diameter of a node in levels I or II should not exceed 1.5 cm, and the minimum transaxial diameter should not exceed 1.1 cm (Figs. 2-13 and 2-15).

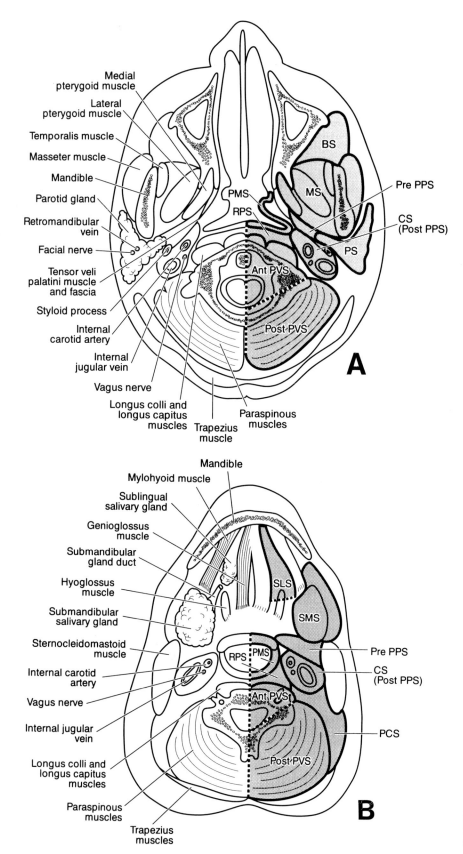

**FIGURE 2-7.** Axial diagrams of the neck to the high suprahyoid (**A**), low suprahyoid (**B**), and infrahyoid.

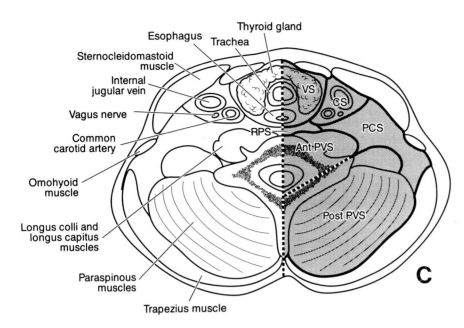

FIGURE 2-7. (*continued*) (C) levels showing the relationships of the sublingual space (SLS); submandibular space (SMS); buccal space (BS); parotid space (PS); prestyloid parapharyngeal space (PrePPS); carotid space (CS) (also known as the poststyloid parapharyngeal space [PostPPS] in the suprahyoid neck); masticator space (MS); pharyngeal mucosal space (PMS); visceral space (VS); retropharyngeal space (RPS); the posterior cervical space (PCS); the anterior compartment of the prevertebral space (AntPVS); and the posterior compartment of the perivertebral space (PostPVS). (Harnsberger HR. The perivertebral space. In: Harnsberger HR. *Head and neck imaging*, 2nd ed. St. Louis: Mosby Year Book, 1995:105–119. Smoker WRK. Normal anatomy of the neck. In: Som PM, Curtin HD, eds. *Head and neck imaging*, 3rd ed. St. Louis: Mosby Year Book, 1996:711–771. Wippold FJ II. Neck. In: Lee JKT, Sagel SS, Stanley RJ, Heiken JP, eds. *Computed body tomography with MRI correlation*, 3rd ed. Philadelphia: Lippincott-Raven, 1998:107–182.)

For levels III to VII, maximum and minimum transaxial diameter should be no greater than 1.0 cm.

- Internal lymph node heterogeneity is one of the most reliable criteria for recognizing lymphadenopathy. Central regions within nodes displaying hypodensity on CT, hypointensity on T1-weighted, and hyperintensity on T2-weighted MR images should be regarded as abnormal and usually signify necrosis (Fig. 2-15). Necrosis generally is proportional to nodal size; however, this finding should be considered abnormal regardless of nodal size. The hilum of a normal node may contain hypodense fat on CT imaging and should not be mistaken for necrosis (Fig. 2-5).
- Clusters are defined as three or more contiguous ill-defined nodes within the same level, ranging from 8 mm to 15 mm in size. Clusters may be seen in inflammation, cancer, or lymphoma (Fig. 2-16). Small cancerous nodes, seemingly normal by size criteria, may be clustered with larger, obviously malignant nodes.

**TABLE 2-1. LOCATION OF ANATOMIC SPACES OF THE NECK**

| Space | Suprahyoid | Infrahyoid |
|---|---|---|
| Buccal | X | |
| Sublingual | X | |
| Submandibular | X | |
| Parotid | X | |
| Parapharyngeal | | |
|   Prestyloid (parapharyngeal) | X | |
|   Poststyloid (carotid) | X | X |
| Masticator | X | |
| Retropharyngeal | X | X |
| Perivertebral | X | X |
| Posterior cervical | X | X |
| Pharyngeal mucosal | X | |
| Visceral | | X |

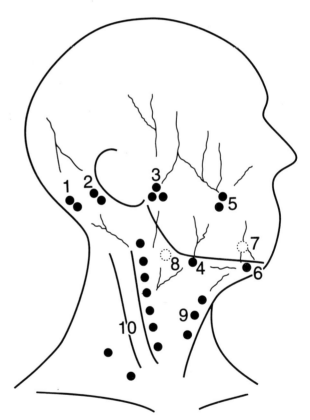

FIGURE 2-8. Diagram of the cervical lymph nodes. Major groups of the cervical lymph nodes include: occipital (1), mastoid (2), parotid (3), submandibular (4), facial (5), submental (6), sublingual (concealed by the deep structures of the neck) (7), retropharyngeal (concealed in the deep structures of the neck) (8), anterior cervical (9), and lateral cervical (10). (Wippold FJ II. Neck. In: Lee JKT, Sagel SS, Stanley RJ, Heiken JP, eds. *Computed body tomography with MRI correlation*, 3rd ed. Philadelphia: Lippincott-Raven, 1998:107–182.)

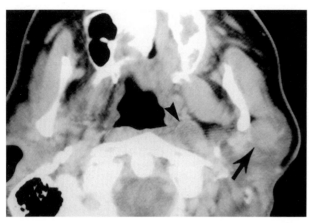

**FIGURE 2-9.** Parotid node. Prominent parotid lymph node (*arrow*) in CT scan of a patient with lymphoma. Note the retropharyngeal lymph node (*arrowhead*). (Wippold FJ II. Neck. In: Lee JKT, Sagel SS, Stanley RJ, et al., eds. *Computed body tomography with MRI correlation*, 3rd ed. Philadelphia: Lippincott-Raven, 1998:107–182, by permission.)

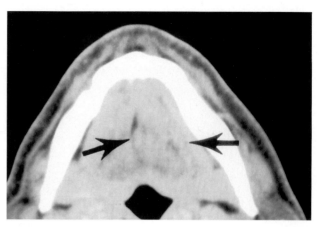

**FIGURE 2-11.** Sublingual lymph nodes. CT scan showing several small lymph nodes (*arrows*) within the sublingual space adjacent to the sublingual salivary glands and mylohyoid muscle. Nodes are also seen in the midline, between the genioglossus muscles. (Wippold FJ II. Neck. In: Lee JKT, Sagel SS, Stanley RJ, et al., eds. *Computed body tomography with MRI correlation*, 3rd ed. Philadelphia: Lippincott-Raven, 1998:107–182, by permission.)

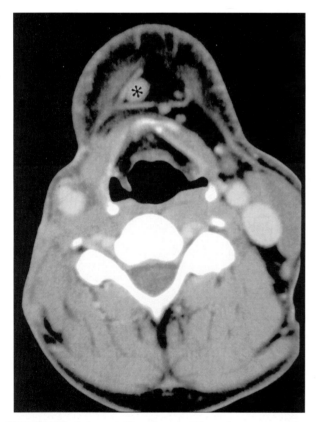

**FIGURE 2-10.** Submental lymph node. CT scan in a cancer patient following right radical neck dissection demonstrating a prominent submental lymph node (*asterisk*). The right sternocleidomastoid muscle, right internal jugular vein, and right cervical lymph nodes have been removed. (Wippold FJ II. Neck. In: Lee JKT, Sagel SS, Stanley RJ, et al., eds. *Computed body tomography with MRI correlation*, 3rd ed. Philadelphia: Lippincott-Raven, 1998:107–182, by permission.)

- Shape is no longer thought to be reliable in differentiating normal from pathologic nodes. Round nodes tend to be neoplastic, whereas elliptical or bean-shaped nodes are generally normal or hyperplastic. However, many exceptions may be encountered.
- Tumor spread beyond the capsule of a node is manifested by capsular enhancement, ill-defined nodal margins, obliterated fat planes surrounding the node, and edema or thickening in the adjacent soft tissues.
- Additional imaging signs of lymphadenopathy are the presence of enhancement and calcification within nodes. Calcification of a node may be seen in granulomatous disease such as tuberculosis, previously radiated neoplastic nodes, and metastatic thyroid carcinoma.

### 2.5. Posttherapy Neck

- Therapy for head and neck cancer may involve surgery, radiation, chemotherapy, and immunotherapy or combined modalities. Surgical treatment can be divided into surgery for the primary lesion (such as laryngectomy for laryngeal cancer), adjunctive surgery for spread of disease (such as neck dissection for cervical lymphadenopathy), and reconstructive surgery (such as construction of myocutaneous flaps).[21,29]
- The imaging evaluation of the posttherapy patient begins with a thorough understanding of the procedures performed coupled and with pretreatment images that identify the original lesion.
- Primary and adjunctive surgery usually entails partial or complete removal of the lesion. Discussion with the surgeon about the extent of the procedure assists in the appreciation of anatomic alterations typically seen on imaging. In these instances, key anatomic structures will be absent

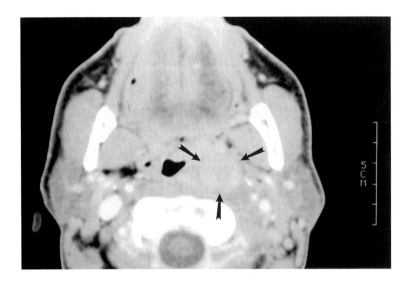

**FIGURE 2-12.** Retropharyngeal node. CT scan showing an enlarged left retropharyngeal lymph node (*arrows*) in a patient with nasopharyngeal carcinoma.

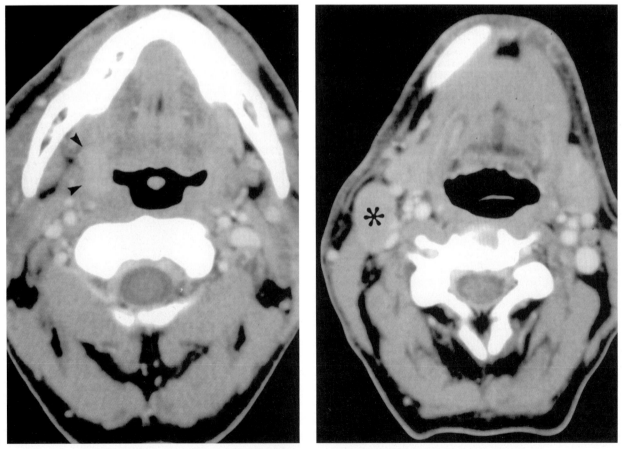

**FIGURE 2-13.** Tonsillar carcinoma with internal jugular lymphadenopathy. **A:** axial CT scan revealing dense right tonsillar mass (*arrowheads*). **B:** enlarged right internal jugular lymph node (asterisk) superior to the hyoid bone (level II lymphadenopathy).

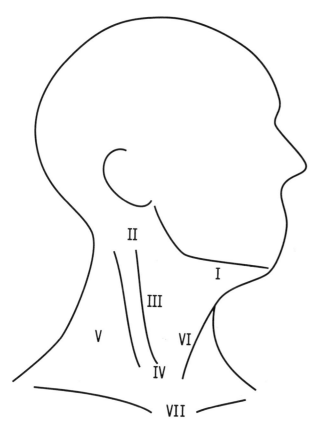

**FIGURE 2-14.** Cervical lymph node levels defined by the American Joint Committee on Cancer (AJCC). Level I consists of the submental and submandibular lymph nodes. Levels II, III, and IV consist of the high, middle, and lower internal jugular chain nodes. Level V corresponds to the spinal accessory and transverse cervical lymph node chains. Level VI consists of pretracheal and paratracheal lymph nodes. Level VII corresponds to the nodes in the tracheo-esophageal groove and upper mediastinum. (Wippold FJ II. Neck. In: Lee JKT, Sagel SS, Stanley RJ, et al., eds. *Computed body tomography with MRI correlation,* 3rd ed. Philadelphia: Lippincott-Raven, 1998:107–182, by permission.)

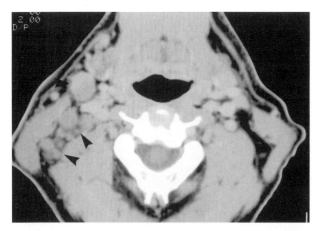

**FIGURE 2-16.** Lymphoma with abnormal lymph node clusters. Axial CT scan in a patient with squamous cell cancer demonstrating multiple small lymph nodes (*arrowheads*) within the lateral cervical chain. Although several of the nodes are normal by size criteria, the multiplicity indicates lymphadenopathy. Clusters are also present in the left neck. (Wippold FJ II. Neck. In: Lee JKT, Sagel SS, Stanley RJ, et al., eds. *Computed body tomography with MRI correlation,* 3rd ed. Philadelphia: Lippincott-Raven, 1998:107–182, by permission.)

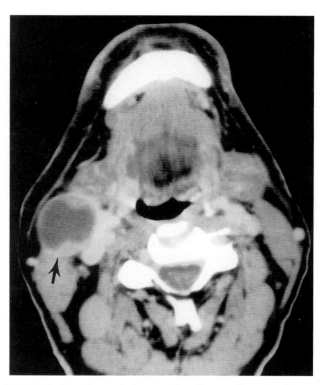

**FIGURE 2-15.** Metastatic internal jugular lymph node. CT scan of an enlarged right internal jugular lymph node (level II) (*arrow*) demonstrating internal inhomogeneity consistent with necrosis.

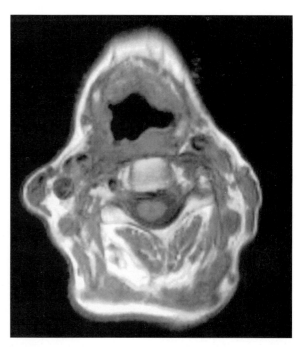

**FIGURE 2-17.** Supraglottic laryngectomy. T1-weighted MR image of a patient with a supraglottic laryngectomy. The neopharyngeal tissues are thickened. Recognition of the surgery depends on the appreciation of absent anatomy (such as the epiglottis).

*CT and MR Imaging of Head and Neck Cancer* **27**

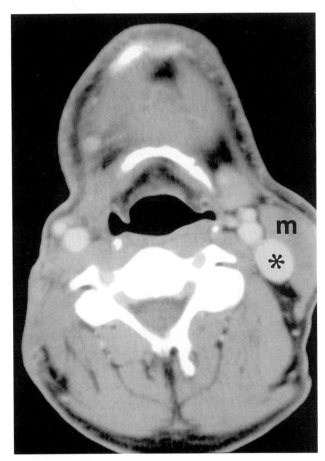

**FIGURE 2-18.** Axial CT scan following a right radical neck dissection. The asymmetry of the neck is striking. Note the absent right jugular vein and sternocleidomastoid muscle compared with the normal left sternocleidomastoid muscle (m) and left internal jugular vein (*asterisk*).

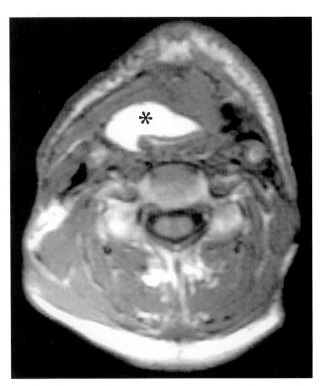

**FIGURE 2-19.** Myocutaneous graft in a patient with hypopharyngeal carcinoma treated with radical neck dissection. T1-weighted MR image revealing the hyperintense fat-containing graft (*asterisk*) and surrounding soft-tissue thickening following a total laryngectomy.

on posttherapy scans (Figs. 2-17 and 2-18). Reconstructive surgery usually entails augmentation of residual tissues or transplanting distant tissues for cosmetic and functional effect. Again, the surgeon can supply essential information about the procedure that facilitates understanding of the anatomic alterations seen on imaging. In these instances, anatomic structures not present on the pretherapy scans will be visible (Fig. 2-19).[21,29–31]

- Patients receiving radiation therapy develop soft-tissue and bony changes on imaging with doses of 6,500 to 7,000 cGy. Depending on the ports and doses of radiation, these changes may include thickening of the skin and platysma; stranding of the subcutaneous fat; fibrosis of the muscles of mastication; enhancement and eventual atrophy of the major and minor salivary glands; stranding of the fat-containing preepiglottic and paraglottic spaces; thickening of the epiglottis, aryepiglottic folds, false vocal cords, and true cords; enhancement of mucosal surfaces; contraction of the thyrohyoid membrane; chondronecrosis and cartilage collapse; fatty infiltration of the radiated bone marrow; osteoradionecrosis of the mandible;

atrophy due to cranial neuropathies; diminished vascular flow due to accelerated atherosclerotic disease; and rarely, sarcomas.[21,31,32] (Fig. 2-20 to 2-22). Three-dimensional radiation port planning may ameliorate posttherapy xerostomia by shielding the parotid glands.[6]

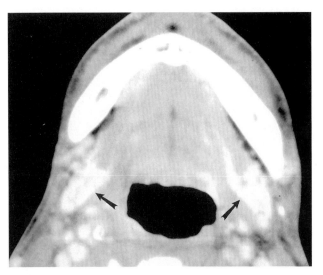

**FIGURE 2-20.** Radiation sialadenitis. Axial CT scan revealing densely enhancing submandibular salivary glands (*arrows*) following radiation for neck carcinoma.

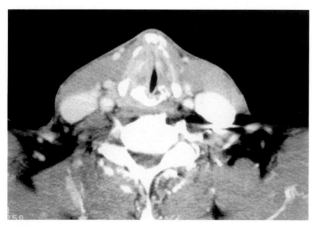

**FIGURE 2-21.** Mucosal edema following radiation therapy. Enhanced CT demonstrates asymmetric thickening of the true vocal cords with irregular enhancement and airway narrowing following radiation therapy for a glottic carcinoma.

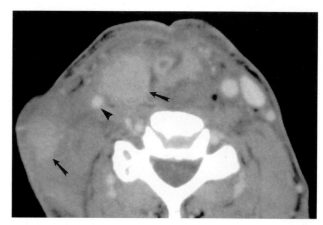

**FIGURE 2-23.** Recurrent carcinoma in a patient with a total laryngectomy. Axial CT scan reveals dense masses (*arrows*) representing recurrent carcinoma within the neck. Note the absent right internal jugular vein following the patient's radical neck dissection. The normal laryngeal structures are absent. Note the small right carotid artery (*arrowhead*). The skin is thickened and the subcutaneous fat is edematous following radiation therapy.

- For patients with successful surgical therapy, scans should remain stable over time, with the exceptions that bulky, fatty reconstruction flaps usually atrophy and fibrotic scar develops. Tissue planes become more defined as postsurgical edema subsides, but they may remain somewhat obscured when compared with the preoperative images. The complete or nearly complete resolution of the primary lesion on imaging is one of the best criteria for a successful radiation response.
- Development of a focal, dense, and necrotic mass within the original surgical bed or the reconstructed tissue or appearance of enlarging lymph nodes draining the surgical site usually indicates recurrent tumor (Fig. 2-23). Residual mass of greater than 50% of the original tumor volume suggests a radiation therapy failure.[33]
- A baseline imaging study in patients who are especially at risk for recurrence should not be performed for at least a month because of the persistence of potentially confusing postsurgical hemorrhage and edema. Scanning at intervals of 4 months to 6 months for the first 1 to 3 years is then appropriate.[30] Annual examinations are then performed unless a change in clinical status prompts a more timely scan.[30]

## REFERENCES

1. Russell E. The radiologic approach to malignant tumors of the head and neck, with emphasis on computed tomography. *Clin Plast Surg* 1985;12:343–374.
2. Wortham D, Hoover L, Lufkin R, et al. Magnetic resonance imaging of the larynx: a correlation with histologic sections. *Otolaryngol Head Neck Surg* 1986;94:123–133.
3. Suojanen J, Mukherji S, Dupuy D, et al. Spiral CT in evaluation of head and neck lesions: work in progress. *Radiology* 1992;183:281–283.
4. Suojanen J, Mukherji S, Wippold F. Spiral CT of the larynx. *Am J Neuroradiol* 1994;15:1579–1582.
5. Zeiberg A, Silverman P, Sessions R, et al. Helical (spiral) CT of the upper airway with three-dimensional imaging: technique and clinical assessment. *Am J Roentgenol* 1996;166:293–299.
6. Emami B, Purdy J, Simpson J, et al. 3-D conformal radiotherapy in head and neck cancer. *Front Radiot Ther Oncol* 1996;29:207–220.
7. Hudgins P, Gussack G. MR imaging in the management of extracranial malignant tumors of the head and neck. *Am J Roentgenol* 1992;159:161–169.
8. Glazer H, Niemeyer J, Balfe D, et al. Neck neoplasms: MR imaging. Part II. Posttreatment evaluation. *Radiology* 1986;160:349–354.
9. Hasso A, Brown K. Use of gadolinium chelates in MR imaging of lesions of the extracranial head and neck. *J Magn Reson Imaging* 1993;3:247–263.
10. Barakos J, Dillon W, Chew W. Orbit, skull base, and pharynx: contrast-enhanced fat suppression MR imaging. *Radiology* 1991;179:191–198.

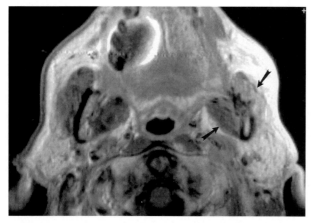

**FIGURE 2-22.** Masticator space changes following radiation therapy. Atrophied and hyperintense, contrast-enhancing changes in the left masseter and medial pterygoid muscles (*arrows*) on enhanced T1-weighted images following radiation therapy.

11. Balaban R, Ceckler T. Magnetization transfer contrast in magnetic resonance imaging. *Magn Reson Q* 1992;8:116–137.

12. Lambre H, Anzai Y, Farahani K, et al. Interventional magnetic resonance imaging of the head and neck and new imaging techniques. *Neuroimaging Clin N Am* 1996;6:461–472.

13. Harris K, Smith T, Cragg A, et al. Nephrotoxicity from contrast material in renal insufficiency: ionic versus nonionic agents. *Radiology* 1991;179:849–852.

14. Haustein J, Niendorf H, Krestin G, et al. Renal tolerance of gadolinium-DTPA/dimeglumine in patients with chronic renal failure. *Invest Radiol* 1992;27:153–156.

15. Som P. The present controversy over imaging method of choice for evaluating the soft tissues of the neck. *Am J Neuroradiol* 1997;18:1869–1872.

16. Grodinsky M, Holyoke E. The fasciae and fascial spaces of the head, neck and adjacent regions. *Am J Anat* 1938;63:367–407.

17. Williams DI. An imager's guide to normal neck anatomy. *Semin Ultrasound CT MR* 1997;18:157–181.

18. Harnsberger H. The perivertebral space. In: Harnsberger H, ed. *Head and neck imaging,* 2nd ed. St. Louis: Mosby Year Book, 1995:105–119.

19. Mukherji S, Castillo M. A simplified approach to the spaces of the suprahyoid neck. *Radiol Clin N Am* 1998;36:761–780.

20. Smoker W. Normal anatomy of the neck. In: Som P, Curtin H, eds. *Head and neck imaging,* 3rd ed. St. Louis: Mosby Year Book, 1996:711–771.

21. Wippold FI. Neck. In: Lee J, Sagel S, Stanley R, et al., eds. *Computed body tomography with MRI correlation,* 3rd ed. Philadelphia: New York: Lippincott-Raven, 1998:107–182.

22. Chong V, Fan Y-F, Mukherji S. Carcinoma of the nasopharynx. *Semin Ultrasound CT MR* 1998;19:449–462.

23. Wippold F. Diagnostic imaging of the larynx. In: Cummings C, Fredrickson J, Harker L, et al., eds. *Otolaryngology–head and neck surgery,* 3rd ed. St. Louis: Mosby, 1998:1895–1919.

24. Rouviere H. *Anatomy of the human lymphatic system.* Ann Arbor, MI: Edwards Bros, 1938.

25. Kaji A, Mohuchy T, Swartz J. Imaging of cervical lymphadenopathy. *Semin Ultrasound CT MR* 1997;18:220–249.

26. Som PM, Curtin HD, Mancuso AA. An imaging-based classification for the cervical nodes designed as an adjunct to recent clinically based nodal classification. *Arch Otolaryngol Head Neck Surg* 1999;125:388–396.

27. Som P. Lymph nodes of the neck. *Radiology* 1987;165:593–600.

28. Van den Brekel M, Stel H, Castelijns J, et al. Cervical lymph node metastasis: assessment of radiologic criteria. *Radiology* 1990;177:379–384.

29. Gore R, Levine M. Postoperative pharynx. In: Gore R, Levine M, eds. *Textbook of gastrointestinal radiology,* 2nd ed. Philadelphia: WB Saunders, 2000:257–270.

30. Som P, Urken M, Biller H, et al. Imaging the postoperative neck. *Radiology* 1993;187:593–603.

31. Wippold JI. Imaging the treated oral cavity and oropharynx. *Eur J Radiol* 2002 In press.

32. Tartaglino L, Rao V, Markiewicz D. Imaging of radiation changes in the head and neck. *Semin Roentgenol* 1994;29:81–91.

33. Mukherji S, Mancuso A, Kotzur I, et al. Radiologic appearance of the irradiated larynx. Part II. Primary site response. *Radiology* 1994;193:149–154.

# 3

# POSITRON-EMITTING TOMOGRAPHY (PET) IMAGING IN HEAD AND NECK CANCER

**WADE L. THORSTAD**
**K.S. CLIFFORD CHAO**

## 1. HISTORY OF ONCOLOGIC PET*

- PET was developed in the 1970s by researchers at Washington University and remained principally a research tool until the mid-1990s.
- Biologic imaging of the brain and heart were the focus of early research.
- Oncologic applications were developed and assumed increasing clinical importance; however, lack of a reimbursement mechanism prevented widespread use in the United States.
- In January 1998, the Health Care Financing Administration (HCFA) developed coverage policies for solitary pulmonary nodules and initial staging of non–small cell lung cancer.
- In July 2001 HCFA provided broad coverage for the diagnosis, staging, and restaging of six malignancies including non–small cell lung cancer, esophageal cancer, colorectal cancer, lymphoma, melanoma, and head and neck cancer.
- The new indications for coverage provided by HCFA in July 2001 specifically require dedicated PET systems.

## 2. RATIONALE

- An increased rate of glucose metabolism in malignant cells was first reported in the 1930s.[1]
- [18]F-fluorodeoxyglucose (FDG) is a glucose analog. FDG is transported into tumor cells and is phosphorylated similar to glucose, but does not undergo glycolysis, nor can it easily escape from the metabolic compartment.
- FDG PET images are based on metabolic activity rather than anatomy. Subclinical tumor and/or normal-sized

lymph nodes ($\leq 1$cm) may be detected with PET due to abnormal metabolism at the molecular level.
- Before mass effect caused by a tumor or a metastatic lymph node, many significant abnormalities have occurred at the molecular level.
- Molecular probes for *in vivo* imaging of oligonucleotides, peptides, enzymes, ligands, receptors, transport substrates, tissue hypoxia, and so on, provide a biological window with which to observe and potentially intervene in the malignant process.
- Labeling molecular probes with standard nuclear medicine tracers (Tc-99m, In-111, Ga-67, etc.) changes the property of the probe, potentially invalidating normal function of the probe.
- Creating positron-emitting isotopes of molecular probes is possible using nitrogen, oxygen, or carbon atoms inherent in the organic structure (with N-13, O-15, or C-11, respectively).
- By definition, isotopes differ only in nuclear constituents; chemical and biochemical reactions among isotopes are identical. A positron-emitting molecular probe of interest can be created and its *in vivo* action observed without perturbing the normal function of the probe.
- Because of the sensitivity with which radioactive events may be detected, it is possible to detect positron-emitting molecular probes at tissue concentrations in the range of picomoles to femtomoles per gram.
- Although almost all experience with imaging head and neck tumors to date has been with FDG, there is intense interest in the development of new molecular probes.
- [11]C-methionine and [11]C-thymidine have recently been used to evaluate amino acid metabolism in head and neck tumors.[2,3]
- Hypoxic specific tracers, including F-18 Misonidazole and Copper diacetyl-bis $N^4$-methylthiosemi carbazone (Cu-64 ATSM), have been developed and hypoxia in human

---

*PET refers to F-18 FDG PET unless otherwise noted.

**TABLE 3-1. PET COMPARED WITH CT/MRI FOR DETECTION OF LYMPH NODE METASTASIS IN HEAD AND NECK CANCER**

| Author/Year | No. of Patients | Sens PET | Spec PET | CT/MRI Sens | CT/MRI Spec |
|---|---|---|---|---|---|
| Rege 1994[14] | 34 | 88% | 89% | 81% (MRI) | 89% (MRI) |
| Laubenbacher 1995[12] | 22 | 90% | 96% | 78% (MRI) | 71% (MRI) |
| McGuirt 1995[13] | 49 | 83% | 82% | 78% (CT) | 86% (CT) |
| Benchaou 1996[9] | 48 | 72% | 99% | 67% (CT) | 97% (CT) |
| Braams 1997[10] | 12 | 91% | 88% | 36% (MRI) | 94% (MRI) |
| Wong 1997[15] | 16 | 67% | 100% | 67% (CT/MRI) | 25% (CT/MRI) |
| Adams 1998[8] | 60 | 90% | 94% | 82% (CT) 80% (MRI) | 85% (CT) 79% (MRI) |
| Myers 1998[31] | 14 | 78% | 100% | 57% (CT) | 90% (CT) |
| Kau 1999[11] | 70 | 87% | 94% | 65% (CT) 88% (MRI) | 47% (CT) 41% (MRI) |

Sens, sensitivity; spec, specificity.

head and neck cancers has been noninvasively imaged *in vivo*.[4-6]

## 3. TECHNIQUE

- FDG is administered after a minimum 4-hour fast.
- Image acquisition from 2 cm above the orbit through the liver will ensure evaluation of the entire upper aerodigestive track to identify metastatic disease or synchronous primary cancer.
- Complete aerodigestive track imaging may also avoid misinterpreting benign pulmonary nodules for metastatic disease and serves as a baseline in the event that future imaging reveals metastatic disease or metachronous cancer.
- Attenuation-corrected (AC) images are recommended for proper interpretation.
- AC corrects for apparent variability in FDG accumulation with the depth due to attenuation by normal tissue.
- Nonattenuation-corrected images may miss superficial tumors and/or lymph nodes due to edge effect distortion.
- Attenuation correction also allows for semiquantitative measurement of FDG uptake via the standardized uptake value (SUV).
- Although discriminatory values are not yet precisely defined for head and neck cancer, SUV in general aids in differentiating malignant from benign tissue and potentially in assessing response to therapy.
- Diabetic patients with elevated fasting glucose may have poor FDG PET images. FDG must compete for tumor uptake with abundant glucose. Diabetics should probably not be imaged unless fasting glucose is less than 150 dl/mg.
- Conversing during the FDG uptake phase may result in significant FDG accumulation in laryngeal musculature, thus complicating interpretation.
- Scalene and sternocleidomastoid muscle uptake may also be elevated in anxious patients or after neck dissection.
- Diazepam may be used to induce muscle relaxation during the FDG uptake phase.[7]

## 4. STAGING HEAD AND NECK CANCER

- Multiple studies suggest that PET is more sensitive and specific in evaluating lymphatic metastasis than such anatomic modalities as CT and MRI (Table 3-1).[8-15]
- Adams et al. evaluated 1,284 lymph nodes in 60 patients with head and neck cancer. Sensitivity and specificity of PET was 90% and 94%, respectively, compared with values of 82% and 85% for CT, and 80% and 79% for MRI.[8]
- Most published studies have been in selected patient groups. The study by Kau et al. compared the diagnostic accuracy of PET with CT and MRI for metastatic lymph node detection in a routine clinical setting at an academic medical center. Sensitivity and specificity for PET were 87% and 94%, respectively, compared with values of 65% and 47% for CT, and 88% and 41% for MRI.[11]
- Virtually all primary tumors identified with CT and/or MRI are also identified with PET.
- PET lacks anatomic detail sufficient for determining the T stage of a tumor. PET strengths are regional nodal and distant metastatic staging (31).

## 5. UNKNOWN PRIMARY CARCINOMA PRESENTING WITH CERVICAL LYMPH NODE METASTASIS

- In 1950, approximately 10% of patients with proven malignancy had no known primary site.[16]
- Improvements in diagnostic imaging and pathologic evaluation (i.e., immunohistochemical staining) have reduced this number to about 2% today.[17,18]
- Patients who present with cervical lymph node metastasis from an unknown primary tumor present difficult management decisions.
- Among patients with cervical metastasis from unknown primary cancers after clinical examination, panendoscopy, and CT/MRI examination, 25% to 30% are found to have a primary head and neck cancer when evaluated with PET.[10,19,20]

## TABLE 3-2. PET COMPARED WITH CT/MRI FOR DETECTION OF RECURRENCE IN HEAD AND NECK CANCER

| Author/Year | No. of Patients | Sens PET | Spec PET | CT/MRI Sens | CT/MRI Spec |
|---|---|---|---|---|---|
| Rege 1994[14] | 17 | 90% | 100% | 60% (MRI) | 57% (MRI) |
| Lapela 1995[23] | 22 | 88% | 86% | 92% (CT) | 50% (CT) |
| Anzai 1996[21] | 12 | 88% | 100% | 25% (CT/MRI) | 75% (CT/MRI) |
| Greven 1997[22] | 31 | 80% | 81% | 58% (CT) | 100% (CT) |

■ PET has been shown to change management in 33% of patients with cervical lymph node metastasis from an unknown primary site.[19]

## 6. DETECTION OF RECURRENCE

■ The clinical outcome of patients with recurrent head and neck cancer is poor.
■ Early identification of recurrence may increase the likelihood of successful salvage treatment.
■ Anatomic evaluation after surgery and irradiation or primary chemoradiotherapy is frequently nonconclusive because of treatment-related disruption of normal anatomy and tissue planes.
■ Several studies demonstrate that PET is superior to clinical examination and CT/MRI imaging for detecting recurrence in head and neck carcinoma (Table 3-2).[14,21–23]
■ Wong et al. showed that PET staged 13 posttreatment necks with an accuracy of 100% as compared with 54% accuracy with CT/MR and 62% accuracy with clinical examination.[15]
■ The appropriate timing of PET after completion of radiation therapy to assess for persistent/recurrent disease is unresolved but may lie between 1 and 4 months.
■ In 16 patients with a normal 1-month posttreatment PET, three eventually failed at the primary site (false-negative rate of 18%). None of 11 patients with a normal 4-month posttreatment PET failed at the primary site (false-negative rate of 0).[22]
■ In six patients with an abnormal 1-month PET, all six eventually failed at the primary site (false-positive rate of 0). In seven patients with an abnormal 4-month PET, six eventually failed at the primary site (false-positive rate of 14%).[22]

## 7. ASSESSMENT OF TREATMENT RESPONSE

■ Although PET has a good track record with detection of recurrence as noted earlier, prediction of ultimate outcome early during treatment would have tremendous implications for the patient.
■ The ability to predict the outcome of chemoradiotherapy for organ-sparing head and neck cancer treatment would allow early use of surgical intervention in those not

responding and more confident avoidance of surgery in those with a good response.
■ Studies with FDG PET for assessing response during radiation therapy are conflicting, showing both decrease and increase in SUV during radiation. Normal tissue inflammation may be related to an increase in SUV during radiation.[24,25]
■ A study using C-11 methionine (MET) during radiation showed a significant reduction in MET uptake after a median dose of 24 Gy but no correlation with ultimate outcome was demonstrated.[26]
■ Research is ongoing to identify a PET tracer correlating early response to radiotherapy with ultimate outcome in head and neck carcinoma.

## 8. IMPACT OF FDG PET ON RADIOTHERAPY TREATMENT PLANNING

■ Rahn et al. evaluated 34 patients with primary or recurrent squamous cell carcinoma of the head and neck that had PET scans in addition to conventional staging procedures before treatment planning. The extent of changes of treatment strategy or target volume due to PET findings was analyzed. In nine of 22 patients with primary tumors and seven of 12 patients with recurrent disease, PET led to changes in treatment strategy or target volume.[27]

## 9. COST-EFFECTIVENESS

■ Hollenbeak et al. demonstrated cost-effectiveness of a treatment strategy that includes PET in the diagnostic work-up of head and neck cancer patients who are N0 clinically. The incremental cost-effectiveness ratio for the PET strategy was more than $8,700 per year of lives saved, or approximately $2,500 per quality-adjusted life-year.[28]
■ Valk et al. demonstrated an incidence of distant metastasis in a group of locally advanced and recurrent head and neck cancer of 31%. The change in management from aggressive to palliative resulted in a savings-to-cost ratio of approximately 2:1.[29]
■ Larger, prospective studies are needed to better assess the cost-effectiveness of PET for various clinical indications in head and neck cancer.

*PET Imaging in Head and Neck Cancer* **33**

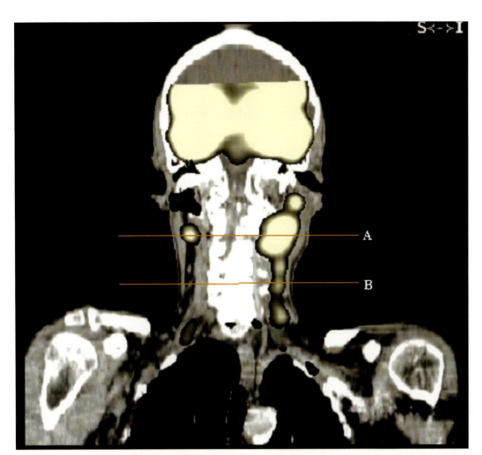

**FIGURE 3-1.** Coronal view of coregistered CT and FDG-PET images showing a large (37 × 28 mm) left-side metastatic lymph node and multiple small lymph nodes on both necks in a patient with tonsillar primary. The small lymph nodes are clearly abnormal on PET but do not meet size criteria for malignancy on CT.

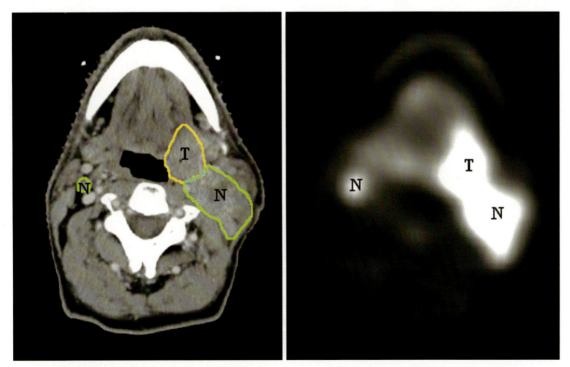

**FIGURE 3-2.** Axial CT and PET images at level A in Fig. 3-1. Outlined on the left is the tonsillar carcinoma and ipsilateral lymph node metastasis. The outlined right lymph node measures 8.3 × 8.8 × 5.6 mm on CT but is hypermetabolic on PET and pathologically involved.

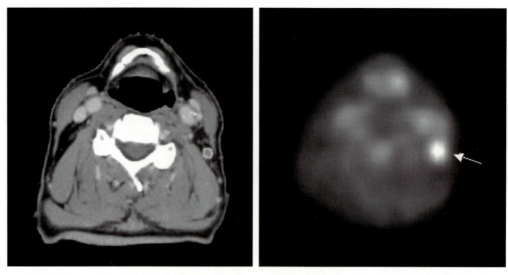

**FIGURE 3-3.** Axial CT and PET images at level B in Fig. 3-1. The outlined left lymph node measures 7.0 × 6.8 × 9 mm on CT but is hypermetabolic on PET and pathologically involved.

## 10. FUSION OF ANATOMIC AND METABOLIC IMAGES

- Anatomic and metabolic image fusion for radiotherapy treatment planning has the potential to more define tumor boundaries and lymph node metastasis accurately than anatomic imaging alone.
- Image fusion has traditionally been performed with software; accuracy and quality assurance issues regarding the "fit" of the image sets remain important concerns.

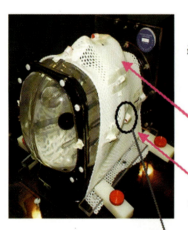
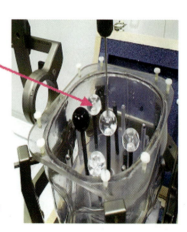
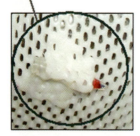

**FIGURE 3-4.** An anthropomorphic head phantom developed to assess the accuracy of image registration and fusion process. Room-in view shows a plastic ampule, serving as fiducial makers for CT-PET coregistration, attached to the surface of thermoplastic mask. (Chao KSC, Bosch WR, Mutic S, et al. A novel approach to overcome hypoxic tumor resistance: ATSM-guided intensity modulated radiation therapy. *Int J Radiat Oncol Biol Phys* 2001;49:1171–1182, by permission.)

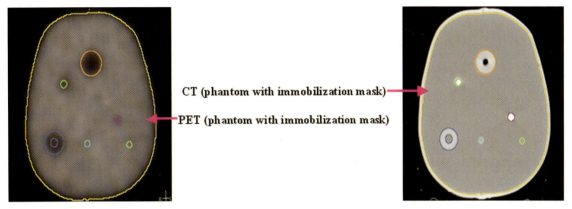

**FIGURE 3-5.** Validation of imaging fusion fidelity. Image registration was verified by contouring balls and rods on the primary CT scan and observing mapped contour locations on the secondary PET images. All contours were within 2 mm of their expected locations on the PET scans. (From Chao KSC, Bosch WR, Mutic S, et al. A novel approach to overcome hypoxic tumor resistance: ATSM-guided intensity modulated radiation therapy. *Int J Radiat Oncol Biol Phys* 2001;49:1171–1182, by permission.)

- Careful immobilization of head and neck cancer patients with thermoplastic devices is reproducible and has been shown to allow acceptable image fusion (Figs. 3-1 to 3-3).[30]
- The ability to accurately immobilize patients with head and neck cancer in thermoplastic devices makes software fusion more straightforward than in other parts of the body (Figs. 3-4 and 3-5).
- New CT/PET hybrid machines are just becoming available. These hybrid-imaging units offer "hardware" fusion that should serve as a benchmark for accurate image fusion.

## 11. FUTURE DEVELOPMENTS

- Studies to date have shown superiority of PET in detecting lymph node metastasis and recurrent disease when compared with CT/MRI. Fusion images allow the strength of anatomic imaging to compensate for the weakness of

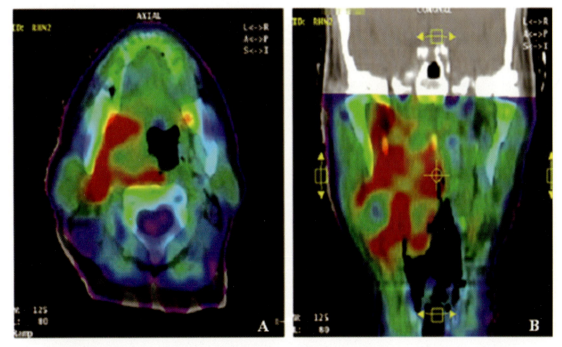

**FIGURE 3-6.** Color-washed images illustrated regions of heterogeneous $^{60}$Cu-ATSM intensity within the gross tumor representing the presence of tumor hypoxia. (Chao KSC, Bosch WR, Mutic S, et al. A novel approach to overcome hypoxic tumor resistance: ATSM-guided intensity modulated radiation therapy. *Int J Radiat Oncol Biol Phys* 2001;49:1171–1182, by permission.)

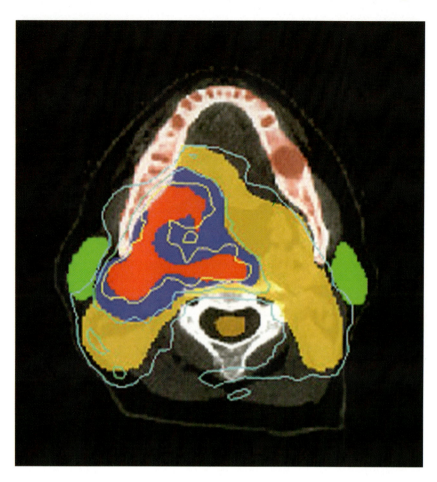

**FIGURE 3-7.** Delineation of the gross tumor volume and its ATSM-avid fraction by CT-PET imaging fusion. (From Chao KSC, Bosch WR, Mutic S, et al. A novel approach to overcome hypoxic tumor resistance: ATSM-guided intensity modulated radiation therapy. *Int J Radiat Oncol Biol Phys* 2001;49:1171–1182, by permission.)

PET imaging and vice versa. Emerging studies with hybrid CT/PET devices will likely demonstrate image fusion to be the new gold standard in head and neck oncologic imaging.

- CT/PET hybrid machines using FDG and a variety of PET molecular probes will provide images with outstanding anatomic detail combined with information related to various molecular abnormalities associated with malignant disease.
- Gene expression has been imaged in animal models. Gene therapy and image confirmation of appropriate expression may guide radiotherapy targeting in the future.
- Monitoring of a therapeutic strategy during treatment may become possible, allowing a shift to a more aggressive approach in the subgroup of patients who prove resistant to a specific approach.
- Studies are underway at Washington University in St. Louis to assess the feasibility of a Cu-ATSM PET image-guided intensity modulated radiation therapy (IMRT) to boost the hypoxic subvolume in head and neck tumors (Figs. 3-6 and 3-7).

## REFERENCES

1. Warburg O. *The metabolism of tumors.* London: Constable, 1930.
2. Eijkeren M, Schryver A, Goethals P, et al. Measurement of short-term $^{11}$C-thymidine activity in human head and neck tumours using positron emission tomography (PET). *Acta Oncol* 1992;31:539–543.
3. Leskinen-Kallio S, Lindholm P, Lapela M, et al. Imaging of head and neck tumors with positron emission tomography and 11-C-methionine. *Int J Radiat Oncol Biol Phys* 1994;30:1195–1199.
4. Chao KSC, Bosch WR, Mutic S, et al. A novel approach to overcome hypoxic tumor resistance: ATSM-guided intensity modulated radiation therapy. *Int J Radiat Oncol Biol Phys* 2001;49:1171–1182.
5. Lewis JS, Sharp TL, Jones LA, et al. Selective 60/64Cu-ATSM uptake in hypoxic tumors correlated with direct tissue oxygen measurement, PET imaging and electronic autoradiography. *J Nucl Med* 2000;41:115P.
6. Rasey JS, Koh WJ, Evans ML, et al. Quantifying regional hypoxia in human tumors with positron emission tomography of [$^{18}$F] fluoromisonidazole: a pretherapy study of 37 patients. *Int J Radiat Oncol Biol Phys* 1996;36:417–428.
7. Barrington S, Maisey M. Skeletal muscle uptake of fluorine-18-FDG: effect of oral diazepam. *J Nucl Med* 1996;37:1127–1129.
8. Adams S, Baum R, Stuckensen T, et al. Prospective comparison of 18F-FDG PET with conventional imaging modalities (CT, MRI, US) in lymph node staging of head and neck cancer. *Eur J Nucl Med* 1998;25:1255–1260.
9. Benchaou M, Lehmann W, Slosman D, et al. The role of FDG-PET in the preoperative assessment of N-staging in head and neck cancer. *Acta Otolaryngol* 1996;116:332–335.
10. Braams J, Pruim J, Kole A, et al. Detection of unknown primary head and neck tumors by positron emission tomography. *Int J Oral Maxillofac Surg* 1997;26:112–115.

11. Kau R, Alexiou C, Laubenbacher C, et al. Lymph node detection of head and neck squamous cell carcinomas by positron emission tomography with fluorodeoxyglucose F-18 in a routine clinical setting. *Arch Otolaryngol Head Neck Surg* 1999;125:1322–1328.
12. Laubenbacher C, Saumweber D, Wagner M, et al. Comparison of fluorine-18-fluorodeoxyglucose PET, MRI and endoscopy for staging head and neck squamous-cell carcinomas. *J Nucl Med* 1995;36:1747–1757.
13. McGuirt WF, Williams DW 3rd, Keyes JJ, et al. A comparative diagnostic study of head and neck nodal metastases using positron emission tomography. *Laryngoscope* 1995;105:373–375.
14. Rege S, Maass A, Chaiken L, et al. Use of positron emission tomography with fluorodeoxyglucose in patients with extracranial head and neck cancers. *Cancer* 1994;73:3047–3058.
15. Wong W, Checretton E, McGurk M, et al. A prospective study of PET-FDG imaging for the assessment of head and neck squamous cell carcinoma. *Clin Otolaryngol Appl Sci* 1997;22:209–214.
16. Abrams H, Spiro R, Goldstein M. Metastases in carcinoma: analysis of 1000 autopsied cases. *Cancer* 1950;3:120–124.
17. Abbruzzese J, Abbruzzese M, Hess K, et al. Unknown primary carcinoma: natural history and prognostic factors in 657 consecutive patients. *J Clin Oncol* 1994;12:1272–1280.
18. Muir C. Cancer of unknown primary site. *Cancer* 1995;75:353–356.
19. Jungehulsing M, Scheidhauer K, Damm M, et al. 2[$^{18}$F]-fluoro-2-deoxy-D-glucose positron emission tomography is a sensitive tool for the detection of occult primary cancer (carcinoma of unknown primary syndrome) with head and neck lymph node manifestation. *Otolaryngol Head Neck Surg* 2000;123:294–301.
20. Kole A, Nieweg O, Pruim J, et al. Detection of unknown occult primary tumors using positron emission tomography. *Cancer* 1998;82:1160–1166.
21. Anzai Y, Carroll W, Quint D, et al. Recurrence of head and neck cancer after surgery or irradiation: prospective comparison of 2-deoxy-2[F-18]fluoro-D-glucose PET and MR imaging diagnoses. *Radiology* 1996;200:135–141.
22. Greven K, Williams DW 3rd, Keyes J, et al. Distinguishing tumor recurrence from irradiation sequelae with positron emission tomography in patients treated for larynx cancer. *Int J Rad Oncol Biol Phys* 1994;29:841–845.
23. Lapela M, Grenman R, Kurki T, et al. Head and neck cancer: Detection of recurrence with positron emission tomography and 2-[18F]fluoro-2-deoxy-D-glucose. *Radiology* 1995;197:205–211.
24. Berlangieri S, Brizel D, Scher R, et al. Pilot study of positron emission tomography in patients with advanced head and neck cancer receiving radiotherapy and chemotheraphy. *Head Neck* 1994;16:340–346.
25. Hautzel H, Muller-Gartner H. Early changes in fluorine-18-FDG uptake during radiotherapy. *J Nucl Med* 1997;38:1384–1386.
26. Nuutinen J, Jyrkkio S, Lehikoinen P, et al. Evaluation of early response to radiotherapy in head and neck cancer measured with [$^{11}$C]methionine-positron emission tomography. *Radiother Oncol* 1999;52:225–232.
27. Rahn A, Baum R, Adamietz I, et al. Value of 18F fluorodeoxyglucose positron emission tomography in radiotherapy planning of head-neck tumors. *Strahlenther Onkol* 1998;174:358–364.
28. Hollenbeak C, Lowe V, Stack B. The cost-effectiveness of fluorodeoxyglucose 18-F positron emission tomography in the N0 neck. *Cancer* 2001;92:2341–2348.
29. Valk P, Pounds T, Tesar R, et al. Cost-effectiveness of PET imaging in clinical oncology. *Nucl Med Biol* 1996;23:737–743.
30. Mutic S, Dempsey J, Bosch W, et al. Multimodality image registration quality assurance for conformal three-dimensional treatment planning. *Int J Radiat Oncol Biol Phys* 2001;51:255–260.
31. Myers L, Wax M, Nabi H, et al. Positron emission tomography in the evaluation of the N0 neck. *Laryngoscope* 1998;108:232–236.

# 4

# DOSE PRESCRIPTION AND TARGET DELINEATION FOR NODAL VOLUMES

## K.S. CLIFFORD CHAO

## 1. INTRODUCTION

- Promising treatment results of head and neck and prostate conformal therapy or intensity modulated radiation therapy (IMRT) have provided significant incentives for the radiation oncology community to incorporate this imaging-based technology into daily clinical practice.
- Protecting critical normal tissue without compromising tumor target coverage requires extensive knowledge of the patterns of tumor extension and spread, and the ability to delineate accurately both the tumor target volumes and normal structures.
- Thorough understanding of the natural course of tumor spread ensures the delineation of clinical target volume that represents the region potentially containing microscopic disease as defined in International Commission on Radiation Units and Measurements (ICRU) reports No. 50 and No. 62.[1,2]
- Ideally, if an imaging modality can provide sufficient information on whether certain nodal regions contain micrometastasis, accurate determination of nodal target volume for head and neck IMRT will be possible. Unfortunately, neither physical examination nor radiologic imaging techniques used in clinical practice are proficient to detect microscopic disease. Sako et al. found that to be clinically detectable the submandibular nodes must measure at least 0.5 cm.[3] Similarly, a deep cervical node located adjacent to muscles must exceed 1 cm in diameter to be clinically palpable.
- Notably, the incidence of occult nodal metastasis ranged from 25% to 60% during the 1950s and 1960s. Even with advances in morphology-based imaging techniques, such as CT or MRI, determination of nodal metastasis based on the size of the lymph node still underestimates between 12% and 60% of micrometastasis. Detection of micrometastasis by functional imaging is an evolving area of research and may not be applicable clinically in the immediate future. Therefore, the current clinical practice to determine target volume for IMRT relies on historic information from surgical pathologic experiences.

- In 1948, Rouviere described the anatomic details of the cervical lymphatic network (Fig. 4-1).[4] Based on this description, the TNM atlas proposed a terminology that divides the head and neck lymph nodes into 12 groups according to their relationship with the adjacent muscles, vessels, and nerves.[5]
- In 1991 a Committee for Head and Neck Surgery and Oncology of the American Academy for Otolaryngology–Head and Neck Surgery postulated a classification (Robbins' classification) that divides the neck into six levels or eight nodal groups for those lymph nodes routinely removed during neck dissection[6] (Fig. 4-2).
- Lymph nodes that are not routinely dissected, such as retropharyngeal, parotid, buccal, or occipital nodes, are not included in Robbins's classification. Both systems describe the boundaries of the node region based on anatomic structures, such as major blood vessels, muscles, nerves, bones and cartilage, and the radiologic boundaries of these nodal levels have been summarized recently[7–11] (Fig. 4-3).

## 2. DETERMINATION OF CLINICAL TARGET VOLUMES

- We used terminology similar to that proposed by Robbins Classification for the determination of clinical target volumes (Table 4-1).[6]
- Determination of CTVs was based on the incidence and location of metastatic neck nodes from various head and neck subsites, which were gathered from the published literatures and summarized in Table 4-2. The distribution of nodal metastasis to different lymph node levels in the head and neck region varies by primary tumor subsite. The number under each column represents the percent of lymph node metastasis in patients with squamous cell carcinoma arising from various head and neck subsides. Because metastatic nodes may manifest in more than one nodal level at presentation, the summation of percentage

*Dose Prescription and Target Delineation for Nodal Volumes*  39

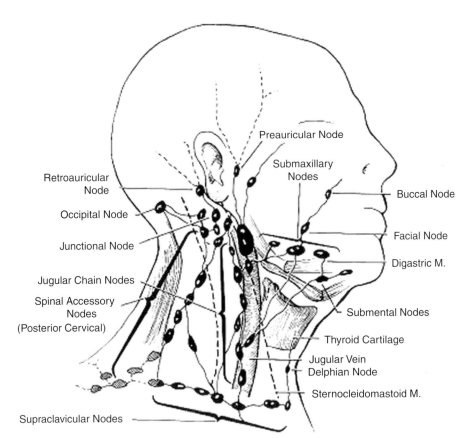

**FIGURE 4-1.** Lymph nodes in the head and neck region. (Redrawn from Rouviere H. *Anatomy of the human lymphatic system.*, Tobias MJ, trans. Ann Arbor, MI: Edwards Brothers, 1938:27, by permission.)

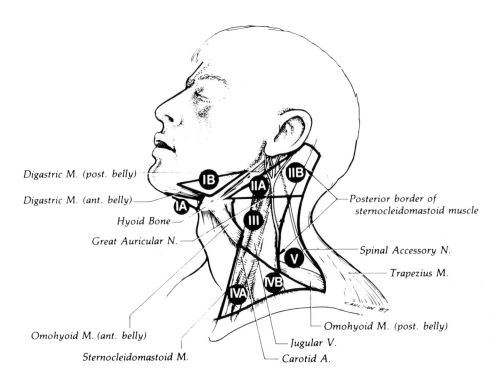

**FIGURE 4-2.** Surgical lymph node groups (levels) in the head and neck region. (Suen JY, Goepfert H. Editorial: Standardization of neck dissection nomenclature. *Head Neck Surg* 1987;10:76, by permission.)

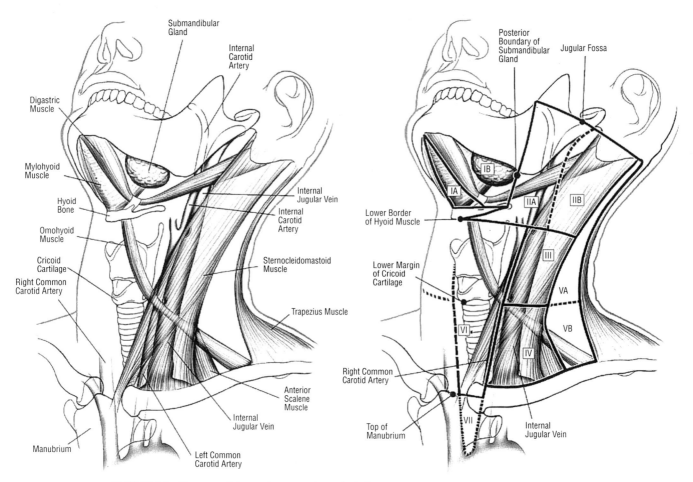

**FIGURE 4-3.** Diagram of the neck as seen from the left anterior view. *Left:* The pertinent anatomy that relates to the nodal classification. *Right:* An outline of the levels of the classification. Note that the line of separation between levels I and II is the posterior margin of the submandibular gland. The separation between levels II and III and level V is the posterior edge of the sternocleidomastoid muscle. However, the line of separation between levels IV and V is an oblique line extending from the posterior edge of the sternocleidomastoid muscle to the posterior edge of the anterior scalene muscle. The posterior edge of the internal jugular vein separates level IIA and IIB nodes. The top of the manubrium separates levels VI and VII. (Som PM, Curtin HD, Mancuso AA. An imaging-based classification for the cervical nodes designed as an adjunct to recent clinically based nodal classifications. *Arch Otolaryngol Head Neck Surg* 1999;125:388–396, by permission.)

from all nodal levels (regions) may exceed 100%, especially in the N+ group.
- Treatment of the contralateral neck remains controversial since there are very few data on the patterns of pathologic node distribution in the contralateral neck. This treatment also is likely to result from clinical judgment rather than from scientific evidence. However, contralateral nodal regions should be included, especially in tumors that tend to spread to the contralateral neck nodes or when tumor arises from or invades a midline structure, such as the soft palate, the base of the tongue, the posterior pharyngeal wall, or the nasopharynx. For example, nodal metastasis exists in 85% to 90% of patients with nasopharyngeal carcinoma, and about 50% of them have bilateral disease; therefore, both necks need to be treated.[12]
- Table 4-3 shows that macroscopic or microscopic bilateral nodal metastases present with more than 30% of tumor residing in the base of tongue, pharyngeal wall, and pyriform sinus.
- The probability of contralateral nodal metastasis can be predicted with better accuracy if these tumor characteristics are taken into account. Table 4-4 shows the tumor factors for oral cavity carcinoma that could influence the incidence of contralateral nodal metastasis.
- On the other hand, tumors arising from the true vocal cord, the paranasal sinuses, and the middle ear have a low risk of lymph node metastasis, and only ipsilateral neck needs to be included in IMRT field.[7]
- If a tumor arises from buccal mucosa and retromolar trigone, which has a lower chance of contralateral neck node metastasis, especially when the primary tumor size is small and no involvement of the ipsilateral neck node is evident, the contralateral neck may not need to be treated.

## TABLE 4-1. CLASSIFICATION AND DEFINITION OF NECK NODES (39)

| Robbins's Classification | | Definition |
|---|---|---|
| Level | Terminology | Surgical/Anatomic Landmarks |
| Ia | Submental group | Contains the submental and submandibular triangles bounded by the |
| Ib | Submandibular group | posterior belly of the digastric muscle, the hyoid bone inferiorly, and the body of the mandible superiorly |
| II | Upper internal jugular group | Contains the upper internal jugular lymph nodes and extends from the level of the hyoid bone inferiorly to the skull base superiorly |
| III | Middle internal jugular group | Contains the middle internal jugular lymph nodes from the hyoid bone superiorly to the cricothyroid membrane inferiorly |
| IV | Lower internal jugular group | Contains the lower internal jugular lymph nodes from the cricothyroid membrane superiorly to the clavicle inferiorly |
| V | Spinal accessory group | Contains the lymph nodes in the posterior triangle bounded by the anterior border of the trapezius posteriorly, the posterior border of the sternocleidomastoid muscle anteriorly, and the clavicle inferiorly (For descriptive purposes, level V may be further subdivided into upper, middle, or lower levels corresponding to the superior and inferior planes that define levels II, III, and IV.) |
| VI | Anterior compartment group | Contains the lymph nodes of the anterior compartment from the hyoid bone superiorly to the suprasternal notch inferiorly. On each side the lateral border is formed by the medial border of the carotid sheath. |
| VII | Upper mediastinal group | Contains the lymph nodes inferior to the suprasternal notch in the upper mediastinum |

*Other groups:* Retropharyngeal, buccinator (facial), intraparotid, preauricular, postauricular, suboccipital

- Having tumor characteristics and clinical/pathologic information in mind, the following guidelines using a simplified but clinical relevant method for target volume determination and delineation were implemented.
  - □ *Clinical target volume 1 (CTV1)* for definitive IMRT patients encompasses the gross tumor and the region adjacent to the gross tumor but not directly involved by tumor based on clinical findings and CT or MRI imaging. Radiologically or clinically involved neck node is also included in CTV1 with 2-cm margins truncating air and bone.
  - □ CTV1 for postoperative IMRT patients encompasses the preoperative gross tumor volume plus 1- to 2-cm margin, including the resection bed with soft-tissue

## TABLE 4-2. INCIDENCE AND DISTRIBUTION OF METASTATIC DISEASE IN CLINICALLY NEGATIVE (N−) AND POSITIVE (N+) NECK NODES (IN PERCENTAGE) (39)

| Clinical Presentation | Radiologically Enlarged Retropharyngeal Nodes | | Pathologic Nodal Metastasis | | | | | | | | | |
|---|---|---|---|---|---|---|---|---|---|---|---|---|
| | | | Level I | | Level II | | Level III | | Level IV | | Level V | |
| | N− | N+ | N− | N+ | N− | N+ | N− | N+ | N− | N+ | N− | N+ |
| Nasopharynx | 40 | 86 | — | — | — | — | — | — | — | — | — | — |
| Oral cavity | | | | | | | | | | | | |
| Oral tongue | — | — | 14 | 39 | 19 | 73 | 16 | 27 | 3 | 11 | 0 | 0 |
| Floor of mouth | — | — | 16 | 72 | 12 | 51 | 7 | 29 | 2 | 11 | 0 | 5 |
| Aveolar ridge and RMT | — | — | 25 | 38 | 19 | 84 | 6 | 25 | 5 | 10 | 1 | 4 |
| Oropharynx | | | | | | | | | | | | |
| Base of tongue | 0 | 6 | 4 | 19 | 30 | 89 | 22 | 22 | 7 | 10 | 0 | 18 |
| Tonsil | 4 | 12 | 0 | 8 | 19 | 74 | 14 | 31 | 9 | 14 | 5 | 12 |
| Hypopharynx | | | | | | | | | | | | |
| Pharyngeal wall | 16 | 21 | 0 | 11 | 9 | 84 | 18 | 72 | 0 | 40 | 0 | 20 |
| Pyriform sinus | 0 | 9 | 0 | 2 | 15 | 77 | 8 | 57 | 0 | 23 | 0 | 22 |
| Larynx | | | | | | | | | | | | |
| Supraglottic larynx | 0 | 4 | 6 | 2 | 18 | 70 | 18 | 48 | 9 | 17 | 2 | 16 |
| Glottic larynx | — | — | 0 | 9 | 21 | 42 | 29 | 71 | 7 | 24 | 7 | 2 |

*Sources:* Complied from McLaughlin 1995,[24] Candela 1990,[25] Shah 1990,[26] Bataini 1985,[27] Byers 1988,[28] Lindberg 1972.[29]
RMT, retromolar trigone.

### TABLE 4-3. INCIDENCE OF CONTRALATERAL OR BI-LATERAL NECK NODE METASTASIS BY PRIMARY TUMOR SITE (39)

| | cN+, Bilateral | cN+, Contralateral Only | cN−, pN+ Bilateral |
|---|---|---|---|
| Oral tongue | 12% | — | 33% |
| FOM | 27% | — | 21% |
| BOT | 37% | — | 55% |
| Tonsil | 16% | 2% | — |
| Pharyngeal wall | 50% | — | 37% |
| Pyriform sinus | 49% | 6% | 59% |
| Supraglottis | 39% | 2% | 26% |
| Glottic larynx | — | — | 15% |

Sources: Compiled from Northrop 1972,[30] Bataini 1985,[27] Byers 1988,[28] Woolgar 1999,[31] Buckley 2000.[32] BOT, base of tongue; FOM, floor of mouth.

### TABLE 4-4. FACTORS INFLUENCING CONTRALATER-AL LN METASTASIS IN ORAL CANCER (39)

| Variable | RR of Contralateral LN Metastasis | 95% CI |
|---|---|---|
| Tumor site | | |
| Tongue | 1.0 | Ref. |
| FOM | 1.5 | 0.9–2.6 |
| RMT | 0.3 | 0.1–1.1 |
| Distance from midline | | |
| >1 cm | 1.0 | Ref. |
| Cross <1 cm | 2.8 | 1.1–7.5 |
| Cross >1 cm | 12.7 | 5.6–29.1 |
| Tumor stage | | |
| T1 | 1.0 | Ref. |
| T2–T3 | 2.2 | 0.7–5.5 |
| T4 | 5.8 | 2.0–16.3 |

Source: Modified from Kowalski 1998.[33] FOM, floor of mouth; RMT, retromolar trigone.

invasion by the tumor, or extracapsular extension by metastatic neck nodes. Preoperative CT imaging, surgical defects, or postsurgical changes seen on postoperative CT scan determine the surgical bed.

☐ *Clinical target volume 2 (CTV2)* for both definitive and postoperative IMRT groups primarily includes the clinically/radiologically or pathologically uninvolved cervical lymph nodes, deemed as elective nodal regions or prophylactically treated neck.

■ Our approach on selective neck treatment is similar to the recommendations proposed by Gregoire et al.[7] These target volume specifications were integrated with the published clinical data shown in Table 4-2. Based on these historical data, we proposed that a treatment of the N0 neck is warranted if the probability of occult cervical metastasis is higher than 5%.

■ Tables 4-5 and 4-6 summarize the target volume (CTV1 and CTV2) specifications for various head and neck tumor subsites for postoperative and definitive IMRT.

■ To facilitate clinical throughput, at our institution IMRT was applied to the upper neck for salivary sparing. The lower neck was treated with a conventional AP lower neck port if indicated. Standard superior border for lower neck field was at the level of thyroid notch. A similar approach

was also implemented elsewhere.[13] In patients with tumor or metastatic lymph node extending below this level, the junction line was adjusted to avoid bisecting gross disease.

## 3. DELINEATION OF CLINICAL TARGET VOLUME

■ Since the definition of neck node level and the anatomic boundaries described in Robbins's Classification were based on specific soft-tissue landmarks for surgical procedures and are not easily seen on CT and MRI slices, we implemented modified guidelines for the delineation of the various node levels in the neck. We supplemented with a retropharyngeal nodal group to Robbins's Classification to assist readers in better understanding nodal target volume determination and delineation for head and neck IMRT. Table 4-7 lists our institutional recommendations for the radiologic boundaries of these nodal levels.

### TABLE 4-5. TARGET VOLUME SPECIFICATION FOR DEFINITIVE AND POSTOPER-ATIVE IMRT (39)

| Target | Definitive IMRT | High-Risk Postoperative IMRT | Intermediate-Risk Postoperative IMRT |
|---|---|---|---|
| CTV1 | Gross tumor and the adjacent soft tissue/nodal regions | Surgical bed with soft-tissue involvement or nodal region with extracapsular extension | Surgical bed without soft-tissue involvement or nodal region without extracapsular extension |
| CTV2 | Elective nodal regions* | Elective nodal regions* | Elective nodal regions* |

Source: Modified from Chao KSC, Wippold FJ, Ozyigit G, et al. Determination and delineation of nodal target volumes for head and neck cancer based on the patterns of failure in patients receiving definitive and postoperative IMRT. Int J Radiat Oncol Biol Phys 2002;53:1174–1184.
*Suggested guidelines for elective nodal regions are shown in Table 4-6.

## TABLE 4-6. CLINICAL TARGET VOLUME DETERMINATION FOR HEAD AND NECK IMRT (39)

| Tumor Site | Clinical Presentation | CTV1 | CTV2 |
|---|---|---|---|
| | | *Oral Cavity* | |
| Buccal RMT | T1–2N0 | P | IN (I–III) |
| | T3–4N+* | P + IN (I–III) | CN (I–III) |
| | N2c | P + IN + CN (I–V) | |
| Oral tongue | T1–2N0 | P | IN ± CN (I–IV) |
| | T3–4N+* | P + IN (I–IV) | CN (I–IV) |
| | N2c | P + IN + CN (I–V) | |
| FOM | T1–2N0 | P | IN + CN (I–III) |
| | T3–4N+* | P + IN (I–III) | CN (I–III) |
| | N2c | P + IN + CN (I–V) | |
| | | *Oropharynx* | |
| BOT | T1–2N0 | P | IN + CN (II–IV, RPLN) |
| | T3–4N+* | P + IN (II–IV, RPLN) | CN (I–V, RPLN) |
| | N2c | P + IN + CN (I–V, RPLN) | |
| Tonsil | T1–2N0 | P | IN ± CN (II–IV, RPLN) |
| | T3–4N+* | P + IN (II–IV, RPLN) | CN (I–V, RPLN) |
| | N2c | P + IN + CN (I–V, RPLN) | |
| | | *Hypopharynx* | |
| | T1–2N0 | P | IN + CN (II–IV) |
| | T3–4N+* | P + IN (II–IV, RPLN) | CN (II–IV) |
| | N2c | P + IN + CN (I–V, RPLN) | |
| | | *Larynx*[†] | |
| | T1–2N0 | P | IN + CN (II–IV) |
| | T3–4N+* | P + IN (II–IV) | CN (II–IV) |
| | N2c | P + IN + CN (I–V) | |
| | | *Nasopharynx* | |
| | T1–2N0 | P | IN + CN (I–V, RPLN) |
| | T3–4N+* | P + IN (I[‡]–V, RPLN) | CN (I–V, RPLN) |
| | N2c | P + IN + CN (I[‡]–V, RPLN) | |

*Source:* Modified from Chao KSC, Wippold FJ, Ozyigit G, et al. Determination and delineation of nodal target volumes for head and neck cancer based on the patterns of failure in patients receiving definitive and postoperative IMRT. *Int J Radiat Oncol Biol Phys* 2002;53:1174–1184.
BOT, base of tongue; CN, contralateral neck nodes (level); FOM, floor of mouth; IN, ipsilateral neck nodes (level); P, gross tumor with margins for definition IMRT or surgical bed for post-op IMRT; RPNL, retropharyngeal lymph nodes; RMT, retromolar trigone.
*N+ = N1–3 except N2c.
[†]T1–2 carcinoma of the true vocal cord excluded.
[‡]Include submandibular node (Level Ib) when level II node involved.

- The recent recommendations proposed by several authors on the locations of the surgical neck compartments were also in good agreement with our system.[7,8,11]
- Following our guidelines, all margins of each specific neck node level could be demarcated on axial CT sections.
- Figures 4-4 and 4-5 depict nodal target volume delineation at different levels of the neck in patients receiving definitive and postoperative IMRT. We operatively demarcate nodal GTV in Fig. 4-4 to provide readers with visual assistance in understanding the location of gross nodal disease and the corresponding design of CTV1 and CTV2.
- Sparing salivary gland function is important in preserving the quality of life of patients. The literature has shown a dose response of parotid gland function after radiation treatment.[14–17] We elected not to spare the deep lobe of parotid gland to prevent marginal failure in the parapharyngeal space. Therefore, only the superficial lobes of parotid glands were demarcated.

- One significant pathologic factor to consider for target volume delineation is the presence of extracapsular extension (ECE). The probability of tumor extending outside the nodal capsule increases as a function of tumor size. When metastatic nodal disease expands and ruptures the capsule of cervical lymph nodes, the incidence of local recurrence increases.
- Huang et al. demonstrated a higher tumor recurrence in patients with ECE (+) neck, while postoperative radiation therapy improved local regional control.[18] Peters et al. defined the resected neck into high- and low-risk groups to which different radiation doses were recommended.[19]
- Therefore, when delineating target volume in the postoperative neck, inclusion of generous soft-tissue margins

## TABLE 4-7. RECOMMENDATIONS FOR RADIOLOGIC BOUNDARIES OF NECK NODE REGIONS (39)

| Level | Recommended Boundary |
|---|---|
| I | *Cranial:* mylohyoid muscle; *caudal:* hyoid bone<br>*Anterior:* symphisis menti; *posterior:* posterior edge of submandibular gland<br>*Lateral:* medial edge of mandible; *medial:* lateral edge of anterior belly of digastric muscle |
| II | *Cranial:* cranial base; *caudal:* bottom edge of hyoid bone<br>*Anterior:* posterior margin of submandibular gland; *posterior:* the posterior edge of SCM<br>*Lateral:* medial edge of SCM; *medial:* medial edge of vessel bundle,* paraspinal muscle |
| III | *Cranial:* bottom edge of hyoid bone; *caudal:* lower margin of cricoid cartilage<br>*Anterior:* posterolateral edge of sternohyoid muscle; *posterior:* the posterior edge of SCM<br>*Lateral:* medial edge of SCM; *medial:* medial edge of vessel bundle,* paraspinal muscle |
| IV | *Cranial:* lower margin of cricoid cartilage; *caudal:* cranial border of clavicle<br>*Anterior:* posterolateral edge of SCM muscle; *posterior:* the anterior edge of paraspinal muscle<br>*Lateral:* lateral border of SCM; *medial:* medial border of vessel bundle, lateral border of thyroid |
| V | *Cranial:* cranial base; *caudal:* cranial border of clavicle<br>*Anterior:* posterior edge of SCM; *posterior:* anterior edge of trapezius muscle<br>*Lateral:* platysma muscle, skin; *medial:* paraspinal muscle |
| Retropharyngeal | *Cranial:* base of skull; *caudal:* cranial edge of the body of hyoid bone<br>*Anterior:* levator veli palatini; *posterior:* prevertebral muscles<br>*Lateral:* medial edge of vessel bundle; *medial:* midline |

SCM, sternocleidomastoid muscle.
*Vessel bundle, internal carotid artery and internal jugular vein.

around the tumor bed is imperative. Should the information regarding which lymph node levels containing ECE (+) node not be available pathologically, a preoperative imaging study (CT or MRI) can assist in determining which regions require a more generous soft-tissue margin for CTV1 delineation.

■ Figure 4-5 differentiates ECE (+) and ECE (−) necks in patients receiving postoperative IMRT. In ECE (+) neck, soft tissues are more generously included, and the CTV1 needs to extend close to the skin surface, especially in the region or level of the ECE (+) node(s) specified by the pathologic examination.

■ When postoperative IMRT is needed for the ECE (−) neck, the target volume should avoid skin surface to decrease acute dermal toxicity. In our experience, sparing 2 to 3 mm of dermal structures in target volume design (Fig. 4-5) clearly results in much better radiation tolerance, less treatment breaks, and no compromise in local regional control.

■ Although the lower neck was treated with conventional techniques in the majority of patients, similar principles were applied to depict CTV delineation in the lower neck region for readers' reference in Figs. 4-4 and 4-5.

■ Also, it needs to be emphasized that margins for organ motion or patient setup error are not included in delineating the target volume, since they need to be determined by individual institutions implementing a head and neck IMRT program. Using reinforced thermoplastic mask for immobilization, our experience indicated that a 3-mm margin was needed for IMRT plan computation to account for patient setup uncertainty.[20,21]

■ The dilemma comes when definitive IMRT is used to treat an undissected neck and no pathologic information is available to determine whether metastatic disease has extended outside the lymph node capsules. In this case, we seek surgical pathologic experience for guidance. Table 4-8 summarizes the incidence of ECE in various sizes of lymph nodes that contain metastatic disease. When nodal size is as small as 1 cm, 17% to 40% may have broken through the capsule. When the size of metastatic node exceeds 3 cm, more than 75% have ECE. This information is pertinent to target volume design because additional soft-tissue margins around the whole nodal level where grossly enlarged nodes reside need to be included in CTV1, which usually provides margins around the gross disease truncating air and bone (Fig. 4-4). CTV volumes

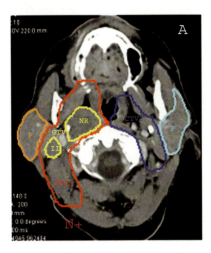 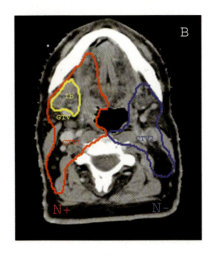
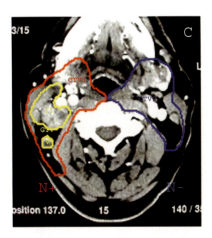 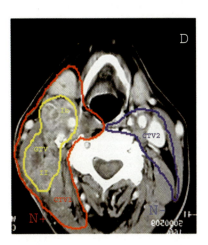
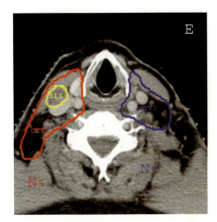 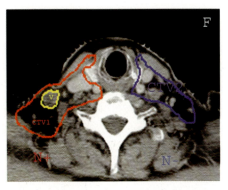

**FIGURE 4-4.** Clinical target volume (CTV) target delineation of clinically N+/N− necks in base-of-tongue cancers receiving definitive IMRT. Axial enhanced CT scans at the level of pterygoid plates (**A**), mandible (**B**), submandibular gland (**C**), hyoid bone (**D**), thyroid cartilage (**E**), and cricoid cartilage (**F**), in a patient with metastatic head and neck cancer. Clinical target volumes with the presence of metastatic lymphadenopathy are compared with those without radiologic evidence of metastatic neck node. The gross tumor was operatively demarcated to provide readers with visual assistance in understanding the location of gross nodal disease and the corresponding target volume. Clinical target volume1 (CTV1): red line; CTV2: blue line; Ib: level Ib node, II: level II node, III: level III node; V: level V node; N+: positive nodes; N−: negative nodes; NR: nodes of Rouviere. GTV: grossly enlarged lymph node. (Chao KSC, Wippold FJ, Ozyigit G, et al. Determination and delineation of nodal target volumes for head and neck cancer based on the patterns of failure in patients receiving definitive and postoperative IMRT. *Int J Radiat Oncol Biol Phys* 2002;53:1174–1184, by permission.)

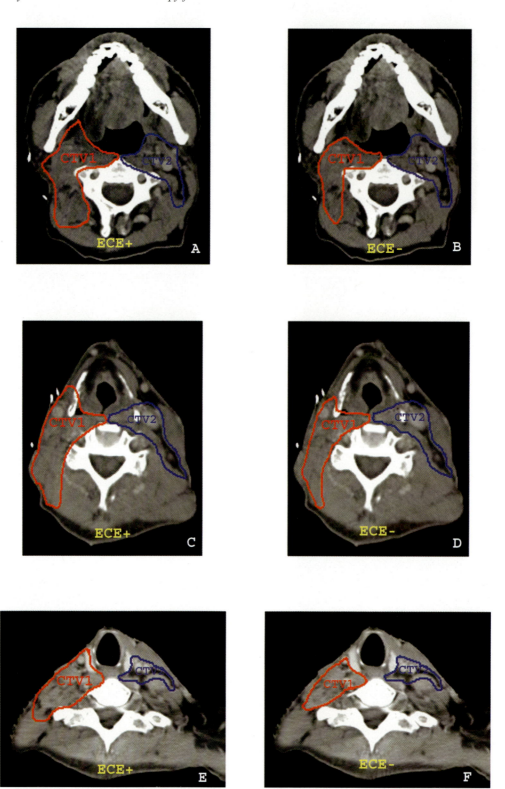

**FIGURE 4-5.** Clinical target volume delineation of pathologically ECE ± necks in base-of-tongue cancers receiving postop IMRT. Axial enhanced postoperative CT scans at the level of mandible (**A,B**), thyroid cartilage (**C,D**), and thyroid gland (**E,F**) in a patient with metastatic head and neck cancer. Clinical target volumes with the presence of extracapsular extension (**A,C,E**) are compared with volumes without extracapsular extension (**B,D,F**). Clinical target volume1 (CTV1): red line; CTV2: blue line; ECE+: presence of extracapsular extension; ECE−: absence of extracapsular extension. GTV: grossly enlarged lymph node. (Chao KSC, Wippold FJ, Ozyigit G, et al. Determination and delineation of nodal target volumes for head and neck cancer based on the patterns of failure in patients receiving definitive and postoperative IMRT. *Int J Radiat Oncol Biol Phys* 2002;53:1174–1184, by permission.)

## TABLE 4-8. INCIDENCE OF EXTRACAPSULAR EXTENSION OF METASTATIC NECK NODE BY SIZE (41)

| Author | Nodal Size | <1 cm | 1–3 cm | >3 cm |
|---|---|---|---|---|
| Annyas 1979[34] | 7 | 23% | 53% | 74% |
| Johnson 1981[35] | 8 | — | 65% | 75% |
| Carter 1987[36] | 9 | 17% | 83% | 95% |
| Hirabayashi 1991[37] | 0 | 43% | — | 81% |

*Source:* Modified from Chao KSC, Wippold FJ, Ozyigit G, et al. Determination and delineation of nodal target volumes for head and neck cancer based on the patterns of failure in patients receiving definitive and postoperative IMRT. *Int J Radiat Oncol Biol Phys* 2002 *(in press).*

that we used for the most part are generous and likely contribute to the high control rates. Since head and neck IMRT is still in its infancy, we elected to be generous in target volume delineation to avoid undesirable marginal failure. When the clinical experience and knowledge continue to advance, these guidelines will be adjusted accordingly.

## 4. DOSE PRESCRIPTION FOR HEAD AND NECK IMRT

- Table 4-9 summarizes the corresponding dose prescriptions for CTV1 and CTV2.[20] CTV1 is considered as a higher-risk volume, and a higher dose is given to this target volume.
- Daily fraction size to CTV has been found to be associated with local regional control rate. Patients receiving 2-Gy fraction doses to primary target volume (CTV1) showed better 2-year DFS survival (94% versus 78%, $p = .05$).[22]
- We also found an association between CTV1 volume and the composite University of Washington head and neck questionnaire (UW-QOL) score assessing the quality of life in 50 IMRT patients.[23]
- There was a significant negative correlation between absolute mean CTV1 volumes and composite UW-QOL scores ($r = -0.36$, $p = .01$). There was a nonsignificant

negative correlation between absolute CTV2 volumes and composite UW-QOL scores. There was also a strong significant correlation between total absolute mean CTV volumes and composite UW-QOL scores ($r = -0.44$, $p = .003$). In multivariate analysis, the only single significant independent predicting variable for composite UW-QOL score was the absolute mean CTV1 volume.

- It substantiates the importance of target volume determination and delineation. Other clinical parameters such as tumor stage and nodal status were also predicting the mean total score of UW-QOL. Chemotherapy adversely affected the health-related QOL in definitive IMRT patients.

## 5. WASHINGTON UNIVERSITY HEAD AND NECK IMRT NODAL CONTROL RESULTS

- Between February 1997 and December 2000, 126 patients were treated with head and neck cancer with curative intent.
- The primary tumor was located at nasopharynx in 12 patients, paranasal sinuses or nasal cavity in nine patients, oral cavity in 15 patients, oropharynx in 63 patients, supraglottic larynx in eight patients, hypopharynx in eight patients, unknown primary in nine patients, and other regions of the head and neck in three patients.
- Fifty-two patients received definitive IMRT, four with stage II disease, nine with stage III disease, and 39 with stage IV tumor. The clinical/radiologic nodal status of these 52 patients was N0 in 12 patients, N1 in nine patients, N2 in 24 patients (nine N2a, 11 N2b, four N2c), and N3 in seven patients. Among them, 17 refused chemotherapy and were treated with RT alone, whereas the remaining 35 were treated with concurrent chemotherapy per an intramural protocol. Chemotherapy was cisplatin-based regimens in all cases.
- Seventy-four patients received postoperative IMRT, five with stage I disease, four with stage II disease, 17 with stage III disease, and 39 with stage IV tumor. The pathologic

## TABLE 4-9. IMRT CLINICAL TARGET VOLUME (CTV) AND NORMAL TISSUE DOSE SPECIFICATION WITH BIOLOGIC EQUIVALENT DOSE (BED) CORRECTION FOR HEAD AND NECK CANCER—WASHINGTON UNIVERSITY GUIDELINE[38]

| Target Volume | Conventional Technique | IMRT | | |
|---|---|---|---|---|
| | | Definitive (35 Fractions) | High-Risk Postoperative (33 Fractions) | Intermediate-Risk Postoperative (30 Fractions) |
| CTV1 | 66–70/2 Gy | 70/2 Gy | 66/2 Gy | 60/2 Gy |
| CTV2 | 50–54/2 Gy | 56/1.66 Gy | 54/1.64 Gy | 52/1.73 Gy |

*Source:* Ozyigit G, Chao KSC. Clinical experience of head and neck IMRT with serial tomotherapy. *Med Dosim* 2002 *(in press).*
*Note:* Normal tissue tolerance for IMRT prescription: Optic nerve and optic chiasm, 55 Gy; retina, 45 Gy; brainstem 50–55 Gy; spinal cord, 45–48 Gy; parotid gland, 20–30 Gy; mandible, 70 Gy.

nodal status of these 74 patients was N0 in 18 patients, N1 in 13 patients, N2 in 37 patients (10 N2a, 19 N2b, eight N2c), and N3 in six patients.

- Extracapsular nodal extension (ECE) was present among 32 patients. Chemotherapy was not routinely given postoperatively; however, five patients with extensive nodal involvement in the lower neck received adjuvant cisplatin-based chemotherapy at the physician's discretion.
- Following our guidelines, the radiation dose (mean ± standard deviation) for 52 definitive IMRT patients was 70.23 ± 3.44 Gy to CTV1 and 60.15 ± 2.87 Gy to CTV2. Mean dose to CTV1 and CTV2 in 74 postoperative cases was 65.05 ± 4.21 Gy and 57 ± 5.58 Gy, respectively.
- Median follow-up was 26 months (range, 12 to 55 months). Persistent disease was defined as the histopathologically proven residual disease within 6 months after the completion of definitive IMRT.
- Dose-volume histograms (DVH) of failures within the IMRT field (excluding low neck recurrence) were calculated on an 8-mm$^3$ isotropic voxel grid using a commercial data analysis software (Mathworks, Matlab). Treatment failures were analyzed and failures were categorized as (a) "in-field," if more than 95% of disease volume was within either CTV1 or CTV2, (b) "marginal," if 20% to 95% of disease volume was within CTV1 or CTV2, or (c) "out-field" if less than 20% of disease volume was within either CTV1 or CTV2.

## 5.1. Patterns of Nodal Failure

- Persistent or recurrent nodal disease was found in six of 52 (12%) patients receiving definitive IMRT. Four failures were "in-field" to the CTV1 and two were in the lower neck outside IMRT volume.
- Seven of 74 (9%) patients receiving postoperative IMRT failed in the nodal region. One failure was "marginal" to the CTV1 but "in-field" to the CTV2. Two failures were marginal to CTV2. Two failures were in the lower neck and outside the IMRT field. Another two failures were in CTV1 but in one of them there was also lower neck failure, which was outside IMRT field.
- Predominant in-field failure denotes the urgent need to discern the radioresistant tumor, such as hypoxic tumor, by functional imaging or molecular markers.

## 6. SEQUELA OF TREATMENT

- Severe acute skin reaction and late fibrosis of subcutaneous tissue can be avoided by providing 2 to 3 mm of space between skin surface and CTV boundary when the risk of dermal soft-tissue extension by the tumor is minimal (Figs. 4-4 and 4-5).

## REFERENCES

1. ICRU 62. *Prescribing, recording, and reporting photon beam therapy* (supplement to ICRU Report 50). Washington, DC: International Commission on Radiation Units and Measurements, 1999.
2. ICRU 50. *Prescribing, recording, and reporting photon beam therapy.* Washington, DC: International Commission on Radiation Units and Measurements, 1993.
3. Sako K, Bradier RN, C. MF, et al. Feasibility of palpation in the diagnosis of metastases to cervical nodes. *Surg Gynecol Obstet* 1964;118:989–990.
4. Rouviere H. *Anatomie humaine descriptive et topographique,* 6th ed. Paris: Masson et Cie., 1948.
5. Spiessl B, Beahrs OH, Hermanek P. *Illustrated guide to the TNM/pTNM classification of malignant tumours,* 2nd ed. Berlin: Springer, 1992.
6. Robbins KT, Medina JE, Wolfe GT, et al. Standardizing neck dissection terminology: official report of the Academy's Committee for Head and Neck Surgery and Oncology. *Arch Otolaryngol Head Neck Surg* 1991;117:601–605.
7. Gregoire V, Coche E, Cosnard G. Selection and delineation of lymph node target volumes in head and neck conformal radiotherapy. Proposal for standardizing terminology and procedure based on the surgical experience. *Radiother Oncol* 2000;56:135–150.
8. Nowak PJ, Wijers OB, Lagerwaard FJ, et al. A three-dimensional CT-based target definition for elective irradiation of the neck. *Int J Radiat Oncol Biol Phys* 1999;45:33–39.
9. Wijers OB, Levendag PC, Tan T, et al. A simplified CT-based definition of the lymph node levels in the node negative neck. *Radiother Oncol* 1999;52:35–42.
10. Martinez-Monge R, Fernandes PS, Gupta N. Cross-sectional nodal atlas: a tool for the definition of clinical target volumes in three-dimensional radiation therapy planning. *Radiology* 1999;211:815–828.
11. Som PM, Curtin HD, Mancuso AA. An imaging-based classification for the cervical nodes designed as an adjunct to recent clinically based nodal classifications. *Arch Otolaryngol Head Neck Surg* 1999;125:388–396.
12. Fletcher GH, Million RR. Malignant tumor in nasopharynx. *Am J Roentgenol Radium Ther Nucl Med* 1965;93:44–55.
13. Hunt MA, Zelefsky MJ, Wolden S, et al. Treatment planning and delivery of intensity-modulated radiation therapy for primary nasopharynx cancer. *Int J Radiat Oncol Biol Phys* 2001;49:623–632.
14. Emami B, Lyman J, Brown A, et al. Tolerance of normal tissue to therapeutic irradiation. *Int J Radiat Oncol Biol Phys* 1991;21:109–122.
15. Eisbruch A, Ten Haken RK, Kim HM, et al. Dose, volume, and function relationships in parotid salivary glands following conformal and intensity-modulated irradiation of head and neck cancer. *Int J Radiat Oncol Biol Phys* 1999;45:577–587.
16. Chao KS, Deasy JO, Markman J, et al. A prospective study of salivary function sparing in patients with head-and-neck cancers receiving intensity-modulated or three-dimensional radiation therapy: initial results. *Int J Radiat Oncol Biol Phys* 2001;49:907–916.
17. Chao KS, Majhail N, Huang C, et al. Intensity-modulated radiation therapy reduces late salivary toxicity without compromising tumor control in patients with oropharyngeal carcinoma: a comparison with conventional techniques. *Radiother Oncol* 2001;61:275–280.
18. Huang DT, Johnson CR, Schmidt-Ullrich R, et al. Postoperative radiotherapy in head and neck carcinoma with extracapsular lymph node extension and/or positive resection margins: a

comparative study. *Int J Radiat Oncol Biol Phys* 1992;23:737–742.

19. Peters LJ, Goepfert H, Ang KK, et al. Evaluation of the dose for postoperative radiation therapy of head and neck cancer: first report of a prospective randomized trial. *Int J Radiat Oncol Biol Phys* 1993;26:3–11.

20. Chao KS, Low DA, Perez CA, et al. Intensity-modulated radiation therapy in head and neck cancers: the Mallinckrodt experience. *Int J Cancer* 2000;90:92–103.

21. Low DA, Chao KS, Mutic S, et al. Quality assurance of serial tomotherapy for head and neck patient treatments. *Int J Radiat Oncol Biol Phys* 1998;42:681–692.

22. Lin M, Ozyigit G, Chao K. Impact of tumor stage and radiation fraction size on tumor control and treatment toxicity in head and neck cancer patients treated with IMRT. *Proceedings of the American Society for Therapeutic Radiation and Oncology,* 44th annual meeting. New Orleans, LA, 2002.

23. Ozyigit G, Chao K. Significant impact of target volume size on the quality of life of head and neck cancer patients treated with IMRT. *Proceedings of the American Society for Therapeutic Radiation and Oncology,* 44th annual meeting. New Orleans, LA, 2002.

24. McLaughlin MP, Mendenhall WM, Mancuso AA, et al. Retropharyngeal adenopathy as a predictor of outcome in squamous cell carcinoma of the head and neck. *Head Neck* 1995;17:190–198.

25. Candela FC, Kothari K, Shah JP. Patterns of cervical node metastases from squamous carcinoma of the oropharynx and hypopharynx. *Head Neck* 1990;12:197–203.

26. Shah JP, Candela FC, Poddar AK. The patterns of cervical lymph node metastases from squamous carcinoma of the oral cavity. *Cancer* 1990;66:109–113.

27. Bataini JP, Bernier J, Brugere J, et al. Natural history of neck disease in patients with squamous cell carcinoma of oropharynx and pharyngolarynx. *Radiother Oncol* 1985;3:245–255.

28. Byers RM, Wolf PF, Ballantyne AJ. Rationale for elective modified neck dissection. *Head Neck Surg* 1988;10:160–167.

29. Lindberg R. Distribution of cervical lymph node metastases from squamous cell carcinoma of the upper respiratory and digestive tracts. *Cancer* 1972;29:1446–1449.

30. Northrop M, Fletcher GH, Jesse RH, et al. Evolution of neck disease in patients with primary squamous cell carcinoma of the oral tongue, floor of mouth, and palatine arch, and clinically positive neck nodes neither fixed nor bilateral. *Cancer* 1972;29:23–30.

31. Woolgar JA. Histological distribution of cervical lymph node metastases from intraoral/oropharyngeal squamous cell carcinomas. *Br J Oral Maxillofac Surg* 1999;37:175–180.

32. Buckley JG, MacLennan K. Cervical node metastases in laryngeal and hypopharyngeal cancer: a prospective analysis of prevalence and distribution. *Head Neck* 2000;22:380–385.

33. Kowalski LP, Medina JE. Nodal metastases: predictive factors. *Otolaryngol Clin North Am* 1998;31:621–637.

34. Anyas AA, Snow GB, van Slooten EA, et al. Prognostic factors of neck node metastasis: their impact on planning a treatment regime. Read before the American Society of Head and Neck Surgeons. Los Angeles, 1979.

35. Johnson JT, Barnes EL, Myers EN, et al. The extracapsular spread of tumors in cervical node metastasis. *Arch Otolaryngol* 1981;107:725–729.

36. Carter RL, Bliss JM, Soo KC, et al. Radical neck dissections for squamous carcinomas: pathological findings and their clinical implications with particular reference to transcapsular spread. *Int J Radiat Oncol Biol Phys* 1987;13:825–832.

37. Hirabayashi H, Koshii K, Uno K, et al. Extracapsular spread of squamous cell carcinoma in neck lymph nodes: prognostic factor of laryngeal cancer. *Laryngoscope* 1991;101:502–506.

38. Ozyigit G, Chao K. Clinical experience of head and neck IMRT with serial tomotherapy. *Med Dosim* 2002;27:91–98.

39. Chao KSC, Wippold FJ, Ozyigit G, et al. Determination and delineation of nodal target volumes for head and neck cancer based on the patterns of failure in patients receiving definitive and postoperative IMRT. *Int J Radiat Oncol Biol Phys* 2002;57:1174–1184.

# 5

# PARANASAL SINUSES AND NASAL CAVITY

**GOKHAN OZYIGIT**
**K.S. CLIFFORD CHAO**

## 1. ANATOMY

- The nasal cavity begins at the limen nasi and ends at the posterior nasal choanae. The bony partitions between the nasal cavity, sinuses, and orbits are quite thin and offer little resistance to cancer spread.
- The posterior choanae communicate directly with the nasopharynx. The nasal cavity is located between the base of the cranium superiorly and the hard palate inferiorly. It is divided into right and left halves by a midline septum. The bones and the cartilages that compose the roof and sides of the external nose are shown in Fig. 5-1.
- The vomer extends from the body of the sphenoid and joins the lower and posterior portion of the septum. The upper and the anterior part of the septum is continuous with the cribriform plate, which is paper thin and no real barrier to tumor invasion. The septum is usually deflected to one side.
- The sections of the nasal cavity and adjacent sinuses are shown in Figs. 5-2 through 5-5. The lateral walls of the nasal cavity are composed of three turbinates (also called the *inferior, middle,* and *superior concha*) that form the roof of a passage or meatus that communicates with the nasal cavity.
- The nasolacrimal duct enters the nasal cavity by the inferior meatus. The frontal sinus and anterior and middle ethmoidal cells communicate with the nasal cavity via the middle meatus. The superior meatus receives the opening of the posterior ethmoid air cells.
- The pterygopalatine fossa is situated inferior to the inferior orbital fissure, and the infraorbital nerve is located superior to this fossa as it enters the foramen rotundum.
- The ethmoid sinus cells are composed of air cells located between the medial walls of the orbit and the lateral walls of the nasal cavity (Figs. 5-4 to 5-7). Those air cells are divided into three groups: anterior, middle, and posterior. The partition between these cavities is thin and gives no resistance to tumor spread. A thin, incomplete bone called the lamina papyracea is also penetrated easily by the tumor.

- The posterior ethmoidal cells are closely related to the optic canal and the optic nerve (Fig. 5-5). The lacrimal bone covers the anterior cells laterally. The roof of the ethmoid sinuses relates to the cranial fossa. The fovea ethmoidalis is the part of the frontal bone that compromises the roof of the anterosuperior ethmoidal cells.
- The olfactory nerve merges with the nasal cavity from the cribriform plate of the ethmoid bone and innervates the upper one-third of the septum. Branches of the olfactory nerve that penetrate the cribriform plate provide a route of tumor invasion and spread to the floor of the anterior cranial fossa (Fig 5-7).
- The sphenoid sinus is a midline structure in the body of the sphenoid bone (Fig 5-6). The hypophysis and optic chiasm are located superiorly; the cavernous sinuses, laterally; the nasal cavity and ethmoid sinuses, anteriorly; and the nasopharynx, inferiorly. The clivus and brainstem are situated posteriorly (Fig 5-8). Each sinus is connected with the nasal cavity in the sphenoethmoid recess by an aperture in the upper part of its anterior wall.
- The right and left sphenoid sinuses are also divided by a septum and are considered as one. Because the septum is often incomplete or, at best, very thin, the septum is rarely in the anatomic midline.
- Each maxillary sinus has four walls: nasal, orbital, facial, and infratemporal. The nasal wall forms the base; the apex extends into the zygomatic process of the maxilla. The sections of maxillary antrum are shown in Figs. 5-7 to 5-8.
- The roots of the first and second molar teeth, and occasionally other teeth, often project into the floor of the sinus. The nasal wall has openings to the meatus under the middle turbinate. The floor of the maxillary sinus is usually caudal to the floor of the nasal cavity in adults and older children.
- Two irregular air cavities separated by a bony septum form the frontal sinuses. The posterior wall of frontal sinuses that separates them from the anterior cranial fossa is usually thick; they are separated from the anterior ethmoid cells by thin, bony walls.

*Paranasal Sinuses and Nasal Cavity* 51

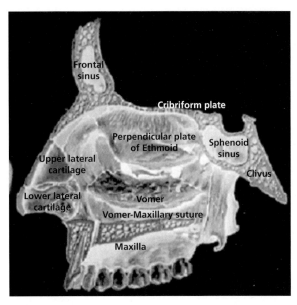

**FIGURE 5-1.** The bones and the cartilages that compose the roof and sides of the external nose, nasal cavity, and paranasal sinuses.

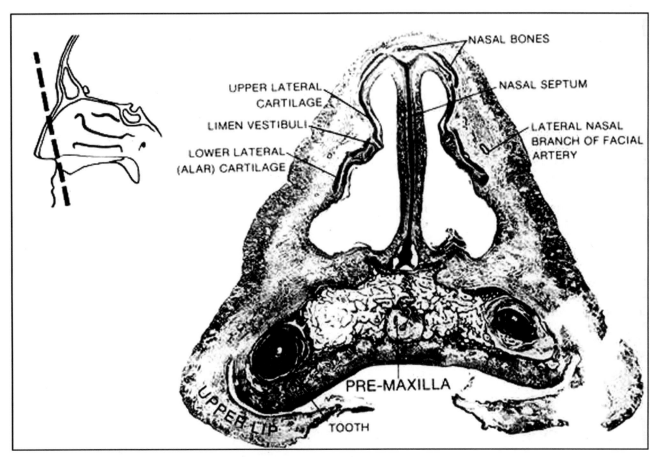

**FIGURE 5-2.** Coronal whole organ section through vestibule. (Bridger MWM, van Nostrand AWP. The nose and paranasal sinuses: applied surgical anatomy—a histologic study of whole organ sections in three planes. *J Otolaryngol* 1978;7[Suppl 6]:4, by permission.)

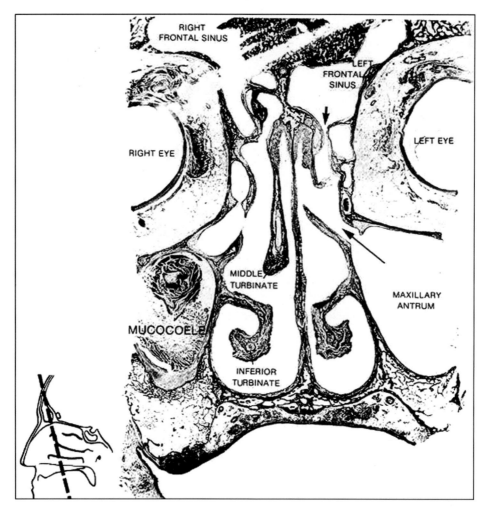

**FIGURE 5-3.** Coronal section through frontal sinuses, midnose, and anterior ethmoids. (Bridger MWM, van Nostrand AWP. The nose and paranasal sinuses: applied surgical anatomy—a histologic study of whole organ sections in three planes. *J Otolaryngol* 1978;7[Suppl 6]:8, by permission.)

## 2. NATURAL HISTORY

- Most lesions are advanced and commonly involve several adjacent sinuses, the nasal cavity, and often the nasopharynx.
- There is often orbital invasion from maxillary sinus or ethmoid sinus cancers (Fig 5-9). Orbital invasion from nasal cavity tumors occurs late.
- The anterior cranial fossa is invaded by way of the cribriform plate and roof of the ethmoid sinuses. The middle cranial fossa is invaded by way of the infratemporal fossa, pterygoid plates, or lateral extension from the sphenoid sinus.
- Lesions involving the olfactory region tend to destroy the septum and may invade through the nasal bone, producing expansion of the nasal bridge and eventually skin invasion.
- Lesions of the anterolateral infrastructure of the maxillary sinus commonly extend through the lateral inferior wall and appear in the oral cavity, where they erode through the maxillary gingiva or into the gingivobuccal sulcus (Fig 5-10). Tumor that extends posteriorly from the maxillary sinus has immediate access to the base of the skull.
- Lymph node metastases generally do not occur until tumor has extended to areas that contain abundant capillary lymphatics (Table 5-1). The submandibular and subdigastric lymph nodes are most commonly involved (Fig 5-11).

## 3. DIAGNOSIS AND STAGING SYSTEM

### 3.1. Signs and Symptoms

- History of recurrent nasal obstruction and recently worsened sinusitis are the common symptoms. Minor and intermittent epitasis may be observed. The mass may protrude from the nose. Obstruction of the nasolacrimal system may cause epiphora. Frontal headache, aberration or loss of smell, diplopia, and proptosis secondary to invasion of the orbit are other signs and symptoms that can be observed in paranasal sinus and nasal cavity tumors.

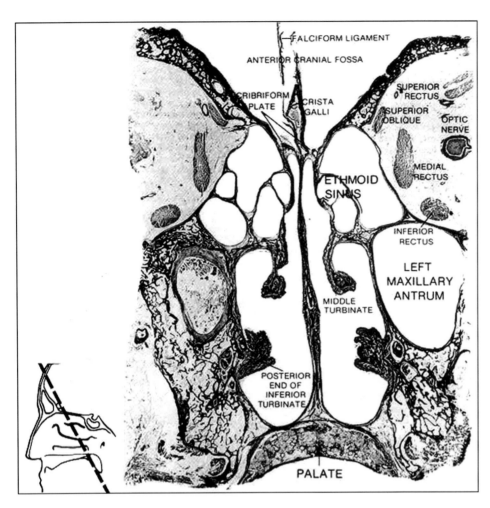

**FIGURE 5-4.** Coronal section through cribriform plate, middle ethmoid sinuses, and posterior inferior turbinates. (Bridger MWM, van Nostrand AWP. The nose and paranasal sinuses: applied surgical anatomy—a histologic study of whole organ sections in three planes. *J Otolaryngol* 1978;7[Suppl 6]:10, by permission.)

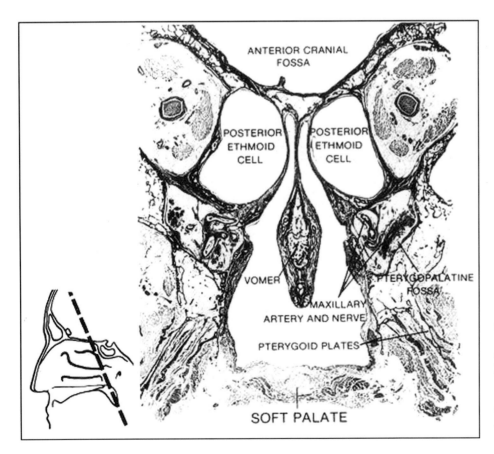

**FIGURE 5-5.** Coronal section just behind the maxillary antrum and just anterior to the sphenoid sinus and nasopharynx. (Bridger MWM, van Nostrand AWP. The nose and paranasal sinuses: applied surgical anatomy—a histologic study of whole organ sections in three planes. *J Otolaryngol* 1978;7[Suppl 6]:12, by permission.)

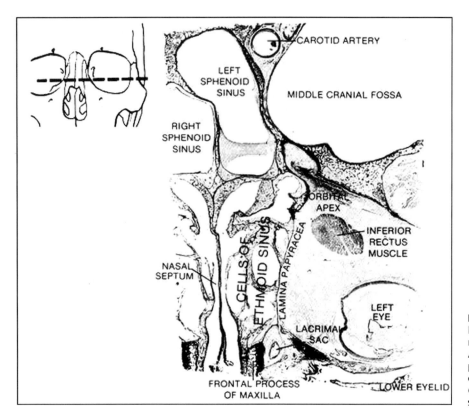

**FIGURE 5-6.** Horizontal section through lacrimal sac, orbit, and ethmoid and sphenoid sinuses. (Bridger MWM, van Nostrand AWP. The nose and paranasal sinuses: applied surgical anatomy—a histologic study of whole organ sections in three planes. *J Otolaryngol* 1978;7[Suppl 6]:26, by permission.)

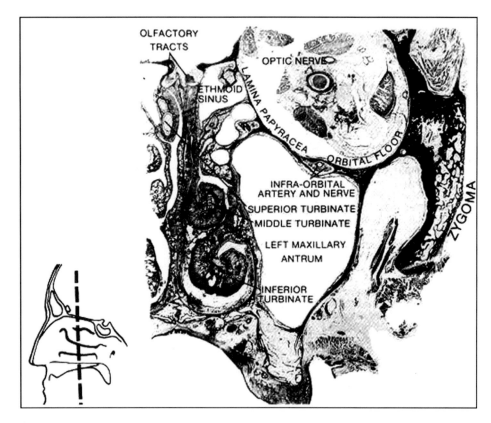

**FIGURE 5-7.** Coronal section through the maxillary antrum. (Bridger MWM, van Nostrand AWP. The nose and paranasal sinuses: applied surgical anatomy—a histologic study of whole organ sections in three planes. *J Otolaryngol* 1978; 7[Suppl 6]:14, by permission.)

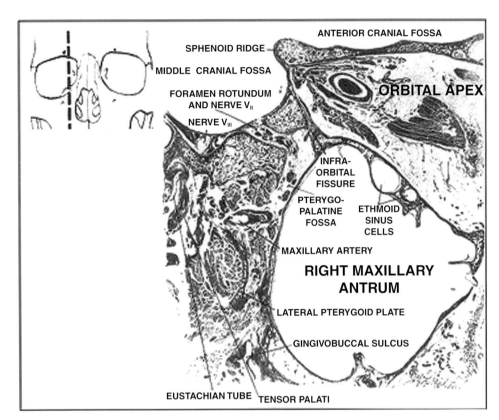

**FIGURE 5-8.** Sagittal section antrum and apex of the orbit. (Bridger MWM, van Nostrand AWP. The nose and paranasal sinuses: applied surgical anatomy—a histologic study of whole organ sections in three planes. *J Otolaryngol* 1978; 7[Suppl 6]:18, by permission.)

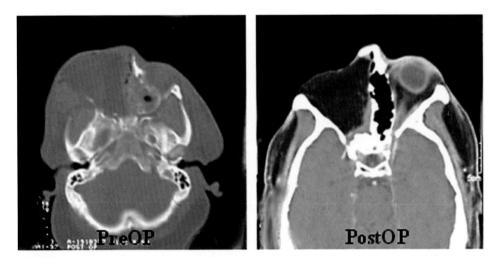

**FIGURE 5-9.** A pathologic T3N0M0 right maxillary sinus carcinoma: preoperative CT scan revealed a large mass originating in the sinus and completely filling it. It extended into the nasal cavity and ethmoid sinus with destruction of the orbital floor. The patient underwent right maxillectomy, right orbital exenteration, and craniofacial resection (postop CT on the right side).

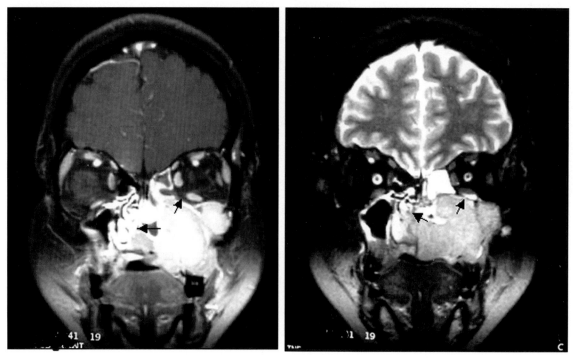

**FIGURE 5-10.** MRI scan of a patient with T4N0 maxillary adenocystic carcinoma. An extensive soft-tissue mass in the left maxillary sinus extending into the ethmoid and orbit with bone destruction (*arrows*).

## 3.2. Physical Examination

- The nasal cavity is inspected using a nasal speculum. A fiber-optic nasoscope can also be used. Cranial nerve examination is very important in paranasal and nasal cavity tumors in order to evaluate the extension of tumor.

## 3.3. Imaging

- Sinonasal CT and MRI should be done both in the axial and coronal planes. The anterior skull base, floor of orbit, and cavernous sinus are evaluated on coronal sections. The orbital apex, pterygopalatine fossa, infratemporal fossa, and face are studied on axial sections. Sections must be 3 mm thick or less.
- Figure 5-12 shows the normal anatomy of paranasal sinuses and nasal cavity as seen on CT slices.

**TABLE 5-1. INCIDENCE OF LYMPH NODE METASTASIS AT PRESENTATION IN PARANASAL SINUS CARCINOMAS**

| Author | No. of Patients | LN (+) in Percentage |
|---|---|---|
| Cheng et al.[9] | 66 | 22 |
| Hopkins et al.[10] | 121 | 21 |
| Jiang et al.[11] | 73 | 8 |
| Kurohara et al.[11] | 924 | 21 |
| Paulino et al.[12] | 42 | 10 |
| Som et al.[13] | 90 | 3 |

- The lymph nodes are not routinely studied in sinonasal cancer. The neck should be examined if soft-tissue, nasopharynx mucosal involvement or high-grade lesions are found.
- The absence of bone on CT is not necessarily an indication of bone invasion, since most of the bony parts are very thin in this region.
- Because of the conical shape of orbit, the maxillary antrum projects into the posteromedial floor of the orbit on axial images.

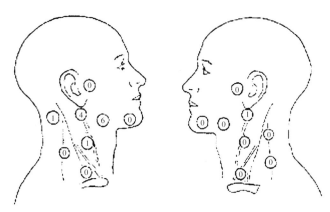

**FIGURE 5-11.** Patterns of neck recurrence in 11 patients without elective neck treatment. (Paulino AC, Fisher SG, Marks JE. Is prophylactic neck irradiation indicated in patients with squamous cell carcinoma of the maxillary sinus? *Int J Radiat Oncol Biol Phys* 1997:39;283, by permission.)

*Paranasal Sinuses and Nasal Cavity* 57

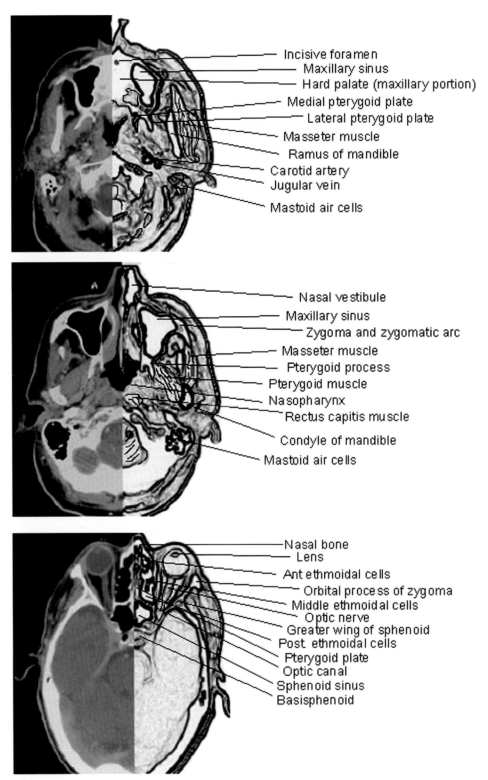

**FIGURE 5-12.** CT slices of the paranasal sinuses and nasal cavity in the axial plane with line diagrams correlating with normal anatomy seen in the same slice.

- Normal perineural enhancement should not be confused with pathologic enhancement of the nerve when evaluating perineural spread of the tumor along the infraorbital nerves.
- CT can detect the intracranial invasion by detecting the bone erosion at the sinodural interface. The overlying dura often appears thickened and is enhanced by invasion of tumor.
- The earliest sign of orbital invasion is erosion of cortical bone and displacement of extraconal orbital fat. Tumor spread to the infratemporal fossa can be detected by erosion of the cortical bone along the posterior wall of the maxillary antrum. This is often seen near the groove of the posterior superior alveolar neurovascular bundle.

### 3.4. Staging

- The staging system of the American Joint Committee on Cancer (AJCC) applies only to maxillary and ethmoid sinus tumors (Table 5-2).[1]
- The University of Florida staging system for tumors of the nasal cavity and ethmoid and sphenoid sinuses is as follows:[2]
    Stage I: limited to site of origin.
    Stage II: extension to adjacent sites (e.g., orbit, nasopharynx, paranasal sinuses, skin, pterygomaxillary fossa).
    Stage III: base of skull or pterygoid plate destruction; intracranial extension.

### 4. PROGNOSTIC FACTORS

- Massive tumor extension to the base of the skull, nasopharynx, posterior wall, or roof of the sphenoid sinus, or cavernous sinus significantly increases surgical morbidity and decreases the likelihood of obtaining clear surgical margins.
- Tumor extension through the periorbita usually requires sacrifice of the eye.

### 5. GENERAL MANAGEMENT

- Table 5-3 summarizes a metaanalysis of data showing the cross-tabulation of site, T stage, and treatment modality according to changes in decades.
- Table 5-4 shows actuarial locoregional control and disease-specific actuarial survival rates according to treatment modality in patients with nasal cavity and paranasal sinus carcinoma.
- Primary surgery followed by postoperative irradiation to a lesser dose than used for irradiation alone is preferred to reduce the risk of unilateral or bilateral optic nerve injury.[2] In most cases, postoperative doses are limited to 60 Gy; 66 to 68 Gy are administered for positive margins.

- For unresectable lesions, high-dose irradiation remains the only alternative, with either once-a-day fractionation of 1.8 to 2.0 Gy to a total dose of 70 Gy or twice-daily treatment of 1.1 to 1.2 Gy per fraction with a 6-hour interfraction interval to total doses of 74 to 79 Gy.[3]

### 5.1. Nasal Cavity

- Inverted papilloma without carcinoma is treated by surgery.
- Traditional intranasal excision, Caldwell-Luc procedure, and ethmoidectomy result in a high recurrence rate.
- Frazell and Lewis observed a 5-year cure rate of 56% for 68 nasal cavity cancers treated surgically.[4]
- In 45 patients with nasal cavity cancers (18 treated with definitive irradiation and 27 with surgery and irradiation), the 5-year disease-specific and overall survival rates were 83% and 75%, respectively.[5]
- No clear role for chemotherapy has been defined.

### 5.2. Ethmoid Sinus

- If the tumor is resectable, surgery is usually performed first. Postoperative irradiation is advised, even if resection margins are negative.
- Removal requires medial maxillectomy and *en bloc* ethmoidectomy. If tumor extends superiorly to involve the fovea ethmoidalis or the cribriform plate, a combined craniofacial approach is required.

### 5.3. Maxillary Sinus

- Most malignancies require radical maxillectomy, including the entire maxilla and ethmoid sinus via a Weber-Fergusson incision. The globe and orbital floor are preserved for inferiorly located tumors.
- Orbital exenteration is indicated when the tumor has spread through the periorbita.
- If the ethmoid roof is involved, craniofacial resection is required.
- Early infrastructure lesions are often cured by surgery alone, but in most cases of maxillary sinus cancer, irradiation is given postoperatively, even if the margins are clear.
- Massive tumor extension to the base of the skull, nasopharynx, or sphenoid sinus may contraindicate surgery.
- Borderline resectable lesions are sometimes treated with full-dose external-beam irradiation, followed by surgery if technically feasible.
- Ninety-six patients with maxillary sinus carcinomas were treated in St. Louis at Washington University from 1960 to 1976; 74 (77%) had squamous cell carcinoma.[6] After preoperative irradiation (mostly 50 to 70 Gy) and surgery, 5-year absolute disease-free survival rates were 60%, 45%, 38%, and 28% in patients with T1, T2, T3, and T4 tumors, respectively.

# TABLE 5-2. AJCC CLASSIFICATION FOR CARCINOMA OF THE PARANASAL SINUSES

### Primary Tumor (T)

| | |
|---|---|
| TX | Primary tumor cannot be assessed |
| T0 | No evidence of primary tumor |
| Tis | Carcinoma *in situ* |

### Maxillary Sinus

| | |
|---|---|
| T1 | Tumor limited to antral mucosa with no erosion or destruction of bone |
| T2 | Tumor causing bone erosion or destruction except for the posterior antral wall, including extension into the hard palate and/or the middle nasal meatus |
| T3 | Tumor invades any of the following: bone of posterior wall of maxillary sinus, subcutaneous tissues, skin of cheek, floor of medial wall of orbit, infratemporal fossa, pterygoid plates, ethmoid sinuses |
| T4 | Tumor invades orbital contents beyond the floor or medial wall, including any of the following: the orbital apex, cribriform plate, base of skull, nasopharynx, sphenoid, frontal sinuses |

### Ethmoid Sinus

| | |
|---|---|
| T1 | Tumor confined to ethmoid with or without bone destruction |
| T2 | Tumor extends into nasal cavity |
| T3 | Tumor extends to the anterior orbit and/or maxillary sinus |
| T4 | Tumor with intracranial extension, orbital extension including apex, involving sphenoid and/or frontal sinus and/or skin of external nose |

### Regional Lymph Nodes (N)

| | |
|---|---|
| NX | Regional lymph nodes cannot be assessed |
| N0 | No regional lymph node metastasis |
| N1 | Metastasis in a single ipsilateral lymph node, <3 cm in greatest dimension |
| N2 | Metastasis in a single ipsilateral lymph node, >3 cm but not >6 cm in greatest dimension; in multiple ipsilateral lymph nodes, none >6 cm in greatest dimension; or in bilateral or contralateral lymph nodes, none >6 cm in greatest dimension |
| N2a | Metastasis in a single ipsilateral lymph node >3 cm but not >6 cm in greatest dimension |
| N2b | Metastasis in multiple ipsilateral lymph nodes, none >6 cm in greatest dimension |
| N2c | Metastasis in bilateral or contralateral lymph nodes, none >6 cm in greatest dimension |
| N3 | Metastasis in a lymph node >6 cm in greatest dimension |

### Distant Metastases (M)

| | |
|---|---|
| MX | Presence of distant metastasis cannot be assessed |
| M0 | No distant metastasis |
| M1 | Distant metastasis |

### Stage Grouping

| | | | |
|---|---|---|---|
| Stage 0 | Tis | N0 | M0 |
| Stage I | T1 | N0 | M0 |
| Stage II | T2 | N0 | M0 |
| Stage III | T3 | N0 | M0 |
| | T1 | N1 | M0 |
| | T2 | N1 | M0 |
| | T3 | N1 | M0 |
| Stage IVA | T4 | N0 or N1 | M0 |
| Stage IVB | Any T | N2 | M0 |
| | Any T | N3 | M0 |
| Stage IVC | Any T | Any N | M1 |

*Source:* Fleming ID, Cooper JS, Henson DE, et al., eds. *AJCC cancer staging manual,* 5th ed. Philadelphia: Lippincott-Raven, 1997:51–52.

## TABLE 5-3. METAANALYSIS DATA: CROSS-TABULATION OF SITE, T STAGE, AND TREATMENT MODALITY

| | Decade (%) | | | |
|---|---|---|---|---|
| | 1960s | 1970s | 1980s | 1990s |
| *Site* | | | | |
| Maxillary sinus | 26 | 31 | 39 | 45 |
| Ethmoid sinus | 27 | 37 | 56 | 51 |
| Nasal cavity | 63 | 54 | 59 | 66 |
| *T Stage* | | | | |
| T1 | 28 | 83 | 87 | 90 |
| T2 | 22 | 53 | 62 | 70 |
| T3 | 10 | 28 | 44 | 44 |
| T4 | 0 | 18 | 19 | 28 |
| *Treatment* | | | | |
| Surgery | 36 | 54 | 57 | 70 |
| Surgery and RT | 33 | 42 | 54 | 56 |
| RT | 21 | 19 | 28 | 33 |
| Chemotherapy* | 0 | 21 | 34 | 42 |
| Number of patients | 3,137 | 3,877 | 5,966 | 3,416 |

*Source:* Modified from Dulguerov P, Jacobsen MS, Allal AS, et al. Nasal cavity and paranasal sinus carcinoma: are we making progress? A series of 220 patients and a systematic review. *Cancer* 2001;92: 3012–3029.
*The chemotherapy data include patients who received chemotherapy as part of their treatment, usually combined with other treatment modalities.

- It is reasonable to expect 5-year survival rates of approximately 60% to 70% for T1 and T2 lesions and 30% to 40% for T3 and T4 lesions after resection and postoperative irradiation. For advanced, unresectable disease, average 5-year survival rates of 10% to 15% are achieved with high-dose irradiation alone.

### 5.4. Sphenoid Sinus

- Irradiation is usually the treatment by default. See "General Management" for radiation dose.

### 5.5. Neck

- Patients with recurrent or poorly differentiated cancers and tumors that extend to an area with dense capillary

## TABLE 5-4. ACTUARIAL LOCOREGIONAL CONTROL AND DISEASE-SPECIFIC ACTUARIAL SURVIVAL RATES ACCORDING TO TREATMENT MODALITY IN PATIENTS WITH NASAL CAVITY AND PARANASAL SINUS CARCINOMA

| | | Survival (%) | | |
|---|---|---|---|---|
| Treatment | No. (%) | 2-Year | 5-Year | 10-Year |
| *ALRC* | | | | |
| Surgery | 44[14] | 74 | 70 | 70 |
| Surgery and radiotherapy | 113[15] | 70 | 63 | 57 |
| Radiotherapy | 61[16] | 47 | 40 | 38 |
| *CSAS* | | | | |
| Surgery | 44[14] | 84 | 79 | 76 |
| Surgery and radiotherapy | 113[15] | 82 | 66 | 60 |
| Radiotherapy | 61[16] | 59 | 57 | 33 |

*Source:* Modified from Dulguerov P, Jacobsen MS, Allal AS, et al. Nasal cavity and paranasal sinus carcinoma: are we making progress? A series of 220 patients and a systematic review. *Cancer* 2001;92:3012–3029.
ALRC, actuarial locoregional control; CSAS, carcinoma-specific actuarial survival.

lymphatics (nasopharynx, oropharynx, oral cavity) have a higher risk of metastasis and are often given elective neck irradiation of 50 Gy over 5 to 6 weeks, administered in 1.8- to 2-Gy daily fractions.

## 6. INTENSITY MODULATED RADIATION THERAPY IN NASAL CAVITY AND PARANASAL SINUS CARCINOMAS

### 6.1. Target Volume Determination

- If chemotherapy was delivered before radiation, the targets should be outlined on the planning CT according to their prechemotherapy extent.
- Table 5-5 summarizes the target volume specification for definitive and postoperative IMRT in paranasal sinus and nasal cavity cancers.
- Table 5-6 summarizes suggested target volume determination for paranasal sinus and nasal cavity cancers.

## TABLE 5-5. TARGET VOLUME SPECIFICATION FOR DEFINITIVE AND POSTOPERATIVE IMRT IN PARANASAL SINUS AND NASAL CAVITY CANCER

| Target | Definitive IMRT | High-Risk Postoperative IMRT | Intermediate-Risk Postoperative IMRT |
|---|---|---|---|
| CTV1 | Soft tissue and nodal regions adjacent to the GTV | Surgical bed with soft-tissue involvement or nodal region with extracapsular involvement | Surgical bed without soft-tissue involvement or nodal region without capsular extension |
| CTV2 | Elective nodal regions* | Elective nodal regions* | Elective nodal regions* |

*See Table 5-6.

## TABLE 5-6. SUGGESTED TARGET VOLUME DETERMINATION FOR MAXILLARY SINUS IMRT

| Tumor Site | Clinical Presentation | CTV1 | CTV2 |
|---|---|---|---|
| Paranasal sinus | T1–2 N0 | P | |
| Nasal cavity | T3–4N+* | P + IN[†] (I–III) | CN (I–III) + RPLN |
| | N2c | P + IN + CN (I – III) + RPLN | |

CN, contralateral neck nodes; IN, ipsilateral neck nodes; P, gross tumor with margins for definition IMRT or surgical bed for postop IMRT; RPLN, retropharyngeal lymph nodes.
*Note: Sphenoid, ethymoid sinuses, and nasal cavity:* Involve posterior structures (nasopharynx, posterior pharyngeal wall). Incidence of LN metastasis commonly goes up. Inclusion of retropharyngeal LN ± bilateral upper neck should be considered.
*N*, ipsilateral N1–3 except N2c
[†]Level Ib only. Level Ia should be included when Ib node is involved.

## 6.2. Target Volume Delineation

■ In patients receiving postoperative IMRT, CTV1 encompasses residual tumor and the region adjacent to it but not directly involved by the tumor, the surgical bed with soft-tissue invasion by the tumor, or extracapsular extension by metastatic neck nodes. CTV2 includes primarily the prophylactically treated neck.

■ In patients receiving definitive IMRT, CTV1 encompasses gross tumor (primary and enlarged nodes) and the region adjacent to it but not directly involved. CTV2 includes primarily the prophylactically treated neck.

■ Figure 5-13 shows CTV1 and CTV2 delineation in a patient with clinically T2N0M0 squamous cell carcinoma of ethmoid sinus receiving definitive IMRT.

■ Figure 5-14 shows CTV1 and CTV2 delineation in a patient with clinically T4N2bM0 squamous cell carcinoma of nasal cavity receiving definitive IMRT.

■ Figure 5-15 shows CTV1 and CTV2 delineation in a patient with clinically T4N0M0 squamous cell carcinoma of maxillary sinus receiving definitive IMRT.

## 6.3. Normal Tissue Delineation

■ Figure 5-16 shows normal tissue delineation.

## 6.4. Suggested Target and Normal Tissue Doses

■ Table 4-9 shows the Washington University guidelines for clinical target volume dose specification with biological equivalent dose correction and normal tissue tolerance for IMRT.

■ To avoid excessive risk of damage to vision, fraction dose to CTV1 may be reduced to 1.8 or 1.9 Gy if CTV1 is in close proximity to the optic nerve or optic chiasm.

## 6.5. IMRT Treatment Results of MIR

■ Following these guidelines, nine paranasal and nasal cavity carcinoma patients were treated with IMRT between February 1997 and December 2000 at Washington University.[7] Three patients were treated postoperatively, and six were treated with definitive IMRT. The T stages were one T1, one T3, and seven T4. The N stages were N0, six; N1, one; and N2, (AJCC staging; one stage I, one stage II, and seven stage IV). Median follow-up time was 36 months (range, 13 to 42 months). We observed no locoregional recurrence or distant metastasis. All patients are alive except one, who died of intercurrent disease.

■ Figure 5-17 shows an example of IMRT dose distribution of a patient receiving definitive IMRT for a T4N0 paranasal sinus cancer. Retropharyngeal nodes and ipsilateral upper jugular nodes were prophylactically treated due to posterior extension of the tumor.

■ A G-tube was placed in two patients during the course of IMRT. One patient developed grade III late xerostomia. Altered vision in two patients and otitis requiring a tympanostomy tube in one patient were other serious late complications of IMRT.

## 7. SEQUELAE OF TREATMENT

## 7.1. Surgery

■ Complications of ethmoid sinus surgery include total blindness, loss of ocular motility, hemorrhage, meningitis, cerebrospinal fluid leak, cellulitis and pansinusitis, brain abscess, stroke, fistula between the cavernous sinus and internal carotid artery, and damage to the frontal lobe.

■ Complications of maxillectomy include failure of the split-thickness graft to heal, trismus, cerebrospinal fluid leak, and hemorrhage.

## 7.2. Radiation Therapy

■ Complications of irradiation of nasal cavity or paranasal sinus tumors include central nervous system damage, unilateral or bilateral loss of vision, serous otitis media, and chronic sinusitis.

■ Long-term complications after irradiation of nasal vestibule cancers have been minimal.

■ The optic nerve or retina may receive a substantial amount of radiation in patients with tumor in the ethmoid or sphenoid sinuses. Radiation retinopathy is rare at 45 Gy after conventional fractions of irradiation. Nakissa et al. reported that all patients who received more than 45 Gy to the posterior pole had recognizable changes; however, most of these did not affect vision.[8] Decreased visual acuity occurred only in patients receiving more than 65 Gy.

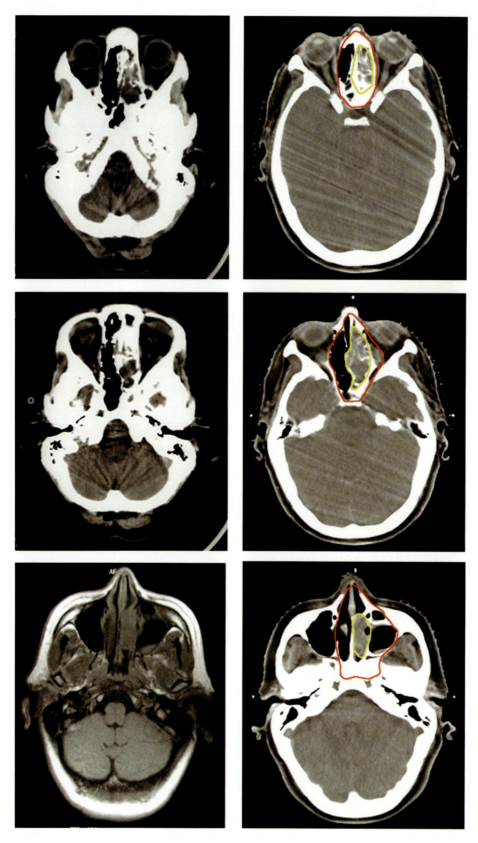

**FIGURE 5-13.** Clinical target volume (CTV) delineation in a patient with T2N0M0 ethmoid sinus carcinoma receiving definitive IMRT. CTV1, red line; gross tumor volume, yellow line.

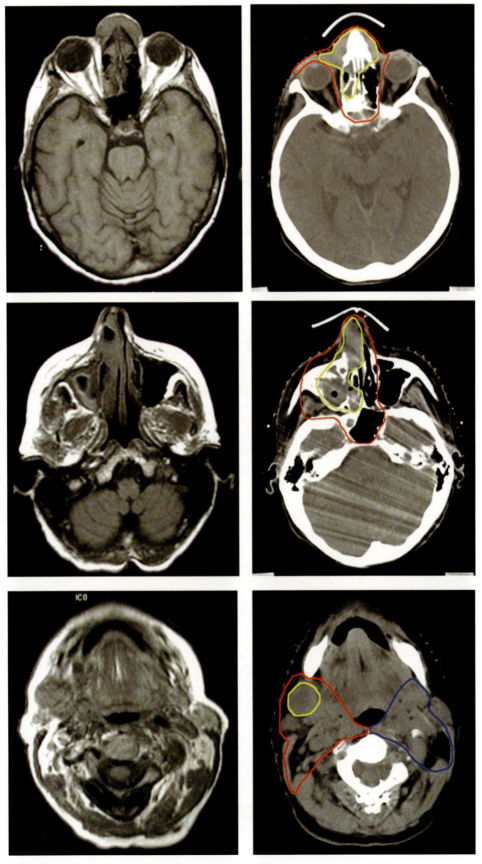

**FIGURE 5-14.** Clinical target volume (CTV) delineation in a patient with T4N2bM0 nasal cavity carcinoma receiving definitive IMRT. A Bolus was used because of skin involvement by tumor. CTV1, red line; CTV2, dark blue line; gross tumor volume, yellow line.

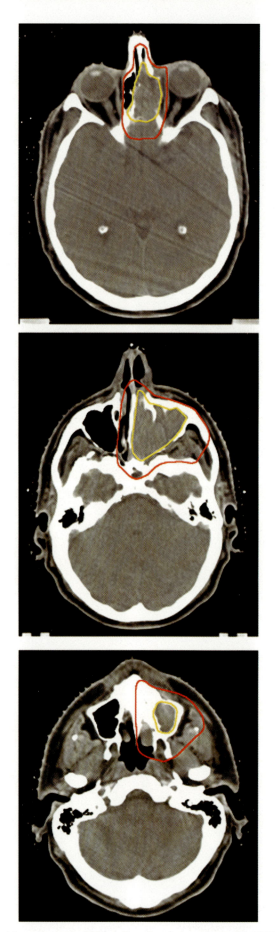

**FIGURE 5-15.** Clinical target volume (CTV) delineation in a patient with T4N0M0 maxillary sinus carcinoma receiving definitive IMRT. CTV1, red line; gross tumor volume, yellow line.

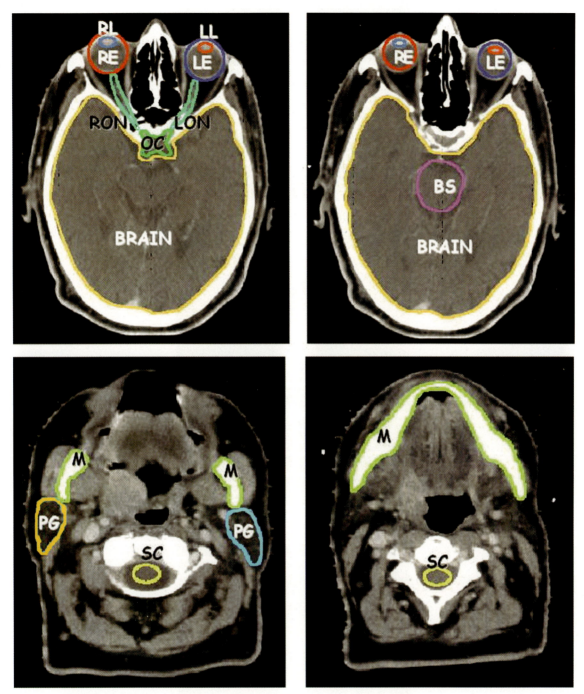

**FIGURE 5-16.** Normal tissue delineation. RL, right lens; LL, left lens; RE, right eye; LE, left eye; RON, right optic nerve; LON, left optic nerve; OC, optic chiasm; M, mandible; PG, parotid gland; SC, spinal cord; BS, brainstem.

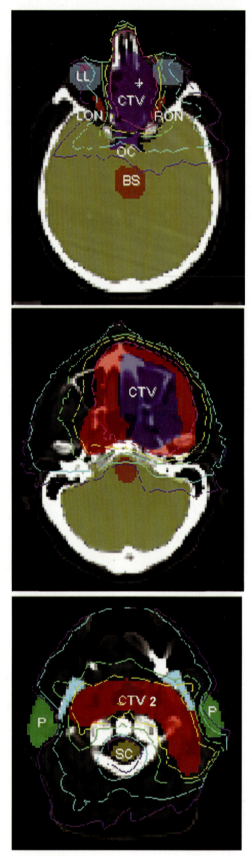

**FIGURE 5-17.** IMRT dose distribution of a patient with T4N0 left maxillary sinus carcinoma receiving definitive IMRT. Ipsilateral left upper lymph nodes were treated prophylactically. CTV, clinical target volume; CTV1, dark blue area; CTV2, red area; LL, left lens; ON, optic nerve; OC, optic chiasm; P, parotid gland; SC, spinal cord. Pink line, 70 Gy; yellow line, 60 Gy; green line, 50 Gy; aqua line, 30 Gy; dark blue, 20 Gy.

Half of all patients displayed some changes at 60 Gy, and 85% to 90% showed changes at 80 Gy. Parsons et al. reported no optic nerve injury in patients receiving more than 59 Gy ($\leq$1.9 Gy/day); however, the 15-year actuarial incidence of optic nerve injury reached 11% for doses above 60 Gy ($\leq$1.9 Gy/day). [3]

## REFERENCES

1. Bridger M, van Nostrand A. The nose and paranasal sinuses: applied surgical anatomy: a histologic study of whole organ sections in three planes. *J Otolaryngol* 1978;7:1–33.
2. Parsons J, Mendenhall W, Stringer S, et al. Nasal cavity and paranasal sinuses. In: Brady L, ed. *Principles and practice of radiation oncology,* 3rd ed. Philadelphia: Lippincott-Raven, 1998:941–959.
3. Parsons J, Bova F, Fitzgerald C, et al. Radiation optic neuropathy after megavoltage external-beam irradiation: analysis of time-dose factors. *Int J Radiat Oncol Biol Phys* 1994;30:755–763.
4. Frazell E, Lewis J. Cancer of the nasal cavity and accessory sinuses: a report of the management of 416 patients. *Cancer* 1963;16:1293–1301.
5. Ang K, Jiang G-L, Frankenthaler R, et al. Carcinomas of the nasal cavity. *Radiother Oncol* 1992;24:163–168.
6. Lee F, Ogura J. Maxillary sinus carcinoma. *Laryngoscope* 1981;91:133–139.
7. Chao K, Wippold F, Ozyigit G, et al. Determination and delineation of nodal target volumes for head and neck cancer based on the patterns of failure in patients receiving definitive and postoperative IMRT. *Int J Radiat Oncol Biol Phys* 2002;53:1174–1184.
8. Nakissa N, Rubin P, Strohl R, et al. Ocular and orbital complications following radiation therapy of paranasal sinus malignancies and review of literature. *Cancer* 1983;51:980–986.
9. Cheng V, Wang C. Carcinomas of the paranasal sinuses: a study of sixty-six cases. *Cancer* 1977;40:3038–3041.
10. Hopkins S, Nag S, Soloway M. Primary carcinoma of the male urethra. *Urology* 1984;23:128–133.
11. Jiang G, Ang K, Peters L, et al. Maxillary sinus carcinomas: natural history and results of postoperative radiotherapy. *Radiother Oncol* 1991;21:193–200.
12. Paulino A, Fisher S, Marks J. Is prophylactic neck irradiaiton indicated in patients with squamous cell carcinoma of the maxillary sinus? *Int J Radiat Oncol Biol Phys* 1997;39:283–289.
13. Som PM, Curtin HD, Mancuso AA. An imaging-based classification for the cervical nodes designed as an adjunct to recent clinically based nodal classification. *Arch Otolaryngol Head Neck Surg* 1999;125:388–396.
14. Bailar J, Gornik H. Cancer undefeated. *N Engl J Med* 1997;336:1569–1574.
15. McCutcheon I, Blacklock J, Weber R, et al. Anterior transcranial (craniofacial) resection of tumors of the paranasal sinuses: surgical technique and results. *Neurosurgery* 1996;38:471–480.
16. Mosesson R, Som P. The radiographic evaluation of sinonasal tumors: an overview. *Otolaryngol Clin North Am* 1995;28:1097–1115.

# 6

# NASOPHARYNX

**K.S. CLIFFORD CHAO**
**GOKHAN OZYIGIT**

## 1. ANATOMY

- The nasopharynx is roughly cuboidal; its borders are the posterior choanae anteriorly, the body of the sphenoid superiorly, the clivus and first two cervical vertebrae posteriorly, and the soft palate inferiorly (Fig. 6-1).
- The lateral and posterior walls are composed of the pharyngeal fascia, which extends outward bilaterally along the undersurface of the apex of the petrous pyramid just medial to the carotid canal. The roof of the nasopharynx slopes downward and is continuous with the posterior wall.
- The eustachian tube opens into the lateral wall; the posterior portion of the eustachian tube is cartilaginous and protrudes into the nasopharynx, making a ridge just posterior to the torus tubarius. Just posterior to the torus is a recess called Rosen Muller's fossa.
- The roof and the posterior wall of nasopharynx are made up of the clivus and basisphenoid, which are the foundation of the central skull base and cavernous sinus: the bony portion of the eustachian tube lies lateral to the carotid canal.
- Many foramina and fissures are located in the base of the skull, through which several structures pass (Table 6-1). Some are potential routes of spread of nasopharyngeal carcinoma (Fig. 6-2).
- The jugular fossa, which lies just posterior to the carotid foramen, is usually larger on the right side. The jugular spur separates the pars nervosa from the pars venosum of the fossa.
- Cranial nerve IX lies within pars nervosa of the jugular fossa, whereas cranial nerves X through XII lie within the pars venosum along with the jugular vein.
- The base of pterygoid plates is part of basisphenoid; the pterygopalatine fossa lies between the pterygoid processes and the maxillary sinus, and is contiguous with the inferior orbital fissure superiorly and the infratemporal fossa laterally. The foramen rotundum can be seen just above the base of the pterygoid processes.
- The upper pharyngeal musculature attaches to the basisphenoid and the styloid process. Levator and tensor veli palatini muscles attachments are visualized along the inferior petrous apex and basisphenoid, respectively.
- An extensive submucosal capillary lymphatic plexus exists in the nasopharyngeal region. This can explain the high incidence of neck node metastasis at initial presentation of patients. The tumor initially spreads to the retropharyngeal lymph nodes, junctional, and jugulodigastric lymph nodes, and then along the internal jugular and spinal accessory chain. Table 6-2 shows incidence and distribution of clinically positive neck nodes in nasopharyngeal carcinoma.[1]
- Lymphatics of the nasopharyngeal mucosa run in an anteroposterior direction to meet in the midline; from there they drain into a small group of nodes lying near the base of the skull in the space lateral and posterior to the parapharyngeal or retropharyngeal space. This group lies close to cranial nerves IX, X, XI, and XII, which run through the parapharyngeal space.
- The retropharyngeal lymph nodes are an important route of spread. The lateral retropharyngeal lymph nodes are located in the retropharyngeal space near the lateral border of the posterior pharyngeal wall and medial to the carotid artery. Directly behind them (Rouviere nodes) are the lateral masses of the atlas (C1). Usually one node occurs in each side, but occasionally two, and very rarely three, are found, and they can be found even at the level of hyoid bone (C3). These nodes atrophy with age and may be absent unilaterally but are rarely absent entirely. Table 6-3 lists the incidence of retropharyngeal lymphadenopathy in nasopharyngeal cancers.
- Lymph nodes of the parotid area may also be involved. This route of spread is possible from the lymphatics of the eustachian tube, which may drain by way of the lymph vessels of the tympanic membrane and external auditory canal to the periparotid lymph nodes.
- Another lymphatic pathway from the nasopharynx leads to the deep posterior cervical node at the confluence of the spinal accessory and jugular lymph node chains.[2]
- A third pathway is to the jugulodigastric node, which is frequently involved in nasopharyngeal carcinoma, according to Lederman.[3]

**TABLE 6-1. FORAMINA OF THE BASE OF SKULL AND ASSOCIATED ANATOMIC STRUCTURES**

| Foramen | Structures |
| --- | --- |
| Cribriform plate (ethmoid) | Olfactory nerve and anterior ethmoidal nerve |
| Optic foramen | Optic nerve and ophthalmic artery |
| Superior orbital fissure | Third (oculomotor), fourth (trochlear), and sixth (abducent) nerves, and ophthalmic division of fifth (trigeminal) nerve; ophthalmic vein; orbital branch of middle meningeal and recurrent branch of lacrimal arteries; sympathetic plexus; some filaments from carotid plexus |
| Foramen rotundum | Maxillary division of trigeminal nerve to pterygopalatine fossa |
| Foramen ovale | Mandibular division of trigeminal nerve; accessory meningeal artery; lesser superficial petrosal nerve |
| Foramen lacerum | Upper portion: internal carotid; sympathetic carotid plexus<br>Lower portion: Vidian nerve; meningeal branch of ascending pharyngeal artery; emissary vein |
| Foramen spinosum | Middle meningeal artery and vein; recurrent branch of mandibular nerve |
| Internal acoustic meatus | Seventh (facial) and eighth (auditory) nerves; internal auditory artery from basilar artery |
| Jugular foramen | Anterior portion: Inferior petrosal sinus<br>Posterior portion: Transverse sinus; meningeal branches from occipital and ascending pharyngeal arteries<br>Intermediate portion: ninth (glossopharyngeal), tenth (vagus), and eleventh (spinal accessory) nerves |
| Hypoglossal canal | Hypoglossal nerve; meningeal branch of ascending pharyngeal artery |
| Foramen magnum | Spinal cord; spinal accessory nerve; vertebral vessels; anterior and posterior spinal vessels |

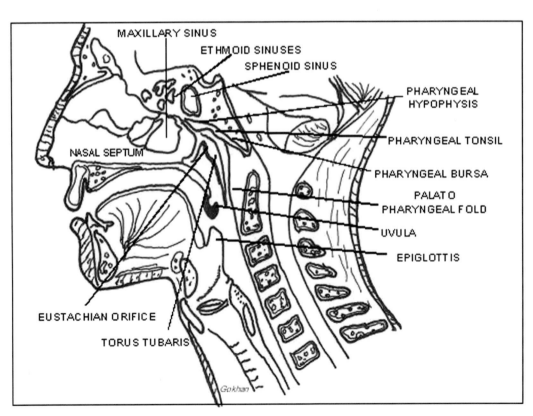

**FIGURE 6-1.** Nasopharynx and related structures in the midsagittal section of the head.

**TABLE 6-2. INCIDENCE AND DISTRIBUTION OF METASTATIC DISEASE IN CLINICALLY POSITIVE (N+)* NECK NODES IN NASOPHARYNX (MIR DATA)1**

|  | Patients with N+ | Clinical Nodal Metastasis ||||||
|---|---|---|---|---|---|---|---|
|  |  | Level I | Level II | Level III | Level IV | Level V | Other[†] |
| Nasopharynx | 115/164 70% | 10/115 8% | 67/115 58% | 11/115 9% | 11/115 9% | 36/115 31% | 3/115 2% |

*Bilateral neck node metastasis was found in 28% and only contralateral neck node metastasis was found in 3% at presentation.
[†]Parotid, postauricular, and buccal nodes.

**TABLE 6-3. INCIDENCE OF RETROPHARYNGEAL LYMPHADENOPATHY IN NASOPHARYNGEAL CANCERS (AFTER CT ERA)**

|  | Incidence of Retropharyngeal Lymph Nodes (Percentage of the Total Number of Patients) |||
|---|---|---|---|
|  | Total | N0 Neck* | N+ Neck[†] |
| McLaughlin et al. 1995[26] | 14/19 (74%) | 2/5 (40%) | 12/14 (86%) |
| Chua et al. 1997[23] | 106/364 (29%) | 21/134 (16%) | 85/230 (37%) |
| Chong et al. 1995[9] | No data | No data | 59/91 (65%) |
| Total | 120/383 (31%) | 23/139 (17%) | 156/335 (47%) |

*Clinically negative nodes in levels I–V.
[†]Clinically positive nodes in levels I–V.

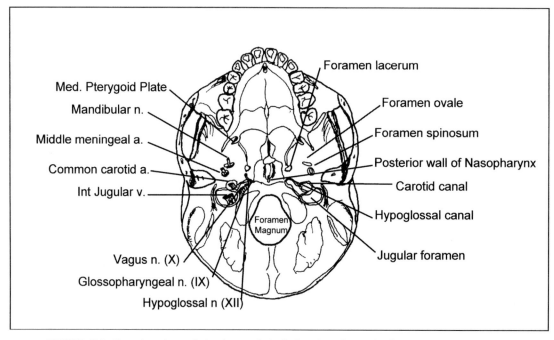

**FIGURE 6-2.** Superior view of the base of skull showing the main foramina and associated anatomic structures.

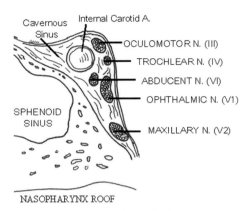

**FIGURE 6-3.** Coronal section through the sphenoid sinus and roof of the nasopharynx showing the relative positions of cranial nerves III to VI.

## 2. NATURAL HISTORY

- Carcinoma of the nasopharynx frequently arises from the lateral wall, with a predilection for the fossa of Rosen Muller and the roof of the nasopharynx.
- Tumor may involve the mucosa or grow predominantly in the submucosa, invading adjacent tissues, including the nasal cavity. In approximately 5% of patients tumor extends into the posterior or medial walls of the maxillary antrum and ethmoids.
- In more advanced stages, tumor may involve the oropharynx, particularly the lateral or posterior wall.
- Upward extension of tumor through the foramen lacerum results in cranial nerve involvement and destruction of the middle fossa (Fig. 6-3).
- Approximately 90% of patients develop lymphadenopathy, which is present in 60% to 85% at initial diagnosis. About 50% of patients have bilateral lymph node involvement.[4]
- Table 6-4 shows the T- and N-stage distribution of nasopharyngeal carcinoma patients at initial presentation according to the AJCC 1988 staging system. Table 6-5 summarizes the T and N distribution of nasopharyngeal cancer patients according to the new AJCC 1997 staging system.
- The incidence of distant metastasis is not related to stage of the primary tumor but correlates strongly with degree of cervical lymph node involvement. In 63 patients with N0 necks, 11 (17%) developed metastatic disease in contrast to 69 of 93 (74%) with N3 cervical lymphadenopathy.[5] The most common site of distant metastasis is bone, followed closely by lung and liver.[6]

## 3. DIAGNOSIS AND STAGING SYSTEM

### 3.1. Signs and Symptoms

- Tumor growth into the posterior nasal fossa can produce nasal stuffiness, discharge, or epitasis. Sometimes the voice has a nasal twang.
- The orifice of the eustachian tube can be obstructed by a relatively small tumor; ear pain or a unilateral decrease in hearing can occur. Sometimes blockage of the eustachian tube produces a middle ear transudate.
- Headache or pain in the temporal or occipital region can occur. Proptosis sometimes results from direct extension of tumor into the orbit.
- Sore throat can occur when tumor involves the oropharynx.
- Although a neck mass elicits medical attention in only 18% to 66% of cases, clinical involvement of cervical lymph nodes on examination at presentation ranges from 60% to 87%.[3,7]
- Some patients present with cranial nerve involvement. In 218 patients, 26% had cranial nerve involvement, but it presented at initial diagnosis in only 3% of patients.[3] Leung et al. reported a 12% incidence of cranial nerve involvement in 564 patients with primary nasopharyngeal carcinoma; it was higher in patients staged with computed tomography (52 of 177, 29%).[8]
- Cranial nerves III through VI are involved by extension of tumor up through the foramen lacerum to the cavernous sinus. Cranial nerves VII, VIII, and I are rarely involved (Fig. 6-4).

**TABLE 6-4. T- AND N-STAGE DISTRIBUTION OF NASOPHARYNGEAL CARCINOMA PATIENTS AT INITIAL PRESENTATION ACCORDING TO AJCC 1988**

| Author | T1 | T2 | T3 | T4 | N0 | N1 | N2 | N3 |
|---|---|---|---|---|---|---|---|---|
| Chua et al.[27] | 92 | 89 | 153 | — | 27 | 46 | 196 | 63 |
| Jian et al.[17] | 5 | 13 | 9 | 13 | 8 | 6 | 20 | 6 |
| Ozyar et al.*[24] | 11 | 23 | 32 | 24 | 18 | 17 | 38 | 17 |
| Wang et al.[28] | 46 | 102 | 46 | 65 | 92 | 23 | 128 | 16 |
| Mesic et al.[29] | 31 | 102 | 45 | 70 | 35 | 30 | 59 | 114 |
| Lee et al.* | 565 | 1,076 | 648 | 2,225 | 1,261 | 600 | 2,403 | 250 |
| Perez et al.[1] | 21 | 33 | 26 | 63 | 48 | 23 | 63 | 8 |
| Total | 771 (14%) | 1,438 (26%) | 959 (17%) | 2,460 (43%) | 1,489 (27%) | 745 (13%) | 2,907 (51%) | 474 (9%) |

**TABLE 6-5. T- AND N-STAGE DISTRIBUTION OF NASOPHARYNGEAL CARCINOMA PATIENTS AT INITIAL PRESENTATION ACCORDING TO AJCC 1997**

| Author | T1 | T2 | T3 | T4 | N0 | N1 | N2 | N3 |
|---|---|---|---|---|---|---|---|---|
| Ozyar et al.[24] | 34 | 32 | 7 | 17 | 18 | 27 | 25 | 20 |
| Lee et al.[11] | 1,641 | 648 | 1,229 | 996 | 1,261 | 1,404 | 785 | 1,064 |
| Chien et al.[30] | 55 | 29 | 14 | 19 | 45 | 40 | 6 | 26 |
| Total | 1,730 (37%) | 709 (15%) | 1,250 (26%) | 1,032 (22%) | 1,324 (28%) | 1,471 (31%) | 816 (17%) | 1,110 (24%) |

## 3.2. Physical Examination

- Fiber-optic nasoscopes and laryngoscopes are the main tools for the examination of nasopharyngeal region. Early lesions occur mostly on the lateral walls or roof. The site of origin is almost never the nasopharyngeal surface of the soft palate and is not often invaded secondarily, even by advanced tumors. In early cases, only slight fullness in Rosen Muller fossa, or a submucosal bulge or asymmetry in the roof may be the only lesions that can be seen. Lymphomas and minor salivary gland tumors tend to remain submucosal until large.
- Nasoscopes may provide help by showing the tumor growth into anterior and superior nasal cavity. Tumor may be seen submucosally infiltrating along the posterior tonsillar pillars, and occasionally down the posterior pharyngeal wall.
- The evaluation of cranial nerves is essential. The fifth and sixth cranial nerves are most commonly involved. Otitis media and decreased hearing can be found on ear examination. Table 6-6 summarizes functions of the cranial nerves, which should be examined in the initial consultation.
- Table 6-7 shows diagnostic work-up for carcinoma of the nasopharynx.

## 3.3. Imaging

- Imaging is required for both staging and treatment planning in all nasopharyngeal carcinomas as well as in the follow-up of the patients.
- The main imaging tools of the nasopharyngeal region are CT and MRI.
- Figure 6-5 shows the normal anatomy of the nasopharynx as seen on CT.
- MRI is the preferred primary examination for disease in

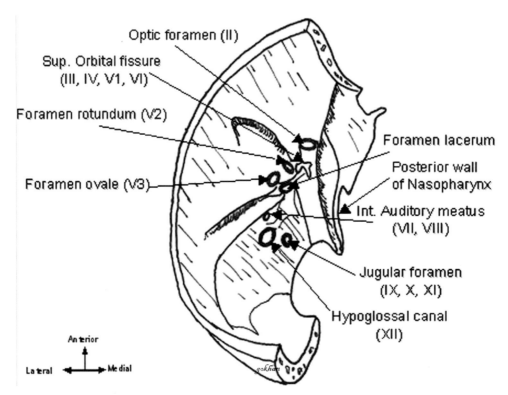

**FIGURE 6-4.** Superomedial view of the base of the skull showing the relations of nasopharynx to foramina of passage of cranial nerves.

**TABLE 6-6. FUNCTIONS OF THE CRANIAL NERVES**

| Cranial Nerve | Function | Abnormality |
|---|---|---|
| I. Olfactory | Smell | Decreased smell sensation |
| II. Optic | Vision | Unilateral amaurosis |
| III. Oculomotor | Eye movement | Ophthalmoplegia |
| | Enervates the striated muscles of the eyelid | Ptosis |
| | Papillary constriction and accommodation of lens for near vision | Loss of accommodation |
| IV. Trochlear | Enervates superior oblique muscle | Limitation in down and inward gazing |
| V. Trigeminal | V1, V2 Cutaneous and proprioceptive sensation from skin, muscles, and joints in face and mouth, and sensory enervation of teeth | Pain and anesthesia in supraorbital and maxillary regions of face |
| | V3: Enervates muscle of mastication, sensory enervation of mandibular region of face | Pain and anesthesia in mandibulary regions of face |
| VI. Abducens | Enervates lateral rectus muscle | Diplopia, limitation of lateral gaze |
| VII. Facial | Enervates muscles of facial expression | Shadowing of nasolabial sulcus |
| | Taste sensation from anterior two-thirds of tongue | Impairment of facial expression |
| | | Loss of taste in anterior two-thirds of the tongue |
| VIII. Vestibulocochlear | Audition | Decreased audition |
| | Equilibrium, postural reflexes, orientation of head in spaces | Vertigo, dizziness |
| IX. Glossopharyngeal | Swallowing | Swallowing difficulty |
| | Enervates the carotid body. | Aberrant sense of taste in posterior one-third of the tongue |
| | Enervates taste buds in posterior two-thirds of tongue | |
| X. Vagus | Enervates striated muscles in larynx and pharynx and controls speech | Hypoesthesia of the mucous membranes in soft palate, pharynx, and larynx |
| | Visceral sensation from pharynx, larynx, thorax, and abdomen | Loss of GAG reflex |
| | | Aspiration symptoms |
| XI. Spinal accessory | Motor enervation of trapezius and Sternocleidomastoid muscle | Paralysis of trapezius and sternocleidomastoid muscles |
| XII. Hypoglossal | Motor enervation of intrinsic muscles of the tongue | Unilateral paralysis and atrophy of the tongue |

the nasopharynx, parapharyngeal space, and infratemporal fossa.

- For skull base invasion, MRI is preferred (Fig. 6-6).
- The neck is always included when CT is performed. Both axial and coronal sections should be performed regardless of whether CT or MRI is the primary examination method.
- The torus tubarius, eustachian tube orifice, and fossa of Rosen Muller are often asymmetric in appearance. Lymphoid tissue tends to atrophy with age and is responsible for superficial contour variation of the nasopharyngeal region. Lymphoid tissue is better visualized with MRI.
- The carotid artery and jugular veins should always be clearly visible in the poststyloid parapharyngeal space, along with at least some surrounding fatty tissue. The intervening cranial nerves IX through XII and the sympathetic chain can sometimes be seen in high-resolution MRI.
- The retropharyngeal lymph nodes are visible on MRI medial to the carotid artery at the border between poststyloid parapharyngeal and retropharyngeal spaces (Fig. 6-7). The nodes are normally 3 to 5 mm in size in adults and 10 to 15 mm in infants and children.
- The fifth nerve ganglion, which lies in the Meckel's

cave, and its branches both within and outside the cavernous sinus are easily recognized on good-quality MRI and CT.

- The third, fourth, and sixth cranial nerves, along with the first division of the trigeminal nerve, are best visualized on coronal MRI as they go through in the wall of the cavernous sinus.
- The fat within nasopharyngeal spaces is normally symmetric, although the size of vessels coursing through the spaces may vary slightly; obliteration of fat is a sign of pathologic involvement in MRI or CT.
- The third division of trigeminal nerve often is seen on MRI exiting the foramen ovale.
- Perineural enhancement within the cranial nerve exit, the foramina, and prominent enhancement of venous plexuses just below the skull base are normal variants.

### 3.4. Staging

- The multiplicity of staging systems makes comparison of results from different institutions extremely difficult.
- The most commonly used staging system is the American Joint Committee tumor-node-metastasis (TNM) system (Table 6-8).

**TABLE 6-7. DIAGNOSTIC WORK-UP FOR CARCINOMA OF THE NASOPHARYNX**

General
　History
　Physical examination, including careful inspection to determine extent of primary tumor and palpation for neck node metastases, testing of cranial nerves, and inspection of tympanic membranes

Special tests
　Indirect and direct nasopharyngoscopy
　Multiple biopsies
　Baseline audiologic testing (as clinically indicated)

Radiographic studies
　Standard
　　Computed tomography or magnetic resonance scans of head and neck
　　Chest radiograph
　Complementary
　　Bone scans: only if indicated by pain or tenderness or elevation of heat-labile fraction of alkaline phosphatase
　　Bone radiographs: only if indicated by abnormal bone scan or symptoms

Laboratories studies
　Blood counts
　Blood chemistry profile
　Liver function studies

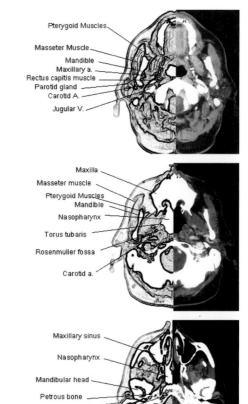

**FIGURE 6-5.** Anatomic line diagrams showing the different levels of the nasopharyngeal region, to correlate with the accompanying CT images at the same level.

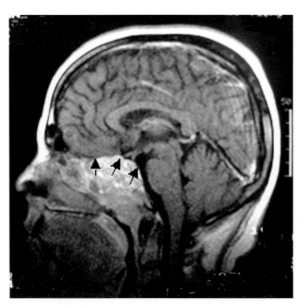
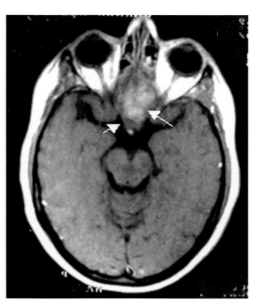

**FIGURE 6-6.** Coronal and sagittal MRI sections showing a T4 nasopharyngeal carcinoma invading the base of skull (*arrows*).

**TABLE 6-8. COMPARISON OF OLD AND NEW AMERICAN JOINT COMMITTEE TNM STAGING SYSTEM FOR NASOPHARYNGEAL CARCINOMA**

| | AJCC 1988 | AJCC 1997 |
|---|---|---|
| | *Primary Tumor* | |
| TX | Primary tumor cannot be assessed | Primary tumor cannot be assessed |
| T0 | No evidence of primary tumor | No evidence of primary tumor |
| Tis | Carcinoma *in situ* | Carcinoma *in situ* |
| T1 | Tumor confined to the one side of nasopharynx | Tumor confined to the nasopharynx |
| T2 | Tumor confined to more than one side of nasopharynx | Tumor extends to soft tissues of oropharynx and/or nasal fossa |
| T2a | | Without parapharyngeal extension |
| T2b | | With parapharyngeal extension |
| T3 | Tumor extends nasal cavity or oropharynx | Tumor invades bony structures and/or paranasal sinuses |
| T4 | Bony erosion, intracranial extension, cranial nerve involvement | Tumor with intracranial extension and/or involvement of cranial nerves, infratemporal fossa, hypopharynx, or orbit |
| | *Neck Nodes*\* | |
| Nx | Regional lymph nodes cannot be assessed | Regional lymph nodes cannot be assessed |
| N0 | No regional lymph node metastasis | No regional lymph node metastasis |
| N1 | Unilateral metastasis in lymph node(s), $\leq 3$ cm in greatest dimension | Unilateral metastasis in lymph node(s), $\leq 6$ cm in greatest dimension, above the supraclavicular fossa |
| N2a | Unilateral, single, $>3$ cm but $\leq 6$ cm | Bilateral metastasis in lymph node(s), $\leq 6$ cm in greatest dimension, above the supraclavicular fossa |
| N2b | Unilateral, multiple, $<6$ cm | |
| N2c | Bilateral but $\leq 6$ cm | |
| N3 | Metastasis in a lymph node(s): $>6$ cm in dimension | Metastasis in a lymph node(s): |
| N3a | | $>6$ cm in dimension |
| N3b | | Extension to the supraclavicular fossa |
| | *Metastases* | |
| MX | Distant metastasis cannot be assessed | Distant metastasis cannot be assessed |
| M0 | No distant metastasis | No distant metastasis |
| M1 | Distant metastasis present | Distant metastasis present |

*Source:* Fleming ID, Cooper JS, Henson DE, et al, eds. *AJCC cancer staging manual,* 5th ed. Philadelphia: Lippincott-Raven, 1997:31–39.
\*The distribution and the prognostic impact of regional lymph node spread from nasopharynx cancer, particularly of the undifferentiated type, are different from those of other head and neck mucosal cancers and justify use of a different N classification scheme.

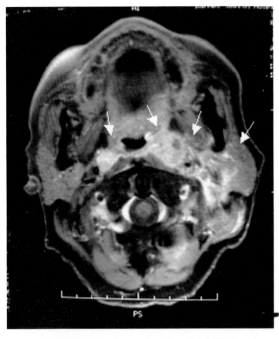
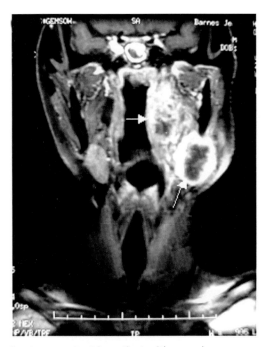

**FIGURE 6-7.** Coronal and sagittal MRI sections showing tumor extent in patient with nasopharyngeal carcinoma.

*Intensity Modulated Radiation Therapy for Head and Neck Cancer*

**TABLE 6-9. MIGRATION OF PATIENT DISTRIBUTION BASED ON AJCC 1988 AND 1997 STAGING SYSTEMS OF NASOPHARYNGEAL CANCER PATIENTS (LITERATURE REVIEW)**

| Center | Stage I | | Stage II | | Stage III | | Stage IV | |
|---|---|---|---|---|---|---|---|---|
| | 1988 | 1997 | 1988 | 1997 | 1988 | 1997 | 1988 | 1997 |
| Cooper et al.[25] | 7 | 19 | 12 | 33 | 13 | 23 | 75 | 32 |
| Cheng et al.[16] | — | — | — | 32 | 12 | 44 | 95 | 31 |
| Ozyar et al.[24] | 2 | 8 | 6 | 21 | 13 | 26 | 69 | 35 |
| Lee et al.[11]* | 156 | 439 | 283 | 929 | 488 | 1,369 | 3,587 | 1,777 |
| Total | 165 | 466 | 301 | 1,015 | 526 | 1,462 | 3,826 | 1,875 |
| | 3% | 10% | 6% | 21% | 12% | 30% | 79% | 39% |

*Unpublished data; actual numbers were given in percent in the original article.

- Table 6-9 shows the comparison of stage distribution of nasopharyngeal carcinoma patients according to the old (AJCC 1988) and new (AJCC 1997) systems. Substantial down-staging was noted with the 1997 staging system, especially for more advanced disease.

## 4. PROGNOSTIC FACTORS

- *Epidemiological factors:* Race, age, and gender have prognostic significance.[9] Perez et al. found that patients younger than 50 years had better survival and better local control.[1] Sham et al. found similar results in their retrospective analysis of 759 patients.[10]
- *Stage:* Sham et al. and Perez et al. showed stage as a significant factor determining the survival and local control.[1,10]
- *Cranial nerve involvement:* Cranial nerve involvement was significantly associated with decreased survival in several series. Lee et al., Sham et al., and Perez et al. found it to be a significant prognostic factor.[1,10,11] However, Chu et al. did not find this to be the case.[12]
- *Lymph node metastasis:* Survival decreases as cervical lymph node involvement progresses from the upper to the middle and lower nodes.[4]

- *Bilateral cervical lymph node involvement:* Lee at al. found bilateral neck node metastasis to be an ominous prognostic factor. They showed that bilaterality was associated with higher risk of nodal failure.[11] However, Sham et al. did not find bilaterality to be a prognostic factor.[10]
- *Histology:* In 122 patients with localized nasopharyngeal carcinoma, histology was the most important prognostic factor for survival. The relative risk of death was 3.4 and 3.2 times greater for nonkeratinizing and squamous cell carcinoma, respectively, than it was for undifferentiated carcinoma.[13] On the other hand, others noted no difference in survival or incidence of distant metastasis between keratinizing and nonkeratinizing squamous cell carcinoma.[1,11]

## 5. GENERAL MANAGEMENT

- Because the nasopharynx is immediately adjacent to the base of the skull, surgical resection with an acceptable margin is often not achievable. Radiation therapy has been the sole treatment for carcinoma of the nasopharynx. Table 6-10 summarizes studies showing the incidence of failure at the primary site correlated with T stage.

**TABLE 6-10. NASOPHARYNGEAL CARCINOMA: INCIDENCE OF FAILURE AT PRIMARY SITE CORRELATED WITH T STAGE (AJCC 1988)**

| Author | Stage | | | |
|---|---|---|---|---|
| | T1 | T2 | T3 | T4 |
| Chu et al.[12] | 24% (25) | 21% (14) | 63% (19) | 45% (22) |
| Hoppe et al.[31] | 13% (38) | 6% (16) | 32% (19) | 56% (9) |
| Kajanti et al.[32] | 13% (71) | 17% (67) | 58% (52) | 100% (64) |
| Lee et al.[33] | 26% (1,527) | 28% (586) | 39% (2,015) | — |
| Mesic et al.[29] | 3% (34) | 15% (102) | 26% (35) | 28% (70) |
| Petrovich et al.[5] | 20% (15) | 32% (34) | 50% (100) | 88% (107) |
| Perez et al.[1] | 20% (23) | 24% (40) | 44% (33) | 60% (68) |
| Average | 25% (1,733) | 26% (859) | 40% (2,273) | 69% (340) |

*Number of patients observed is in parentheses.

**TABLE 6-11. NASOPHARYNGEAL CARCINOMA: INCIDENCE OF FAILURE IN THE NECK CORRELATED WITH N STAGE (AJCC 1988)**

| Author | Stage | | |
|--------|-------|-------|-------|
| | N1 | N2 | N3 |
| Hoppe et al.[31] | 8% (25) | 13% (15) | 11% (18) |
| Kajanti et al.[32] | 22% (76) | 30% (61) | 0% (63) |
| Perez et al.[1] | 12% (28) | 25% (74) | 22% (13) |
| Average | 9% (229) | 20% (191) | 0–30% (186) |

Number of patients is in parentheses.

- Rarely, radical neck dissection has been performed for treatment of neck node metastasis, but it is not superior to irradiation alone. Table 6-11 shows the incidence of failure in the neck correlated with N stage.
- A randomized phase III intergroup trial that compared chemoradiotherapy with radiotherapy alone in patients with stage III and IV nasopharyngeal cancers revealed the advantage of chemotherapy. Radiotherapy was administered in both arms for a total dose of 70 Gy by conventional techniques. The investigational arm received chemotherapy with cisplatin 100 mg/m$^2$ on days 1, 22, and 43 during radiotherapy, and after the completion of radiotherapy patients received additional postradiotherapy chemotherapy with cisplatin 80 mg/m$^2$ on day 1 and fluorouracil 1,000 mg/m$^2$/d on days 1 to 4 every 4 weeks for three courses.[14] The 3-year progression-free survival rate was 24% versus 69% in favor of chemotherapy arm ($p < .001$). The 3-year overall survival rate was 47% versus 78%, respectively ($p = .005$).
- Only a few articles are available that show their treatment results according to the new AJCC staging system. Table 6-12 are overall survival rates of some studies at 3 years based on the new AJCC 1997 system is shown in.

## 6. CHEMOTHERAPY

- Neoadjuvant or adjuvant chemotherapy has been used to treat primary or recurrent nasopharyngeal cancer with complete response rates of 10% to 20% and partial response rates of 40%; recently, significant impact on long-term survival has been reported.
- The results of a recent randomized phase III study showed that adjuvant chemotherapy in advanced nasopharyngeal carcinoma patients has no benefit for overall survival or relapse-free survival.[15]
- In a study from Taiwan, Cheng et al. demonstrated that concurrent chemotherapy followed by radiation therapy produced effective treatment in advanced nasopharyngeal cancer: an 84% 5- year overall survival rate, a 74% disease-free survival rate, and a 90% locoregional control rate. The experience of this study substantiates the intergroup trial's conclusion.[16]
- Table 6-13 summarizes the results of some phase III combined chemotherapy and radiotherapy studies.
- These phase III studies showed that concurrent chemotherapy followed by adjuvant chemotherapy yielded better therapeutic results in advanced nasopharyngeal carcinoma. Another important conclusion is that concurrent use of cisplatin during radiotherapy is essential, and chemotherapy, which is given either neoadjuvant or adjuvant to radiotherapy, has only a little or no benefit in advanced nasopharyngeal carcinoma if given without concomitant cisplatin.

## 7. INTENSITY MODULATED RADIATION THERAPY IN NASOPHARYNGEAL CARCINOMA

### 7.1. Target Volume Determination

- If chemotherapy was delivered before radiation, the targets should be outlined on the planning CT according to their prechemotherapy extent.

**TABLE 6-12. OVERALL SURVIVAL RATES AT 3 YEARS BASED ON AJCC 1997 SYSTEM (LITERATURE REVIEW)**

| Center | Number of Pts | RT | CT | Stage I | Stage II | Stage III | Stage IV |
|--------|---------------|-----|-----|---------|----------|-----------|----------|
| Cooper et al.[25] | 107 | 70 Gy | — | 70% | 65% | 61% | 56% |
| Cheng et al.[16*] | 107 | 70 Gy | + | — | 100% | 93% | 69% |
| Ozyar et al.[24†] | 90 | 66 Gy | + | 100% | 72% | 65% | 55% |
| Lee et al.[11‡] | 4,514 | 60 Gy | + | 94% | 83% | 76% | 50% |
| Chien et al.[30§] | 117 | | + | 88% | 86% | 61% | 48% |
| | 4,935 | 60–70 Gy | | 70–100% | 65–100% | 61–93% | 48–69% |

*CDDP + 5FU concomitant followed by two cycles of CDDP + 5FU in stages II, III, IV.
†Neoadjuvant or concomitant cisplatin in N2–N3 patients
‡Chemotherapy in patients with advanced disease and incomplete remission after radiotherapy.
§Three cycles of adjuvant cisplatin and 5FU in stage III–IV patients.

## TABLE 6-13. PHASE III COMBINED CHEMOTHERAPY AND RADIOTHERAPY STUDIES (LITERATURE REVIEW)

| | Stage (AJCC 1988) | Treatment | Number of Patients | LRR (%) | DFS (%) | Year |
|---|---|---|---|---|---|---|
| Milan[34] | I–IV | RT 60 Gy | 116 | 27 | 56 | 4 |
| | | RT + 6 cycles VCA | 113 | 24 | 58 | |
| INSG[35,36] | IV | RT 70 Gy | 168 | 23 | 31 | 3 |
| | | 3 cycles BEP + RT 70 Gy | 171 | 15 | 47 | |
| Hong Kong[37] | N size ≥ 4 cm or N3 | RT (66 Gy + Boost) | 40 | 15 | 78 | 2 |
| | | 2 cycles PF + RT + 3 cycles PF | 37 | 16 | 68 | |
| AOCOA[27] | N size ≥ 3 cm N2–N3 or | RT 66–74 Gy | 134 | 31 | 46 | 3 |
| | T3 | 2–3 cycles PE + RT | 152 | 25 | 58 | |
| Intergroup Study[14] | III–IV | RT 70 Gy | 69 | 41 | 24 | 3 |
| | | RT and 3 cycles P + 3 cycles PF | 78 | 14 | 69 | |

AJCC, American Joint Committee on Cancer; AOCA, Asian-Oceanian Clinical Oncology Association; BEP, bleomycin, epirubicin and cisplatin; DFS, disease-free survival; INSG, International Nasopharynx Group; LRR, locoregional recurrence; PE, cisplatin and epirubicin; PF, cisplatin and 5-fluorouracil; RT, radiotherapy; VCA, vincristine, cyclophosphamide, and doxorobucin; P, platin.

- Because of the high likelihood of cervical metastases, most authors recommend electively treating all the cervical lymphatics in N0 patients. Contrary to this universal philosophy is a randomized study by Ho showing that survival of N0 patients having prophylactic irradiation of the cervical lymphatics was not better than that of N0 patients not receiving neck irradiation.[17] However, Lee et al. reported in 384 patients with clinically negative necks, 11% (44 patients) of those receiving elective neck irradiation had regional failure compared with 40% (362 of 906) of those not electively treated.[7] This study strongly supports elective irradiation of the neck in patients with clinically negative neck nodes.
- Lymph node groups at risk in the nasopharyngeal region include the following:
  a. Submandibular nodes (surgical level I): if level II node is involved.
  b. Upper deep jugular (junctional, parapharyngeal) nodes: all cases.
  c. Subdigastric (jugulodigastric) nodes, midjugular, lower neck, and supraclavicular nodes (levels II through IV): all cases, bilaterally.
  d. Posterior cervical nodes (level V): all cases, bilaterally.
  e. Retropharyngeal nodes: all cases.

- Table 6-14 summarizes the target volume specification for definitive and postoperative IMRT in nasopharyngeal cancer.
- Table 6-15 shows suggested target volume determination for nasopharyngeal carcinoma.

### 7.2. Target Volume Delineation

- Figure 6-8 shows CTV1 and CTV2 delineation in a patient with clinically T2N1 (AJCC 1997) squamous cell carcinoma of nasopharynx receiving definitive IMRT.
- Figure 6-9 shows CTV1 and CTV2 delineation in a patient with clinically T4N2 (AJCC 1997) squamous cell carcinoma of the nasopharynx receiving definitive IMRT.

### 7.3. Normal Tissue Delineation

- See Chapter 5 for normal tissue delineation (Fig 5-16).

### 7.4. Suggested Target and Normal Tissue Doses

- See Chapter 4 for suggested target and normal tissue doses (Table 4-9).

## TABLE 6-15. SUGGESTED TARGET VOLUME DETERMINATION FOR NASOPHARYNX IMRT (47)

| Clinical Presentation | CTV1 | CTV2 |
|---|---|---|
| T1–2 N0 | P | IN + CN (I–V, RPLN) |
| T3–4N+* | P + IN (I†–V, RPLN) | CN (I–V, RPLN) |
| N2c | P + IN + CN (I†–V, RPLN) | |

Source: Modified from Chao KSC, Wippold FJ, Ozyigit G, et al. Determination and delineation of nodal target volumes for head and neck cancer based on the patterns of failure in patients receiving definitive and postoperative IMRT. *Int J Radiat Oncol Biol Phys* 2002;53:1174–1184.
CN, contralateral neck nodes; IN, ipsilateral neck nodes; P, gross tumor with margins for definition IMRT; RPLN, retropharyngeal nodes.
*N+ = N1–3 except N2c, including Ib node if level II node involved.
†Include submandibular node (level Ib) when level II node involved.

## TABLE 6-14. TARGET VOLUME SPECIFICATION FOR DEFINITIVE IMRT IN NASOPHARYNGEAL CANCER (47)

| Target | Definitive IMRT |
|---|---|
| GTV | Gross tumor by CT, MRI, and physical examination |
| CTV1 | Soft tissue and nodal regions adjacent to the GTV |
| CTV2 | Elective nodal regions* |

Source: Modified from Chao KSC, Wippold FJ, Ozyigit G, et al. Determination and delineation of nodal target volumes for head and neck cancer based on the patterns of failure in patients receiving definitive and postoperative IMRT. *Int J Radiat Oncol Biol Phys* 2002;53:1174–1184.
*See Table 6-15.

Nasopharynx 79

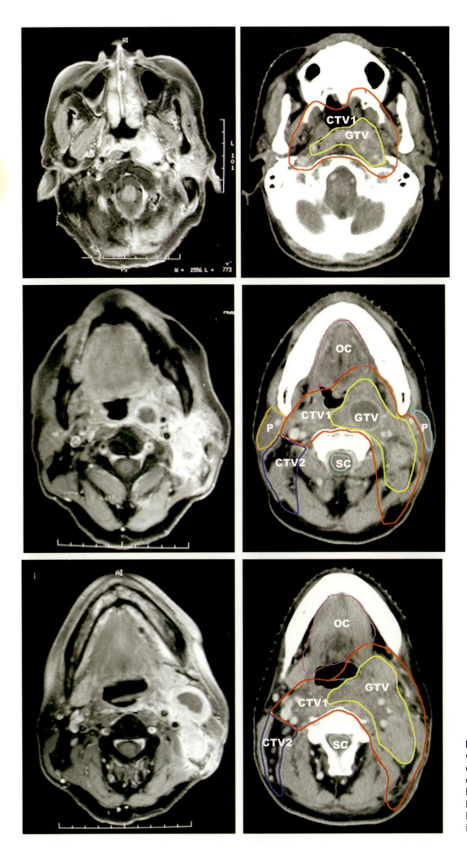

**FIGURE 6-8.** CTV delineation in a patient with a T2N1M0 (AJCC 1997) nasopharyngeal carcinoma receiving definitive IMRT. CTV, clinical target volume; CTV1, red; CTV2, dark blue; GTV, gross tumor volume (yellow line); P, parotid gland; right parotid gland, rust line; left parotid gland, aqua line; oral cavity, magenta line; SC, spinal cord, green line.

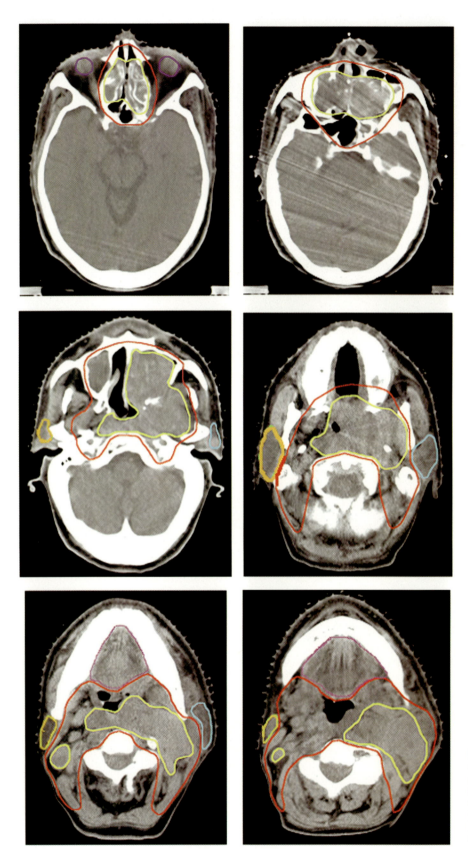

**FIGURE 6-9.** CTV delineation in a patient with a T4N2M0 (AJCC 1997) nasopharyngeal carcinoma receiving definitive IMRT. CTV, clinical target volume; CTV1, red; CTV2, dark blue; GTV, gross tumor volume (yellow line); right parotid gland, rust line; left parotid gland, aqua line; oral cavity, magenta line.

### 7.5. IMRT Treatment Results

- Cheng et al. showed that target coverage of the primary tumor was maintained and nodal coverage was improved in 17 nasopharyngeal carcinoma patients, as compared with conventional beam arrangements.[18] Moreover, the ability of IMRT to spare the parotid gland was exciting. Hunt et al. reported similar results with 23 primary nasopharyngeal carcinoma patients.[19]
- Sultanem et al. showed that in 67 patients treated with IMRT, the 4-year local progression-free survival, local-regional progression-free survival, distant metastases recurrence-free survival, and overall survival were 100%, 97%, 94%, and 94%, respectively, with a median follow-up of 28 months.[20] The 4-year distant metastases recurrence-free rate was 79%. Excellent local-regional control for nasopharyngeal carcinoma was achieved with intensity-modulated radiotherapy. IMRT provided excellent tumor target coverage and allowed the delivery of a high dose to the target with significant sparing of the salivary glands and other nearby critical normal tissues.
- Chao and associates previously presented their institutional results.[21] One hundred and three patients were treated with conventional external beam radiation therapy only (MIR-RT). Twenty-two patients received external beam irradiation with concomitant chemotherapy according to the Intergroup Study 0099 regimen. Among them, 13 patients were treated by conventional beam arrangement (MIR-CRT), and nine patients were treated with IMRT (MIR-IMRT). Three-year progression-free survival for radiation therapy alone was 51% for MIR patients as compared with 24% in IGS ($p < .05$). Progression-free survival at 3 years after chemoradiotherapy was 90% for MIR patients and 69% in IGS ($p < .05$).
- In an updated report, 12 nasopharyngeal carcinoma patients were treated with IMRT between February 1997 and December 2000.[22] The T stages were one T1, three T2, three T3, and five T4. The N stages were one N0, three N1, four N2, and four N3 (AJCC staging; two stage II, two stage III, eight stage IV). Patients received chemotherapy according to the intergroup 0099 regimen. Median follow-up time was 31 months (range, 19 to 52 months). We observed one neck recurrence. Three patients developed distant metastasis. One patient died of distant metastasis. No patient failed at nasopharynx.
- Figure 6-10 shows pre- and post-IMRT MRI sections of a T4N3 nasopharyngeal carcinoma patient and the complete regression of the tumor.
- Figure 6-11 shows an example of IMRT dose distribution of a patient receiving definitive IMRT for a T2N2M0 nasopharyngeal cancer.
- A G-tube was placed in two patients during the course of IMRT. We observed no grade 3 or grade 4 late complications in our patients treated with IMRT. Six grade 2 and four grade 1 late xerostomia were observed. Decreased hearing was common with cisplatin chemotherapy.

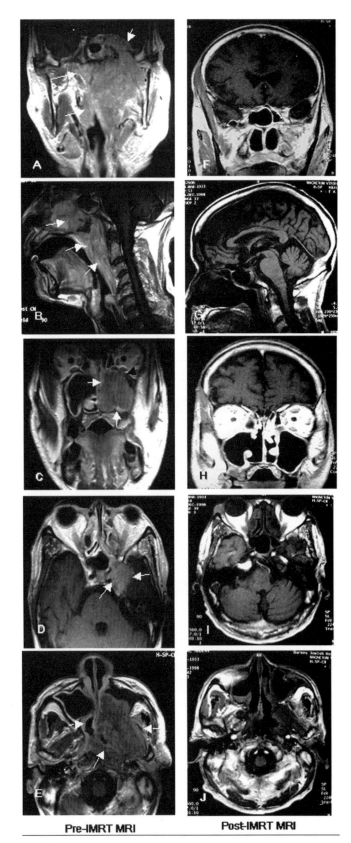

**FIGURE 6-10.** Pre-IMRT (**A–E**) and post-IMRT (**F–J**) MRI sections of a patient with T4N3 nasopharyngeal carcinoma patient showing complete regression of the tumor after a total IMRT dose of 70 Gy with concurrent platinum-based chemotherapy.

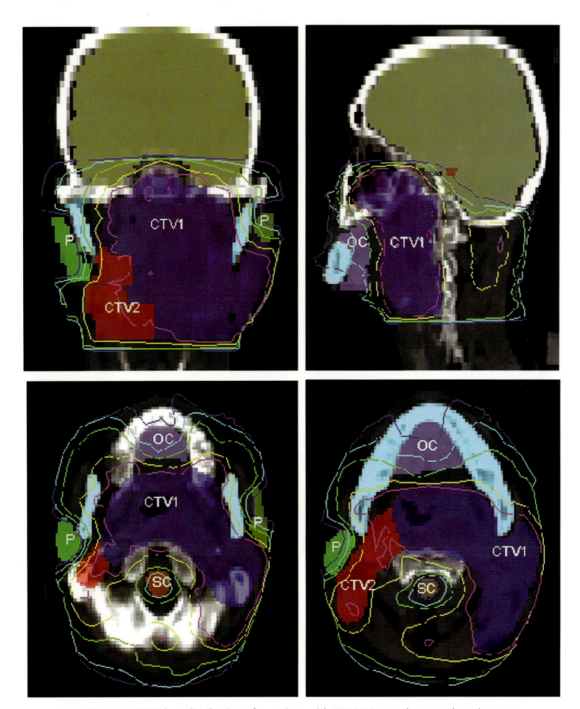

**FIGURE 6-11.** IMRT dose distribution of a patient with T2N2M0 nasopharyngeal carcinoma receiving definitive IMRT. CTV, clinical target volume; CTV1, dark blue area; CTV2, red area; P, parotid gland; SC, spinal cord. Pink line, 70 Gy; yellow line, 60 Gy; green line, 50 Gy; aqua line, 30 Gy; dark blue, 20 Gy.

## 8. SEQUELAE OF TREATMENT

- Xerostomia (moderate to severe) occurs in approximately 75% of patients treated with conventional beam arrangement. IMRT can significantly reduce this in around 25% of patients.[21]

- The incidence of cranial and cervical sympathetic nerve palsy is 0.3% to 6% (median, 1%).[24]
- In one study the incidence of brainstem or cervical spine myelopathy was 1%; the reported incidence is 0.2% to 18%, with a median of 2%.[25] Some complications are correlated with a high dose to the spinal cord or

overlap at the junction of lateral portals and upper neck fields.

- Hypopituitarism causing significant clinical signs and symptoms is not commonly reported in most series of adults but has been described in children. Sham et al.[13] concluded that shielding of the pituitary/hypothalamus is feasible in a significant proportion of patients and that this technique may improve tolerance to treatment without compromising local tumor control.
- Ophthalmologic side effects, after tumor doses of 60 Gy, include opacities in the lens that develop several years after irradiation, similar to radiation cataract.[2]
- Four of 11 patients (36%) with nasopharyngeal carcinoma treated with 70 Gy developed retinopathy 24 to 108 months after treatment.[16]
- The reported incidence of deafness is 1% to 7%; 8% of patients have significant hearing impairment, and 3% had bilateral deafness.[24]
- Osteonecrosis of the mandible or maxilla can be kept to a minimum (1%) by avoiding unnecessarily high doses to these structures. Avoidance of elective dental extractions before irradiation, a vigorous program of oral hygiene and fluoride applications, and a close working relationship between radiation oncologist and dentist are equally important in reducing this complication.
- Dental decay frequently occurs. Dental caries may be reduced with prophylactic fluoride treatment and appropriate dental care. Dental extractions or restorations should be performed before initiation of irradiation to allow adequate time for healing of the gingiva and tooth canal. If dental care is required after irradiation, coverage with antibiotics should be instituted 1 week before dental extractions, and trauma should be minimized.
- Severity and incidence of trismus (5% to 10%) can be reduced by using high-energy x-rays (>18 MeV) or an anterior field for the nasopharynx boost.
- Fibrosis of subcutaneous tissues of the neck can be minimized by providing a 2- or 3-mm space between skin surface and CTV boundary when there is minimal risk of dermal or soft-tissue extension.

## REFERENCES

1. Perez C, Venkata R, Victor M, et al. Carcinoma of the nasopharynx: factors affecting prognosis. *Int J Radiat Oncol Biol Phys* 1991;23:271–280.
2. Fletcher G, Healey JJ, McGraw J, et al. Nasopharynx. In: MacComb W, Fletcher G, eds. *Cancer of the head and neck.* Baltimore: Williams & Wilkins, 1967:152–178.
3. Lederman M.*Cancer of the nasopharynx: its natural history and treatment.* Springfield, IL: Charles C Thomas, 1961.
4. Qin D, Hu Y, Yan J, et al. Analysis of 1379 patients with nasopharyngeal carcinoma treated with radiation. *Cancer* 1988;61:1117–1124.

5. Petrovich Z, Cox J, Middleton R, et al. Advanced carcinoma of the nasopharynx. II. Pattern of failure in 256 patients. *Radiother Oncol* 1985;4:15–20.
6. Valentini V, Balducci M, Ciarniello V, et al. Tumors of the nasopharynx: review of 132 cases. *Rays* 1987;12:77–88.
7. Fletcher G, Million R.*Nasopharynx,* 3rd ed. Philadelphia: Lea & Febiger, 1980.
8. Leung S, Tsao S, Teo P, et al. Cranial nerve involvement by nasopharyngeal carcinoma: response to treatment and clinical significance. *Clin Oncol* 1990;2:138–141.
9. Chong V, Fan V, Khoo J. Retropharyngeal lymphadenopathy in nasopharyngeal carcinoma. *Eur J Radiol* 1995;21:100–105.
10. Sham J, Choy D. Prognostic factors of nasopharyngeal carcinoma: a review of 759 patients. *Br J Radiol* 1990;63:51–58.
11. Lee A, Foo W, Law S, et al. Staging of nasopharyngeal carcinoma: from Ho's to the new UICC system. *Int J Cancer* 1999;84:179–187.
12. Chu A, Flynn M, Achino E, et al. Irradiation of nasopharyngeal carcinoma: correlations with treatment factors and stage. *Int J Radiat Oncol Biol Phys* 1984;10:2241–2249.
13. Kaasa S, Kragh-Jensen E, Bjordal K, et al. Prognostic factors in patients with nasopharyngeal carcinoma. *Acta Oncol* 1993;32:531–536.
14. Al-Sarraf M, LeBlanc M, Giri PGS, et al. Chemoradiotherapy versus radiotherapy in patients with advanced nasopharyngeal cancer: phase III randomized intergroup study 0099. *J Clin Oncol* 1998;16:1310–1317.
15. Chi K, Change Y, Guo W. Phase III study of adjuvant chemotherapy in advanced nasopharyngeal carcinoma patients. *Int J Radiat Oncol Biol Phys* 2002;52:1238–1244.
16. Cheng S, Jian J, Tsai S, et al. Long-term survival of nasopharyngeal carcinoma following concomitant radiotherapy and chemotherapy. *Int J Radiat Oncol Biol Phys* 2000;48:1323–1330.
17. Jian J, Cheng S, Prosnitz L, et al. T classification and clivus margin as risk factors for determining locoregional control by radiotherapy of nasopharyngeal carcinoma. *Cancer* 1998;82:261–267.
18. Cheng JCH, Chao KSC, Low D. Comparison of IMRT techniques for nasopharyngeal carcinoma. *Int J Cancer* 2001;96:126–132.
19. Hunt MA, Zelefsky MJ, Wolden S, et al. Treatment planning and delivery of intensity-modulated radiation therapy for primary nasopharynx cancer. *Int J Radiat Oncol Biol Phys* 2001;49:623–632.
20. Sultanem K, Shu HK, Xia P, et al. Three-dimensional intensity-modulated radiotherapy in the treatment of nasopharyngeal carcinoma: the University of California–San Francisco experience. *Int J Radiat Oncol Biol Phys* 2000;48:711–722.
21. Chao K, Cengiz M, Perez C. Intensity-modulated radiotherapy (IMRT) yields superior functional outcome in locally advanced nasopharyngeal carcinoma: comparison with intergroup study 0099. *Proceedings of the American Society of Clinical Oncology,* 36th annual meeting. New Orleans, LA, 2000.
22. Ozyigit G, Chao K. Clinical experience of head and neck IMRT with serial tomotherapy. *Medical Dosimetry* 2002;27:91–98.
23. Chua D, Sham J, Kwong D. Retropharyngeal lymphadenopathy in patients with nasopharyngeal carcinoma: a computed tomography-based study. *Cancer* 1997;79:869–877.
24. Ozyar E, Yildiz F, Akyol F, et al. Comparison of AJCC 1988 and 1997 classifications for nasopharyngeal carcinoma. *Int J Radiat Oncol Biol Phys* 1999;44:1079–1087.
25. Cooper J, Cohen R, Stevens R. A comparison of staging systems for nasopharyngeal carcinoma. *Cancer* 1998;83:213–219.
26. McLaughlin M, Mendelhall W, Mancuso A, et al. Retropharyngeal adenopathy as a predictor of outcome in squamous cell carcinoma of the head and neck. *Head Neck* 1995;17:190–198.

27. Chua D, Sham J, Choy D, et al. Preliminary report of the Asian-Oceanian clinical oncology association randomized trial comparing cisplatin and epirubicin followed by radiotherapy versus radiotherapy alone in the treatment of patients with locoregionally advanced nasopharyngeal carcinoma. *Cancer* 1998;83:2270–2283.

28. Wang C. Carcinoma of the oropharynx. In: Wang C, ed. *Radiation therapy for head and neck neoplasms.* New York: Wiley-Liss, 1997.

29. Mesic J, Fletcher G, Goepfert H. Megavoltage irradiation of epithelial tumors of the nasopharynx. *Int J Radiat Oncol Biol Phys* 1981;7:447–453.

30. Chien C, Chen S, Hsieh C, et al. Retrospective comparison of the AJCC 5th edition classification for nasopharyngeal carcinoma with the AJCC 4th edition: an experience in Taiwan. *Jpn J Clin Oncol* 2001;31:363–369.

31. Hoppe R, Goffinet D, Bagshaw M. Carcinoma of the nasopharynx: eighteen years' experience with megavoltage radiation therapy. *Cancer* 1976;37:2605–2612.

32. Kajanti M, Mäntylä M. Carcinoma of the nasopharynx: a retrospective analysis of treatment results in 125 patients. *Acta Oncol* 1990;29:611–614.

33. Lee A, Law S, Foo W, et al. Nasopharyngeal carcinoma: local control by megavoltage irradiation. *Br J Radiol* 1993;66:528–536.

34. Rossi A, Molinari R, Borracchi P, et al. Adjuvant chemotherapy with vincristine, cyclophosphamide and doxorubicin after radiotherapy in local-regional nasopharyngeal cancer: results of a 4-year multicenter randomized trial. *J Clin Oncol* 1988;6:1401–1410.

35. Cvitkovic E. Neoadjuvant chemotherapy with epirubicin, cisplatin, bleomycin in undifferentiated nasopharyngeal cancer: preliminary results of international phase III trial (abstr). *Proceed Am Soc Clin Oncol* 1994;13:283.

36. Group INCS. Preliminary results of a randomized trial comparing neoadjuvant chemotherapy (cisplatin, epirubicin, beomycin) plus radiotherapy versus radiotherapy alone in stage IV (≥N2, M0) undifferentiated nasopharyngeal carcinoma. A positive effect on progression free survival. International Nasopharynx Cancer Study Group. VUMCA I trial. *Int J Radiat Oncol Biol Phys* 1996;35:463–469.

37. Chan A, Teo P, TWT L, et al. A prospective randomized study of chemotherapy adjunctive to definitive radiotherapy in advanced nasopharyngeal carcinoma. *Int J Radiat Oncol Biol Phys* 1995;33:569–577.

# 7

# ORAL CAVITY

**GOKHAN OZYIGIT**
**K.S. CLIFFORD CHAO**

## 1. ANATOMY

- The oral cavity consists of the upper and lower lips, gingivobuccal sulcus, buccal mucosa, upper and lower gingiva (including alveolar ridge), hard palate, floor of the mouth, and the anterior two-thirds of the mobile tongue.

- The *lips* are composed of the orbicularis muscle, which is covered by skin and mucous membrane on the inner surface; the transitional area between the two is the vermilion border. The blood supply comes from the labial artery, a branch of the facial artery. The motor nerve branches come from the facial nerve. The sensory nerve to the upper lip is the infraorbital branch of the maxillary nerve and, to the lower lip, branches of the mental nerve, which originates in the inferior alveolar nerve. The commissure is partially innervated by the buccal branch of the mandibular nerve.

- The *alveolar ridge of the maxilla,* which is covered by mucosa and the teeth and continues medially with the hard palate, forms the upper gingiva. The *lower gingiva* covers the mandible from the gingivobuccal sulcus to the mucosa of the floor of the mouth. It continues posteriorly with the retromolar trigone and above with the maxillary tuberosity. There are no minor salivary glands in the mucous membrane over the alveolar ridges.[1]

- The *buccal mucosa* is made up of the mucous membrane covering the internal surface of the lips and cheeks (buccinator muscle), extending from the line of attachment of the upper and lower alveolar ridges to the point of contact of the lips posteriorly and the orbicularis anteriorly. The masseter muscle lies posterior and lateral to the buccinator muscle. The blood supply comes from the facial artery. The buccal nerve, a branch of the mandibular nerve, supplies sensory fibers. The motor nerve to the buccinator muscle is derived from the facial nerve.

- The *floor of the mouth,* bounded by the lower gingiva anteriorly and laterally, extends to the insertion of the anterior tonsillar pillar into the tongue posteriorly (Fig. 7-1). It is divided into halves by the lingual frenulum and is covered by a mucous membrane with stratified squamous epithelium. The sublingual glands lie below the mucous membrane and are separated by the midline genioglossus and geniohyoid muscles. The genial tubercles are bony protuberances occurring at the point of insertion of these two muscle groups on the symphysis.[1] Muscles include the mylohyoid and digastric muscles. The submaxillary glands are located on the external surface of the mylohyoid muscle, between its insertion to the mandible. The submaxillary duct (Wharton's duct) is about 5 cm long and courses between the sublingual gland and genioglossus muscle; its orifice is in the anterior floor of the mouth, near the midline. The sensory nerve is the lingual nerve, a branch of the submaxillary nerve. The arterial supply is the lingual artery, a branch of the external carotid.

- The *tongue* is a muscular organ composed of the styloglossus, hyoglossus, and hyoid muscles (Fig.7-2). It is covered by a mucous membrane with stratified squamous epithelium. The circumvallate papillae, situated posteriorly with a V-shaped configuration, separate the base of the tongue from the mobile tongue. The *oral tongue* consists of the tip, dorsum, lateral borders, and undersurface. The blood supply is the lingual artery, a branch of the external carotid artery.[2] The sensory nerve is the lingual nerve, a branch of the maxillary nerve; the hypoglossal nerve is the motor nerve. The chorda tympani branch of the sensory root of the facial nerve innervates the taste buds.

### 1.1. Lymphatics

- Lymphatics of the upper lip drain mostly to the submandibular lymph nodes; the periauricular and parotid lymph nodes occasionally receive lymphatic channels from the upper lip. Lower lip lymphatics drain to the submandibular and posteriorly to the subdigastric lymph nodes. Lymphatics of the lower gingiva drain to the submandibular and subdigastric lymph nodes.

- The first echelon of lymph node drainage of the floor of the mouth is to the submandibular and subdigastric lymph nodes.

- Primary lymphatic drainage in the oral tongue is to the subdigastric and submandibular lymph nodes. Rouviere described the lymphatic trunks that bypass this primary lymphatic drainage and go directly to the midjugular

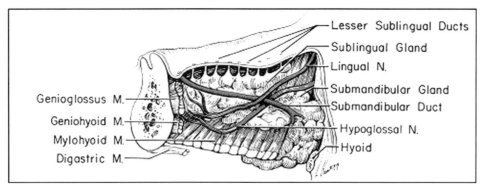

**FIGURE 7-1.** The floor of the oral cavity. (Million RR, et al. Cancer of the head and neck. In: DeVita VT Jr, Hellman S, Rosenberg SA, eds. *Cancer: principles and practice of oncology,* 3rd ed. Philadelphia: JB Lippincott, 1989:506, by permission.)

- lymph nodes, which probably accounts for the relative frequency of metastatic lymph nodes in these locations (Fig. 7-3).[3]
- Lymphatic drainage of the buccal mucosa is primarily to the submandibular and subdigastric lymph nodes.
- Clinically detected nodal metastases on admission by T stage vary according to subsites of the oral cavity (Table 7-1). Incidence and distribution of metastatic disease in clinically negative and positive neck nodes also change according to subsites of the cancer in the oral cavity (Tables 7-2 to 7-4).
- Several factors influence contralateral nodal metastasis in oral cavity cancer (Table 7-5). Except for lesions arising from the tip of the tongue or extending across the midline, metastatic disease usually occurs in the ipsilateral cervical lymph nodes.[4]
- Lymph node involvement in lesions of the lip is relatively rare, although 5% to 10% of patients with clinically negative necks later develop lymph node metastases.[5]
- The incidence of lymph node metastases of the upper gingiva is 15% to 20% on admission. There is about the same incidence of later development of clinical cervical lymph node metastases in initially clinically negative necks.[4]

- About 30% to 65% of patients with cancer of the oral tongue and floor of the mouth have clinically positive neck nodes on presentation (Figs. 7-4 and 7-5).
- Figure 7-6 shows the incidence of clinically evident metastatic lymph nodes in patients with carcinoma of the retromolar trigone and anterior faucial pillar on admission.
- For cancers of the buccal mucosa, the incidence of clinically positive cervical lymph nodes on admission is 10% to 30%.
- Of patients with clinically negative nodes, approximately 40% have pathologically positive nodes. Of all patients with negative nodes at presentation, the incidence of eventual development of a nodal metastasis without treatment is about 20% to 35%. Submental lymph nodes are involved in fewer than 5% of patients.[4]
- The distribution of pathologically positive neck nodes after elective modified neck dissection in patients with carcinomas in the oral cavity, the floor of mouth, and the retromolar trigone is shown in Figs. 7-7, 7-8, and 7-9, respectively.

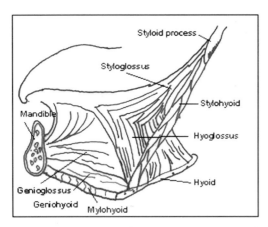

**FIGURE 7-2.** Musculature of the tongue. (Adapted from Clemente CD. *Anatomy: a regional atlas of the human body.* Baltimore: Urban & Schwarzenberg, 1987, by permission.)

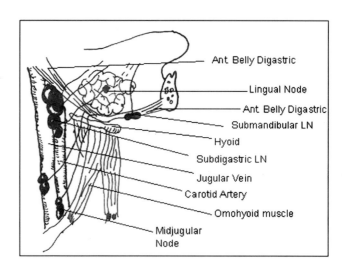

**FIGURE 7-3.** Lymphatics of the tongue. (Adapted from Rouviere H. *Anatomy of the human lymphatic system.* Ann Arbor, MI: Edwards Brothers, 1938:44, by permission.)

## TABLE 7-1. CLINICALLY DETECTED NODAL METASTASES (%) ON ADMISSION BY T STAGE

|  | N0 | N1 | N2–3 |
|---|---|---|---|
| *Oral Tongue* | | | |
| T1 | 86 | 10 | 4 |
| T2 | 70 | 19 | 11 |
| T3 | 52 | 16 | 31 |
| T4 | 24 | 10 | 66 |
| *Floor of Mouth* | | | |
| T1 | 89 | 9 | 2 |
| T2 | 71 | 18 | 10 |
| T3 | 66 | 20 | 24 |
| T4 | 46 | 10 | 43 |
| *RMT or Anterior Tonsillar Pillar* | | | |
| T1 | 88 | 2 | 9 |
| T2 | 62 | 18 | 20 |
| T3 | 46 | 21 | 33 |
| T4 | 32 | 18 | 50 |

*Source:* Compiled from the data of MD Anderson.[12]

- Byers et al. reported the incidence of nodal metastasis by T stage and subsite in oral cavity cancer after elective nodal dissection (Table 7-6).
- The incidence of bilateral lymph node involvement is relatively high for floor-of-mouth cancers because many lesions are near or cross the midline.
- Five percent to 10% of oral tongue cancers have bilateral lymph node metastases (Fig. 7-4).

## 2. NATURAL HISTORY

- Early lesions of the lip invade adjacent skin and the orbicularis muscle. More advanced lesions extend the adjacent commissures of the lip, mandible, and mental nerve. Perineural invasion is related to large tumor size, mandibular invasion, and poorly differentiated histology.
- Floor-of-mouth cancers mostly originate within 2 cm of the anterior midline. They invade early beneath the mucosa into the sublingual gland and the midline genioglossus and geniohyoid muscles. The mylohyoid muscles act as a barrier in early stages. Even small and early le-

sions may extend into periosteum. But mandible invasion occurs late in the course of the disease. Submandibular ducts may be obstructed by the tumor.

- Oral tongue cancers mostly originate on the lateral and undersurfaces of the tongue. They tend to remain in the tongue in early stages. Perineural invasion is rare. Tip-of-the-tongue cancers are diagnosed in early stages. Advanced lesions invade the floor of the mouth and the root of the tongue, producing fixation. Posterior lesions usually grow into musculature of the tongue, the anterior tonsillar pillar, the base of the tongue, and the mandible.
- Most of the buccal mucosa lesions developed on the lateral walls. Advanced lesions invade the underlying muscles and eventually penetrate to the skin and the infratemporal fossa. Advanced lesions may also involve the parotid gland and facial nerve.
- The lesions of the retromolar trigone spread to adjacent buccal mucosa, anterior tonsillar pillar, lower gum, and maxilla; this occurs early. Invasion of the periosteum of the mandible may be seen early, but invasion of the underlying mandible tends to be a late manifestation. The cortex of the mandible is dense, which explains the infrequent bone invasion in the region of the retromolar trigone.
- Most of the tumors originate on the gingival and spread secondarily to the hard palate, soft palate, and underlying bone. Perineural spread occurs by way of the greater and lesser palatine foramina.

## 3. DIAGNOSIS AND STAGING SYSTEM

### 3.1. Signs and Symptoms

- Lip cancer may present as a slowly enlarging, exophytic lesion with an elevated border that is nontender. Minor bleeding may be seen. Erythema of the adjacent skin suggests dermal lymphatic invasion. Paresthesia of the skin of the lip indicates mental nerve invasion.
- Floor-of-mouth tumors are noticed first when the patient feels a lump in the floor of mouth with the tip of the tongue. Pain, bleeding, foul breath, loose teeth, a painful mass in the submandibular region, and a change in speech are other symptoms that can be seen in advanced lesions.

## TABLE 7-2. INCIDENCE AND DISTRIBUTION OF METASTATIC DISEASE IN CLINICALLY NEGATIVE (N−) AND POSITIVE (N+) NECK NODES (IN PERCENTAGE)

|  | Radiologically Enlarged Retropharyngeal Nodes | | Pathologic Nodal Metastasis | | | | | | | | |
|---|---|---|---|---|---|---|---|---|---|---|---|
|  |  |  | Level I | | Level II | | Level III | | Level IV | | Level V |
| Clinical presentation | N− | N+ | N− | N+ | N− | N+ | N− | N+ | N− | N+ | N− | N+ |
| Oral tongue | — | — | 14 | 39 | 19 | 73 | 16 | 27 | 3 | 11 | 0 | 0 |
| Floor of mouth | — | — | 16 | 72 | 12 | 51 | 7 | 29 | 2 | 11 | 0 | 5 |
| Alveolar ridge and retromolar trigone | — | — | 25 | 38 | 19 | 84 | 6 | 25 | 5 | 10 | 1 | 4 |

*Source:* Modified from Chao KSC, Wippold FJ, Ozyigit G, et al. Determination and delineation of nodal target volumes for head and neck cancer based on the patterns of failure in patients receiving definitive and postoperative IMRT. *Int J Radiat Oncol Biol Phys* 2002;53:1174–1184.

## TABLE 7-3. INCIDENCE OF NECK NODE METASTASES BY PRIMARY TUMOR SITE

| Tumor Site | cN+ at Presentation (%) | cN0, pN + Pathologically (%) | cN−, N+ with N0 Neck Treatment (%) |
|---|---|---|---|
| FOM | 30–59 | 21–50 | 20–35 |
| Gingiva | 18–52 | 12–19 | 17 |
| Hard palate | 13–24 | No data | 22 |
| Buccal mucosa | 9–31 | 0/10 | 16 |
| Oral tongue | 34–65 | 25–54 | 38–52 |

*Source:* Modified from Chao KSC, Wippold FJ, Ozyigit G, et al. Determination and delineation of nodal target volumes for head and neck cancer based on the patterns of failure in patients receiving definitive and postoperative IMRT. *Int J Radiat Oncol Biol Phys* 2002;53:1174–1184.
c, clinical; FOM, floor of mouth; p, pathologic.

- Irritation and the sensation of a lump are the most frequent symptoms in tongue cancer. The pain becomes progressively worse and may be referred to the external ear canal. Bleeding is uncommon. Speech and swallowing may be affected in advanced lesions.
- Leukoplakia is present in half of the cases in buccal mucosa tumors. Obstruction of Stensen's duct may cause swelling of the parotid gland. Extension into pterygoids, masseter, or buccinator muscles may cause trismus. Intermittent bleeding may be seen during chewing.
- Local pain and pain referred to the external auditory canal and preauricular area can be produced by retromolar trigone lesions. Trismus may be seen if the lesion invades pterygoid muscles.

## 3.2. Physical Examination

- The extent of disease in oral cavity lesions is determined by visual examination and palpation. Topical anesthesia may be required for examination.
- Bimanual palpation determines the extent of induration and the degree of fixation to the periosteum. Large lesions bulge into the submental or submandibular space. The submandibular duct and gland as well as parotid duct and gland are evaluated by bimanual palpation.

## TABLE 7-4. INCIDENCE OF CONTRALATERAL OR BILATERAL NECK NODE METASTASES BY PRIMARY TUMOR SITE

| Tumor Site | cN+, Bilateral (%) | cN+, Contralateral Only | cN−, pN+ Bilateral (%) |
|---|---|---|---|
| Oral tongue | 12 | — | 33 |
| FOM | 27 | — | 21 |

*Source:* Modified from Chao KSC, Wippold FJ, Ozyigit G, et al. Determination and delineation of nodal target volumes for head and neck cancer based on the patterns of failure in patients receiving definitive and postoperative IMRT. *Int J Radiat Oncol Biol Phys* 2002;53:1174–1184.
c, clinical; FOM, floor of mouth; p, pathologic.

## 3.3. Imaging

### 3.3.1. Lip

- Diagnostic imaging is generally used for locally advanced, deeply infiltrating, or recurrent lip lesions.
- Computed tomography scanning is useful for showing bone invasion. It can detect the abnormalities along the buccal surface of maxilla and mandible. Magnetic resonance imaging is of little or no use for detecting bone erosion.
- The entire course of the infraorbital and mandibular nerves must be studied for patients with deeply infiltrative recurrent tumor or signs or symptoms of perineural invasion. Computed tomography slices beginning at the infraorbital and mental foramina and following the course of each nerve back to the cavernous sinus should be used for those patients, since they are also at risk for bone erosion. Contrast-enhanced MRI may be further used for highly selected patients to detect subtle perineural spread of tumor. Regional lymph nodes must also be included in the slices, since the risk of lymphatic metastasis is high for those patients.

## TABLE 7-5. FACTORS INFLUENCING CONTRALATERAL LN METASTASIS IN ORAL CANCER

| Variable | RR of Contralateral Metastasis | 95% CI |
|---|---|---|
| *Tumor Site* | | |
| Tongue | 1.0 | Ref |
| FOM | 1.5 | 0.9–2.6 |
| RMT | 0.3 | 0.1–1.1 |
| *Distance from Midline* | | |
| >1 cm | 1.0 | Ref |
| Cross <1 cm | 2.8 | 1.1–7.5 |
| Cross >1 cm | 12.7 | 5.6–29.1 |
| *Tumor Stage* | | |
| T1 | 1.0 | Ref |
| T2–3 | 2.2 | 0.7–5.5 |
| T4 | 5.8 | 2.0–16.3 |

*Source:* Modified from Kowalski 1998.
FOM, floor of mouth; RMT, retromolar trigone.

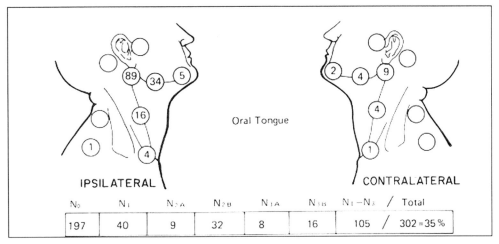

**FIGURE 7-4.** Incidence of clinically evident metastatic lymph nodes in patients with carcinoma of the oral tongue on admission. (Lindberg RD. Distribution of cervical lymph node metastases from squamous cell carcinoma of the upper respiratory and digestive tracts. *Cancer* 1972;29:1446, with permission.)

### 3.3.2. Floor of the Mouth

- The floor of the mouth is seen as a fat-containing space lying between the paired bellies of the genioglossus and geniohyoid muscles on CT and MRI axial images.
- The mylohyoid muscle is seen better on coronal sections as it extends from the mylohyoid line of the mandible to the hyoid. The sublingual spaces are usually symmetric. The submandibular space is separated from the floor of the mouth by the mylohyoid muscle and located in the suprahyoid part of the neck. Since these spaces contain glandular and fat tissue, they are easily distinguished from adjacent muscles on both CT and MRI. The lingual vessel bundle is seen coursing these spaces. The hypoglossal and lingual nerves are normally invisible.
- The hyoglossus muscle is visible on axial and coronal images coursing within the glandular and fatty tissue of the sublingual space.

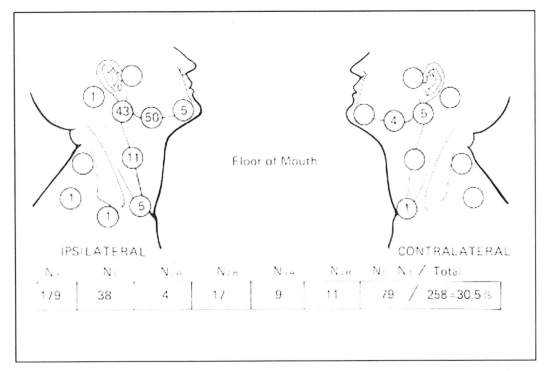

**FIGURE 7-5.** Incidence of clinically evident metastatic lymph nodes in patients with carcinoma of the floor of the mouth on admission. (Lindberg RD. Distribution of cervical lymph node metastases from squamous cell carcinoma of the upper respiratory and digestive tracts. *Cancer* 1972;29:1446, with permission.)

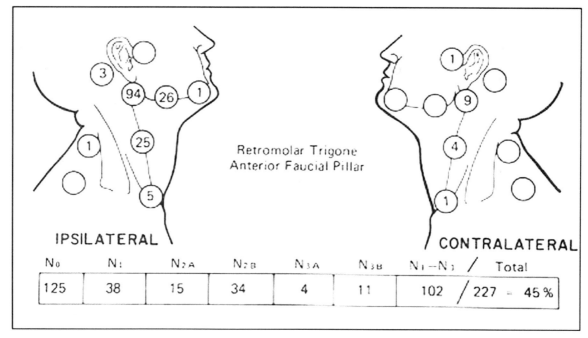

**FIGURE 7-6.** Incidence of clinically evident metastatic lymph nodes in patients with carcinoma of the retromolar trigone and anterior faucial pillar on admission. (Lindberg RD. Distribution of cervical lymph node metastases from squamous cell carcinoma of the upper respiratory and digestive tracts. *Cancer* 1972;29:1448, by permission.)

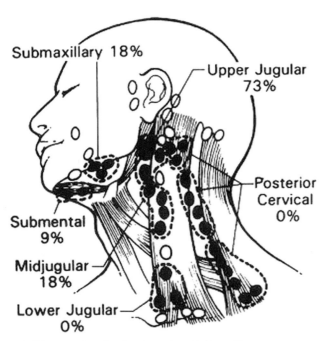

**FIGURE 7-7.** The distribution of pathologically positive neck nodes after elective modified neck dissection in 48 patients with oral tongue carcinoma. (Byers RM, Wolf PF, Ballantyne AJ. Rationale for elective modified neck dissection. *Head Neck Surg* 1988;10:162, by permission.)

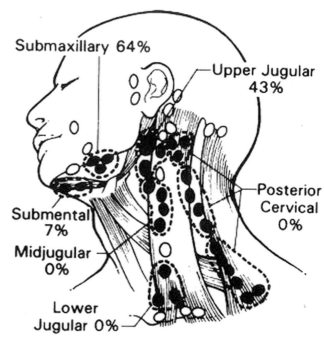

**FIGURE 7-8.** The distribution of pathologically positive neck nodes after elective modified neck dissection in 62 patients with floor of mouth carcinoma. (Byers RM, Wolf PF, Ballantyne AJ. Rationale for elective modified neck dissection. *Head Neck Surg* 1988;10:162, by permission.)

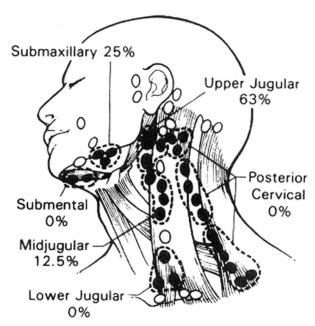

**FIGURE 7-9.** The distribution of pathologically positive neck nodes after elective modified neck dissection in patients with retromolar trigone carcinoma. (Byers RM, Wolf PF, Ballantyne AJ. Rationale for elective modified neck dissection. *Head Neck Surg* 1988;10:163, by permission.)

- The small space lying between the digastric muscles next to their insertion on the mandible is the submental space. The submandibular space contains the submandibular gland, facial vessels, and lymph nodes, which are normally small (less than 5 mm) in the submental space as well.

### 3.3.3. Oral Tongue

- It is difficult to differentiate the zone between the floor of the mouth and ventral surface of the oral tongue in axial images. This is much easier on coronal or sagittal sections of MRI or coronal CT sections. In the sagittal plane of MRI, various intrinsic muscle bundles and the fat tissue can be easily seen. The styloglossus muscle interdigitates with the hyoglossus muscle within the posterior aspect of the tongue.

**TABLE 7-6. ELECTIVE NODAL DISSECTION: INCIDENCE OF NODAL METASTASIS BY T CLASSIFICATION AND SITE IN ORAL CANCER**

| Primary Site | Tx, T1, T2 (%) | T3, T4 (%) | Total (%) |
|---|---|---|---|
| Oral tongue | 21 | 32 | 25 |
| Floor of mouth | 19 | 26 | 21 |
| Lower gum | 12 | 13 | 12 |
| Buccal mucosa | 0 | 0 | 0 |
| Retromolar trigone | 36 | 33 | 35 |

*Source:* Modified from Byers et al. Rationale for elective modified neck dissection. *Head Neck Surg* 1988;10:165.

- The muscles and spaces medial and lateral to the styloglossus muscle are potential places of tumor spread toward the skull base from the floor of the mouth and tongue base.
- Although CT and MRI cannot detect microscopic spread beyond palpable margins of tumor, they can help map the gross tumor boundary before surgical or radiation therapy.

### 3.3.4. Retromolar Trigone

- CT is the choice of imaging, since a detailed study of bony structures, soft tissues, and regional nodes is required. Spread to the lingual muscles can be recognized better on MRI than on CT. Occult spread anteriorly along the attachment of the mylohyoid muscle may be visible on CT or MRI when not palpable or visible by clinical examination. Supplemental MRI may be useful in looking for such perineural spread and in determining extension into the nasal cavity or soft palate.

## 3.4. Staging

- Table 7-7 shows the American Joint Committee on Cancer staging system for carcinoma of the oral cavity and lip.

## 4. GENERAL MANAGEMENT

- Various therapeutic measures are available for managing localized carcinomas of the oral cavity, including surgery, radiation therapy, laser excision, and combinations of these methods.

## 4.1. Lip

- Small cancers (<2 cm) can be cured in more than 90% of patients with surgery or irradiation, with excellent cosmetic and functional results.[6]
- Larger lesions (2 to 4 cm) can also be treated with either surgery or irradiation. However, reconstruction with a flap is often necessary with the surgical approach. The reconstructed lip often presents a significant functional problem.
- Postoperative irradiation is recommended for positive margins or perineural invasion.
- Lesions larger than 4 cm, uncommon lesions with poorly differentiated histology, and tumors involving the commissure are best treated with radiation therapy, with surgery reserved for salvage.
- Regional nodes are not treated in patients with small tumor; however, level I and II nodes should be included in a locally advanced lesion.
- The target volume includes the primary tumor with a 1.5-cm margin, if there is no indication for nodal irradiation and the lesion is well differentiated.

## TABLE 7-7. TNM CLASSIFICATION FOR CARCINOMA OF THE ORAL CAVITY AND LIP

*Primary Tumor (T)*

| | |
|---|---|
| TX | Primary tumor cannot be assessed |
| T0 | No evidence of primary tumor |
| Tis | Carcinoma *in situ* |
| T1 | Tumor <2 cm in greatest dimension |
| T2 | Tumor >2 cm but not >4 cm in greatest dimension |
| T3 | Tumor >4 cm in greatest dimension |
| T4 | (Lip) Tumor invades adjacent structures (inferior alveolar nerve, floor of mouth, skin of face) |
| T4 | (oral cavity) Tumor invades adjacent structures (cortical bone, into deep intrinsic muscles of tongue, maxillary sinus, skin. Superficial erosion alone of bone/tooth socket by gingival primary is not sufficient to classify as T4.) |

*Regional Lymph Nodes (N)*

| | |
|---|---|
| NX | Regional lymph nodes cannot be assessed |
| N0 | No regional lymph node metastasis |
| N1 | Metastasis in a single ipsilateral lymph node, <3 cm in greatest dimension |
| N2 | Metastasis in a single ipsilateral lymph node, >3 cm but not >6 cm in greatest dimension; in multiple ipsilateral lymph nodes, none >6 cm in greatest dimension; or in bilateral or contralateral lymph nodes, none >6 cm in greatest dimension |
| N2a | Metastasis in a single ipsilateral lymph node >3 cm but not >6 cm in greatest dimension |
| N2b | Metastasis in multiple ipsilateral lymph nodes, none >6 cm in greatest dimension |
| N2c | Metastasis in bilateral or contralateral lymph nodes, none >6 cm in greatest dimension |
| N3 | Metastasis in a lymph node >6 cm in greatest dimension |

*Distant Metastases (M)*

| | |
|---|---|
| MX | Presence of distant metastasis cannot be assessed |
| M0 | No distant metastasis |
| M1 | Distant metastasis |

*Stage Grouping*

| | | | |
|---|---|---|---|
| Stage 0 | Tis | N0 | M0 |
| Stage I | T1 | N0 | M0 |
| Stage II | T2 | N0 | M0 |
| Stage III | T3 | N0 | M0 |
| | T1 | N1 | M0 |
| | T2 | N1 | M0 |
| | T3 | N1 | M0 |
| Stage IVA | T4 | N0 or N1 | M0 |
| | Any T | N2 | M0 |
| Stage IVB | Any T | N3 | M0 |
| Stage IVC | Any T | Any N | M1 |

*Source:* Fleming ID, Cooper JS, Henson DE, et al., eds. *AJCC cancer staging manual,* 5th ed. Philadelphia: Lippincott-Raven, 1997:29.

- External-beam irradiations of 100 to 200 keV and/or electron beam of a suitable energy (6 to 9 MeV with 1- to 1.5-cm bolus) are used.
- Individually designed and constructed lead shields in the gingivobuccal sulcus are always used to protect the underlying gum and mandible.
- Doses of 50 Gy in 4 to 4.5 weeks for smaller lesions and 60 Gy in 5 to 6 weeks for larger lesions are usually recommended.
- In smaller lesions, interstitial irradiation alone has been recommended.
- Some institutions have used external-beam irradiation of about 50 Gy followed by an interstitial boost of 15 Gy.

- Table 7-8 summarizes treatment results for carcinoma of the lip.

### 4.2. Buccal Mucosa

- Primary surgery is effective for small, superficial T1 lesions without involvement of the commissure. The procedure removes the malignancy and eradicates any adjacent leukoplakia.
- For intermediate T2 lesions and those involving the commissure, irradiation, which produces a high cure rate with good functional and cosmetic results, is preferred.
- For T3 and T4 tumors with deep muscular invasion, cure rates after radiation therapy are poor. These lesions

## TABLE 7-8. TREATMENT RESULTS: CARCINOMA OF THE LIP

| Author | No. of Patients | Treatment | Local Control | 5-Year CSS |
|---|---|---|---|---|
| MacKay et al.[5] | 2,854 | 92% RT | <2 cm 97% | 65% |
| Baker et al.[13] | 279 | 47% RT | <3 cm 90% | 94% |
| | | 53% surgery | >3 cm 80% | 71% |
| Petrovic et al.[14] | 250 | RT | 94% | |
| Wang et al.[15] | 105 | RT | 90% | 90% |
| De Visscher et al.[16] | 108 | RT | 98% | 75% |
| Fitzpatrick et al.[17] | 361 | 57% RT | 92% | |
| | | 23% surgery | | |
| | | 20% surgery + RT | | |
| MacComb et al.[18] | 444 | 83% surgery | 96% | 94% |
| Mohs et al.[19] | 1,119 | Mohs surgery | <2 cm 97% | 94% |
| | | | >2 cm 60% | |

CSS, cause-specific survival; RT, radiotherapy.

are usually treated with radical surgery, reconstruction, and postoperative irradiation. Some authors have recommended preoperative irradiation followed by *en bloc* excision and a reconstructive procedure, if needed.[7]

- For T1 and most T2 lesions without nodal involvement, results with irradiation are best when photon or electron beam therapy is combined with interstitial implant or intraoral cone therapy.
- For moderately advanced lesions, with or without positive nodes, appropriate radiation therapy must include the primary site and regional lymph nodes. This is best achieved with external-beam irradiation through ipsilateral and anterior wedged-pair fields for a tumor dose of 55 to 60 Gy in 6 weeks, followed by boost irradiation, sparing the mandible, with interstitial implant, intraoral cone, or electron beam for an additional 20 Gy.
- Table 7-9 summarizes the treatment results for carcinoma of the buccal mucosa in.

### 4.3. Gingiva

- Approximately 80% of gingival carcinomas arise from the lower gingiva; 60% of these are posterior to the bicuspid.

- Because bony involvement by carcinoma compromises results of irradiation, careful radiographic examination of the mandible, including panorex and polytomes, is essential as a minimal pretreatment work-up.
- Intraoral dental radiographs or CT scans may better reveal minimal bony involvement of the mandible.
- Small T1 exophytic lesions without bony involvement can be managed by external-beam therapy alone.
- Radical surgery is preferred for advanced lesions associated with destruction of the mandible, with or without metastases, because partial mandibulectomy with radical neck dissection provides good survival rates.[8]
- Radiation portals must include the entire segment of the hemimandible from the mental symphysis to the temporomandibular joint.
- The ipsilateral neck is irradiated if nodes are positive or if lesions are advanced.

### 4.4. Oral Tongue

- Management of carcinoma of the oral tongue is difficult and controversial and depends on the primary lesion's size, location, and growth pattern and the nodal status in the neck.

### TABLE 7-9. TREATMENT RESULTS: BUCCAL MUCOSA

| Author | No. of Patients | Treatment | Local Control (%) | | 5-Year Cause-Specific Survival Rate (%) | |
|---|---|---|---|---|---|---|
| Bloom et al.[20] | 121 | S | — | | Stage I | 77 |
| | | | | | II | 65 |
| | | | | | III | 27 |
| | | | | | IV | 18 |
| Urist et al.[21] | 105 | S | | | Stage I | 95 |
| | | | | | II–III | 80 |
| | | | | | IV | 55 |
| MacComb et al.[18] | 115 | RT ± S | Stage I | 90 | | |
| | | | II–III | 88 | | |
| | | | IV | 38 | | |
| Wang et al.[22] | 60 | RT | | | 45% (3-year NED) | |

S, surgery; RT, radiation therapy.

**TABLE 7-10. TREATMENT RESULTS: ORAL TONGUE**

| Author | No. of Patients | | Therapy | Local Control (%) | | 5-Year Cause-Specific Survival Rate (%) | |
|---|---|---|---|---|---|---|---|
| | T1–2 | T3–4 | | T1–2 | T3–4 | T1–2 | T3–4 |
| Million et al.[2] | 45 | 29 | I + E | 80–60 | 42–0 | 80–76 | 42*–20 |
| Decroix et al.[23] | 382 | 220 | E + I | 86–78 | 71–** | 80–56 | 25–** |
| Gilbert et al.[24] | 20 | 36 | I + E | 91–63 | 36–** | 73–37 | 19–** |
| Wang et al.[22] | 116 | 87 | E | 86–43 | 17–18 | 64–36 | 19–5(3-year NED) |

E, external radiotherapy; I, interstitial.
*Stage III.
**No T4 data.

## 4.5. T1 and T2 Tongue Lesions

- Although surgery or irradiation is effective in controlling small cancers, it is not unreasonable to consider transoral surgical resection for small, well-defined lesions involving the tip and anterolateral border of the tongue.[9] These lesions can be cured by resection without risk of functional morbidity, particularly in aged and feeble patients.
- Radiation therapy (60 to 65 Gy in 6 to 7 weeks) is preferred for small, posteriorly situated, ill-defined lesions inaccessible for surgical excision through the peroral route.
- Superficial, exophytic T1 and T2 lesions with little muscle involvement are amenable to successful treatment with irradiation (70 Gy in 7 weeks).
- For moderately advanced, medium-sized T2 tumors involving the adjacent floor of the mouth, surgical treatment must include partial glossectomy, partial mandibulectomy, and radical neck dissection. Comprehensive irradiation (70 to 75 Gy in 7 to 8 weeks) with progressively decreasing fields to the primary site and neck nodes is preferred. Surgery is reserved for salvage of residual or recurrent disease.

## 4.6. T3 and T4 Tongue Lesions

- Advanced disease with deep muscle invasion, often associated with cervical lymph node metastases, is unlikely to be cured with irradiation alone.
- These lesions are best managed by planned combined irradiation (50 to 60 Gy in 5 to 6 weeks) and surgery.
- Excisional biopsy, even of a small lesion, is usually inadequate for carcinoma of the oral tongue.
- Wide local excision is the treatment of choice for well-circumscribed lesions that can be excised transorally with at least 1-cm margin.
- Wide local excision of lesions of the posterior part of the mobile tongue is difficult and, without reconstruction, can result in serious functional deficits in swallowing and speech. External irradiation combined with interstitial implant may be used for these patients.
- The extent of surgery for larger lesions is usually hemi- or total glossectomy.

- Postoperative irradiation is recommended for larger lesions, close or positive margins, and perineural invasion. It is also recommended for patients with initially positive surgical margins who later have negative surgical margins on reexcision.[10]
- Table 7-10 summarizes the results of treatment for carcinoma of the oral tongue.

## 4.7. The Floor of the Mouth

- In floor-of-mouth lesions that are tethered or fixed to the mandible, resection of the inner table is often recommended, which results in reasonable speech and swallowing.
- Postoperative irradiation is usually recommended because of associated negative prognostic factors.
- For advanced lesions due to bone invasion, wide local excision of tumor along with segmental resection of the mandible is often followed by reconstruction of the floor of the mouth and mandible.
- For very advanced disease involving the floor of the mouth, tongue, and mandible and massive neck disease, the chance of cure with any aggressive treatment is low and is often associated with formidable complications; a course of irradiation should strongly be considered.
- When the tumor is small or limited to the mucosa, it is highly curable by surgery or irradiation alone.
- For extensive, infiltrative T3 and T4 lesions with marked involvement of the adjacent muscle of the tongue and mandible, radical surgery followed by plastic closure and postoperative irradiation is the procedure of choice.
- Very small superficial lesions can be treated with interstitial implant (60 to 65 Gy) or intraoral cone (45 Gy over 3 weeks) alone.
- T1 and early T2 lesions must be treated with external-beam irradiation and various boost techniques such as interstitial implant (45 Gy external plus 25 Gy with implant) or intraoral cone (45 Gy external plus 20 Gy intraoral cone).
- For advanced T3 and T4 lesions, external-beam irradiation is given through large opposing lateral portals with equal loading covering the primary lesion and nodal areas

## TABLE 7-11. TREATMENT RESULTS: FLOOR OF MOUTH

| | No. of Patients | | | Local Control (%) | | 5-Year Cause-Specific Survival Rate (%) | |
|---|---|---|---|---|---|---|---|
| Author | T1–2 | T3–4 | Therapy | T1–2 | T3–4 | T1–2 | T3–4 |
| Wang et al.[22] | 174 | 61 | RT | 90–72 | 23–24 | 85–56 | 7–13 |
| Rodgers et al.[25] | 73 | 25 | RT | 86–69 | 55–40 | 96–70 | 67–1/5 |
| | 22 | 2 | S | 90–75 | 62 | 83–66 | — |
| Fu et al.[26] | 153 | — | RT | 90–81 | 67– | 83–71 | 43–10 |
| Nason et al.[27] | 114 | 75 | S | — | — | 69–64 | 46–26 |
| Gilbert et al.[24] | 40 | 15 | RT | 85–50 | 20 | 73–37 | 25 |

S, surgery; RT, external radiotherapy.

to a dose of approximately 45 Gy in 4.5 to 5 weeks, followed by two- or three-step reduced fields to a total dose of 70 to 74 Gy.

- Table 7-11 summarizes treatment results for carcinoma of the floor of the mouth.

## 4.8. Management of Neck Nodes

- In patients with small lesions resected with adequate margins, thickness of less than 2 mm, and no poor prognostic factors, no further treatment is needed if the neck is clinically and radiographically negative; the neck can be observed.
- In patients with resected primary lesions of the oral tongue or floor of the mouth more than 2 to 3 mm thick and/or poor prognostic factors such as perineural or perilymphatic invasion, the neck needs to be treated.
- Any form of bilateral neck dissection has worse cosmetic results than a moderate dose of irradiation (45 to 50 Gy).
- If neck dissection reveals only one positive node with no extracapsular extension, we usually recommend no radiation therapy to the neck.[6] If neck dissection shows more than one node, and especially metastases at more than one nodal station or extracapsular extension of a single or multiple nodes, a course of postoperative irradiation to the neck is indicated.
- In patients with clinically or radiographically positive neck nodes (by CT scan with contrast), the treatment of choice for the neck is ipsilateral neck dissection followed by bilateral postoperative neck irradiation.
- Contralateral prophylactic neck dissection is a serious disservice to the patient.[6]

## 5. INTENSITY MODULATED RADIATION THERAPY FOR CARCINOMAS OF THE ORAL CAVITY

### 5.1. Target Volume Determination

- If chemotherapy was delivered before radiation, the targets should be outlined on the planning CT according to their prechemotherapy extent.

- Lymph node groups at risk in the oral cavity include the following:
  a. Submandibular nodes (surgical level I): all cases
  b. Upper deep jugular (junctional, parapharyngeal) nodes: all cases (at the neck side ipsilateral to the primary tumor)
  c. Subdigastric (jugulodigastric) nodes, midjugular, lower neck, and supraclavicular nodes (levels II through IV): all cases, bilaterally
  d. Posterior cervical nodes (level V): all cases, at the neck side where there is an evidence of jugular nodal metastases
  e. Retropharyngeal nodes: all cases, if there is evidence of jugular nodal metastases
- Table 7-12 summarizes the target volume specification for definitive and postoperative IMRT in oral cavity cancer.
- Table 7-13 summarizes the suggested target volume determination for oral cavity carcinoma.

### 5.2. Target Volume Delineation

- In patients receiving postoperative IMRT, CTV1 encompasses residual tumor and the region adjacent to it but not directly involved by the tumor, the surgical bed with soft-tissue invasion by the tumor, or extracapsular extension by metastatic neck nodes. CTV2 includes primarily the prophylactically treated neck.
- In patients receiving definitive IMRT, CTV1 encompasses gross tumor (primary and enlarged nodes) and the region adjacent to it but not directly involved. CTV2 includes primarily the prophylactically treated neck.
- Figure 7-10 shows CTV1 and CTV2 delineation in a patient with clinically T3N2bM0 squamous cell carcinoma of the retromolar trigone receiving definitive IMRT.
- Figure 7-11 shows CTV1 and CTV2 delineation in a patient with pathologic T2N2bM0 squamous cell carcinoma of the tongue receiving postoperative IMRT.

### 5.3. Normal Tissue Delineation

- Figure 5-16 shows normal tissue delineation.

**TABLE 7-12. TARGET VOLUME SPECIFICATION FOR DEFINITIVE AND POSTOPERATIVE IMRT IN ORAL CAVITY CANCERS**

| Target | Definitive IMRT | High-Risk Postoperative IMRT | Intermediate-Risk Postoperative IMRT |
|---|---|---|---|
| CTV1 | Soft-tissue and nodal regions adjacent to the GTV | Surgical bed with soft-tissue involvement or nodal region with extracapsular involvement | Surgical bed without soft-tissue involvement or nodal region without capsular extension |
| CTV2 | Elective nodal regions* | Elective nodal regions* | Elective nodal regions* |

*Source:* Modified from Chao KSC, Wippold FJ, Ozyigit G, et al. Determination and delineation of nodal target volumes for head and neck cancer based on the patterns of failure in patients receiving definitive and postoperative IMRT. *Int J Radiat Oncol Biol Phys* 2002;53:1174–1184.
*See Table 7-13.

## 5.4. Suggested Target and Normal Tissue Doses

- Table 4-9 gives the Washington University guideline for clinical target volume dose specification with biological equivalent dose correction and normal tissue tolerance for IMRT.

## 5.5. IMRT Treatment Results of MIR

- Following these guidelines, 15 oral cavity carcinoma patients were treated with IMRT between February 1997 and December 2000 at Washington University.[11] Two patients were treated postoperatively, whereas 13 patients were treated with definitive IMRT. The T stages were T1 in three, T2 in five, T3 in three, and T4 in four. The N stages were N0 in five, N1 in two, and N2 in eight (two stage I, two stage II, two stage III, and nine stage IV, according to AJCC staging system). Median follow-up was 19 months (range, 9 to 44 months). We observed five locoregional recurrences and one patient developed dis-

tant metastasis. Two patients died of cancer; all others are alive.

- Figure 7-12 shows an example of IMRT dose distribution of a patient receiving postoperative IMRT for a T2N0M0 oral tongue cancer.
- A gastrostomy tube was placed in two patients during treatment. We observed no grade 3 or grade 4 late complications in our patients treated with IMRT. Five grade 1 and three grade 2 xerostomias were observed in our patients as late sequelae.

## 5.6. Sequelae of Treatment

- Minor sequelae such as xerostomia, loss of sense of taste, and dental caries may follow curative radiation therapy. Major complications are soft-tissue ulceration, orocutaneous fistula, and osteoradionecrosis of mandible. Osteoradionecrosis may be affected by the proximity of growth, recent dental extractions, radiation dose, and integrity of mucous membrane.

**TABLE 7-13. SUGGESTED TARGET VOLUME DETERMINATION FOR ORAL CAVITY IMRT**

| Tumor Site | Clinical Presentation | CTV1 | CTV2 |
|---|---|---|---|
| Buccal | T1–2 N0 | P | IN (I–III) |
| RMT | T3–4 N+* | P + IN† (I–III) | CN (I–III) |
| | N2c | P + IN + CN† (I–V) | |
| Oral tongue | T1–2 N0 | P | IN ± CN (I–IV) |
| | T3–4 N+* | P + IN (I–IV) | CN (I–IV) |
| | N2c | P + IN + CN (I–V) | |
| FOM | T1–2 N0 | P | IN + CN (I–III) |
| | T3–4 N+* | P + IN (I–III) | CN (I–III) |
| | N2c | P + IN + CN (I–V) | |

*Source:* Modified from Chao KSC, Wippold FJ, Ozyigit G, et al. Determination and delineation of nodal target volumes for head and neck cancer based on the patterns of failure in patients receiving definitive and postoperative IMRT. *Int J Radiat Oncol Biol Phys* 2002;53:1174–1184.
CN, contralateral neck nodes; IN, ipsilateral neck nodes; P, gross tumor with margins for definition IMRT or surgical bed for postop IMRT.
*N, N1-3 except N2c.
†Level Ib only. Include Ia node when Ib node was involved.

Oral Cavity 97

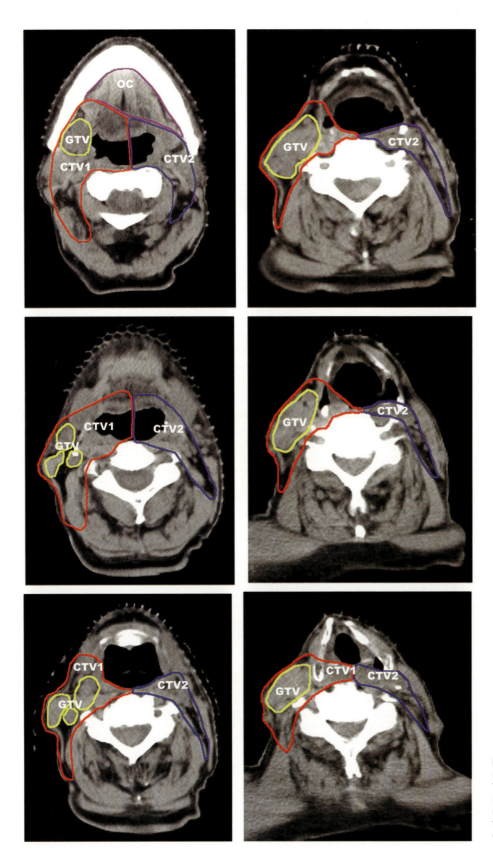

**FIGURE 7-10.** Clinical target volume (CTV) delineation in a patient with T3N2bM0 retromolar trigone carcinoma receiving definitive IMRT. CTV1, red line; CTV2, dark blue line; Gross tumor volume (GTV), yellow line; Oral cavity (OC), magenta line.

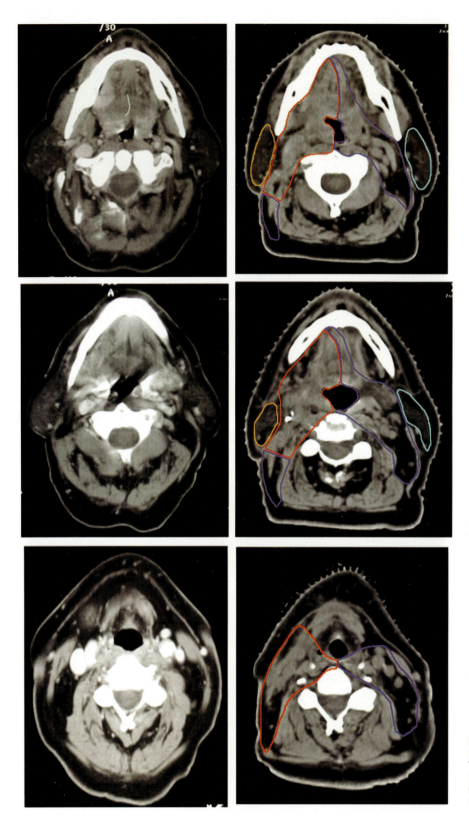

**FIGURE 7-11.** Clinical target volume (CTV) delineation in a patient with T2N2bM0 oral tongue carcinoma receiving postoperative IMRT. CTV1, red line; CTV2, dark blue line; right parotid gland, rust line; left parotid gland, aqua line.

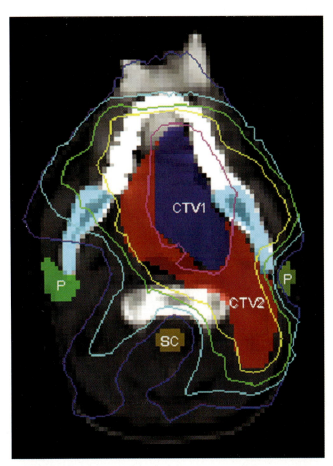

**FIGURE 7-12.** IMRT dose distribution of a patient with T2N0M0 oral tongue carcinoma receiving postoperative IMRT. CTV, clinical target volume; CTV1, dark blue area; CTV2, red area; P, parotid gland; SC, spinal cord. Pink line, 68 Gy; yellow line, 52 Gy; green line, 42 Gy; aqua line, 30 Gy; dark blue, 20 Gy.

## REFERENCES

1. Marks J, Lee F, Smith P, et al. Floor of mouth cancer: patient selection and treatment results. *Laryngoscope* 1983;93:475–480.
2. Million R, Cassisi N. Oral cavity. In: Million R, Cassisi N, eds. *Management of head and neck cancer: a multidisciplinary approach.* Philadelphia: JB Lippincott, 1984.
3. Rouviere H. *Anatomy of the human lymphatic system.* Ann Arbor, MI: Edwards Bros., 1938.
4. Lindberg R. Distribution of cervical lymph node metastases from squamous cell carcinoma of the upper respiratory and digestive tracts. *Cancer* 1972;29:1446–1448.
5. MacKay E, Sellers A. A statistical review of carcinoma of the lip. *Can Med Assoc J* 1964;90:670–672.
6. Emami B. Oral cavity. In: Perez C, Brady LW, eds. *Principles and practice of radiation oncology,* 3rd ed. Philadelphia: Lippincott-Raven, 1998:981–1002.
7. Campos J, Lampe I, Fayos J. Radiotherapy of carcinoma of the floor of the mouth. *Radiology* 1971;99:677–682.
8. Cady B, Catlin D. Epidermoid carcinoma of the gum: a 20-year survey. *Cancer* 1969;23:551–569.
9. Spiro R, Spiro J, Strong E. Surgical approach to squamous carcinoma confined to the tongue and the floor of the mouth. *Head Neck Surg* 1986;9:27–31.
10. Scholl P, Byers R, Batsakis J, et al. Microscopic cut-through of cancer in the surgical treatment of squamous carcinoma of the tongue: prognostic and therapeutic implications. *Am J Surg* 1986;152:354–360.
11. Chao K, Ozyigit G, Cengiz M, et al. Patterns of failure in patients receiving definitive and post-operative IMRT for head and neck cancer. *Int J Radiat Oncol Biol Phys* 2002 *(in press).*
12. Lindberg R. Distribution of cervical lymph node metastases from squamous cell carcinoma of the upper respiratory and digestive tracts. *Cancer* 1972;29:1446–1449.
13. Baker S, Krause C. Carcinoma of the lip. *Laryngoscope* 1980;90:19–27.
14. Petrovich Z, Parker R, Luxton G, et al. Carcinoma of the lip and selected sites of head and neck skin: a clinical study of 896 patients. *Radiother Oncol* 1987;8:11–17.
15. Wang C. *Radiation therapy for head and neck neoplasms: indications, techniques and results.* New York: Wiley, 1987.
16. De Visscher J, Grond S, Botke G, et al. Results of radiotherapy for squamous cell carcinoma of the vermilion border of the lower lip: a retrospective analysis of 108 patients. *Radiother Oncol* 1996;39:9–14.
17. Fitzpatrick P. Cancer of the lip. *J Otolaryngol* 1984;13:32–36.
18. MacComb W, Fletcher G. *Cancer of the head and neck.* In: Baltimore: Williams & Wilkins, 1967:179–212.
19. Mohs F, Snow S. Microscopically controlled surgical treatment for squamous cell carcinoma of the lower lip. *Surg Gynecol Obstet* 1985;160:37–41.
20. Bloom N, Spiro R. Carcinoma of the cheek mucosa: a retrospective analysis. *Am J Surg* 1980;140:556–560.
21. Urist M, O'Brien C, Soong S, et al. Squamous cell carcinoma of the buccal mucosa: analysis of prognostic factors. *Am J Surg* 1987;154:411–414.
22. Wang C. Radiation therapy for head and neck cancers. *Cancer* 1975;36:748.
23. Decroix Y, Ghossein N. Experience of the Curie Institute in treatment of cancer of the mobile tongue. *Cancer* 1981;47:496.
24. Gilbert E, Goffinet D, Bagshaw M. Carcinoma of the oral tongue and floor of mouth. *Cancer* 1975;35:1517–1524.
25. Rodgers L, Stringer S, Mendenhall W, et al. Management of squamous cell carcinoma of the floor of mouth. *Head Neck* 1993;15:16–19.
26. Fu K, Lichter A, Galante M. Carcinoma of the floor of mouth: an analysis of treatment results and the sites and causes of failures. *Int J Radiat Oncol Biol Phys* 1976;1:829–837.
27. Nason RW, Sako K, Beecroft WA, et al. Surgical management of squamous cell carcinoma of the floor of mouth. *Am J Surg* 1989;158:292–296.

# 8

# TONSILLAR FOSSA AND FAUCIAL ARCH

**K.S. CLIFFORD CHAO**
**GOKHAN OZYIGIT**

## 1. ANATOMY

- The oropharynx is the posterior continuation of the oral cavity; it communicates with the nasopharynx above and the laryngopharynx below. It can be subdivided into the palatine (faucial) arch and oropharynx proper (Fig. 8-1).
- The palatine arch, a junctional area between the oral cavity and the laryngopharynx, is formed by the soft palate and the uvula above, the anterior tonsillar pillar and glossopalatine sulcus laterally, and the glossopharyngeal sulcus and the base of the tongue inferiorly.
- Figure 8-2 shows the coronal section of oropharynx with relationships in the parapharyngeal regions.
- The retromolar trigone has been included in the structures of the faucial arch, although it is actually located within the oral cavity. Its apex is in line with the tuberosity of the maxilla (behind the last upper molar). The lateral border extends upward into the buccal mucosa. Medially, it blends with the anterior tonsillar pillar, its base formed by the distal surface of the last lower molar and the adjacent gingivolingual sulcus.[1]
- The lateral walls of the oropharynx are limited posteriorly by the tonsillar fossa and posterior tonsillar pillar (pharyngopalatine folds). These pillars are folds of mucous membrane that cover the underlying glossopalatine and pharyngopalatine muscles.[1] Deep to the lateral wall of the tonsillar fossa are the superior constrictor muscle of the pharynx, the upper fibers of the middle constrictor, the pharyngeus and stylopharyngeus muscles, and the glossopalatine and pharyngopalatine muscles. The tonsillar fossa continues into the lateral and posterior pharyngeal walls.
- The tonsillar fossa and faucial arch have a rich submucosal lymphatic network that is laterally grouped in four to six lymphatic ducts that drain into the subdigastric, upper cervical, and parapharyngeal lymph nodes. Submaxillary lymph nodes may be involved in lesions involving the retromolar trigone, buccal mucosa, or even base of the tongue.

## 2. NATURAL HISTORY

- Many are keratinizing squamous cell carcinomas, which can be graded I to IV, depending on degree of differentiation.
- Carcinomas arising in the faucial arch tend to be keratinizing and more differentiated than those of the tonsillar fossa.
- Lymphoepithelioma is much rarer in the tonsil (<1.5%) than in the nasopharynx.
- Malignant lymphomas, usually non-Hodgkin's type, constitute 10% to 15% of malignant tumors of the tonsil.
- Tumors of the salivary gland type are uncommon in the tonsil or faucial arch.
- Tonsillar fossa lesions tend to be infiltrative, often involving the adjacent retromolar trigone, soft palate, and base of the tongue. At Washington University in St. Louis, primary tumor was confined to the tonsillar fossa in only 5.4% of 384 patients; 65% had involvement of the soft palate, and 41% had extension into the base of the tongue (Fig. 8-3).[2]
- Tumors of the faucial arch can be superficially spreading, exophytic, ulcerative, or infiltrative; the last two types are frequently combined. They become extensive and involve the adjacent hard palate or buccal mucosa in fewer than 20% of patients.
- Mandibular involvement was noted in 14% of 110 patients with primary retromolar trigone carcinomas.[3]
- Tumors of the tonsillar fossa have a high incidence of lymph node metastases (60% to 70%). Most are in the subdigastric lymph nodes, midjugular chain, and submaxillary lymph nodes (in lesions extending anteriorly); 5% to 10% involve the posterior cervical lymph nodes (Fig. 8-4, Table 8-1).[2]
- Metastases in the low cervical chain occur in about 5% to 15% of patients with upper cervical lymph node involvement.
- The incidence of metastatic lymph nodes in the neck increases with tumor stage. Fewer than 10% of T1 lesions,

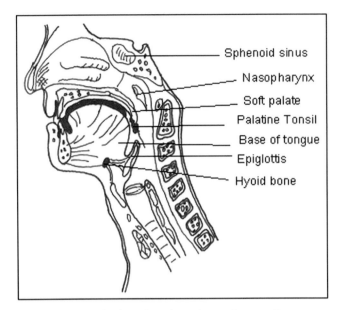

**FIGURE 8-1.** Sagittal section through oropharynx. Because no anatomic landmark demarcates oropharynx from laryngopharynx on the posterior pharyngeal wall, a line drawn from hyoid bone to the posterior wall may be used.

30% of T2 lesions, and 65% to 70% of T3 and T4 lesions have metastatic cervical lymph nodes (Fig. 8-5).[2]
- Contralateral lymphadenopathy in tonsillar tumors is noted in 10% to 15% of patients with positive ipsilateral lymph nodes, more frequently if the primary tumor extends to or beyond the midline (Table 8-2).
- Retromolar trigone, tonsillar pillar, and soft palate lesions have an overall metastatic rate of about 45%. Initially, the most frequent site of nodal involvement is the jugulodigastric lymph nodes. About 10% of patients have submaxillary lymph node involvement. Tumors of the retromolar trigone, anterior faucial pillar, and soft palate rarely metastasize to the posterior cervical lymph nodes. Contralateral spread is infrequent (10%) (Table 8-3).

## 3. DIAGNOSIS AND STAGING SYSTEM

### 3.1. Signs and Symptoms

- Sore throat is the most frequent symptom. Asymptomatic lesions are frequently found on routine examination.
- Difficulty in swallowing or pain in the ear is related to the anastomotic-tympanic nerve of Jacobson.
- Trismus may be a late manifestation if the masseter or pterygoid muscle is involved.
- Invasion of the tongue will eventually limit tongue mobility and, when there is a ulceration at the junction of the anterior tonsillar pillar and oral tongue, causes a great deal of pain.
- Tumors of the tonsillar fossa have similar signs and symptoms except that the lesions tend to be larger before symptoms develop. Ipsilateral sore throat and ear pain are the hallmark of the lesions.
- Lymphomas of the tonsil tend to be large submucosal masses but may ulcerate and appear similar to carcinomas.

### 3.2. Physical Examination

- Indirect mirror examination and digital palpation are needed for diagnosis.
- In addition to a complete history and physical examination, a complete examination of the head and neck is mandatory (Table 8-4).

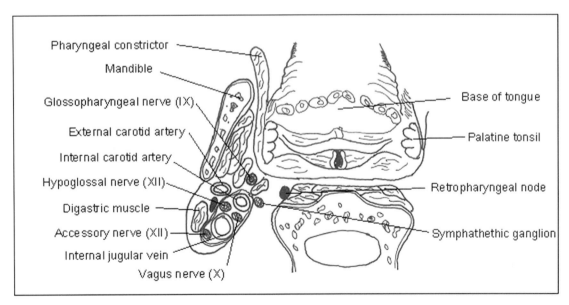

**FIGURE 8-2.** A coronal section of oropharynx showing relationships in the parapharyngeal regions.

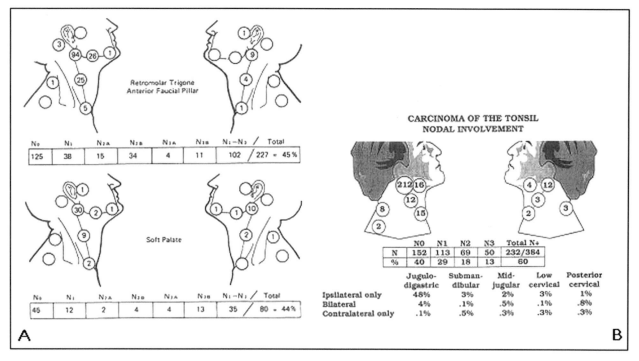

**FIGURE 8-3.** Nodal distribution on admission of patients with carcinoma of faucial arch (**A**) and tonsil (**B**). (**A**, From Lindberg RD: Distribution of cervical lymph node metastasis from squamous cell carcinoma of the upper respiratory and digestive tracts. *Cancer* 29:1466–1449, 1972, by permission. **B**, Unpublished data, Washington University.)

### 3.3. Imaging

- Imaging of the oropharyngeal region is described with all details in Chapter 9.

### 3.4. Staging

- Table 8-5 shows the American Joint Committee staging classification for carcinoma of the oropharynx, including lymph node involvement.

### 4. PROGNOSTIC FACTORS

- *Epidemiologic factors:* Gender may play a role in outcome. But in most of the studies it has no effect on outcome.
- *Stage:* Stage of primary tumor and presence of involved cervical lymph nodes have a significant correlation with local control and 5-year survival.[4-6]
- *Base-of-tongue invasion:* Tumor extension into the base of the tongue is associated with decreased survival.
- *Age:* Age at the time of diagnosis had no effect on survival in several studies.

### 5. GENERAL MANAGEMENT

- Tables 8-6 and 8-7 show the initial local control rates for carcinoma of the tonsil according to T stages with different treatment strategies.
- Table 8-8 summarizes the disease-specific survival of patients with carcinoma of the tonsil.

**TABLE 8-1. INCIDENCE AND DISTRIBUTION OF METASTATIC DISEASE IN NEGATIVE (N−) AND POSITIVE (N+) NECK NODES (IN PERCENTAGE)**

| | Radiologically Enlarged Retropharyngeal Nodes | | Pathologic Nodal Metastasis | | | | | | | | |
|---|---|---|---|---|---|---|---|---|---|---|---|
| | | | Level I | | Level II | | Level III | | Level IV | | Level V | |
| Clinical presentation | N− | N+ | N− | N+ | N− | N+ | N− | N+ | N− | N+ | N− | N+ |
| Tonsil | 4 | 0 | 19 | 14 | 9 | 5 | 4 | 0 | 19 | 14 | 9 | 5 |
| MIR data | 4 | 12 | 8 | 19 | 19 | 74 | 14 | 31 | 9 | 14 | 5 | 12 |

*Source:* Modified from Chao KSC, Wippold FJ, Ozyigit G, et al. Determination and delineation of nodal target volumes for head and neck cancer based on the patterns of failure in patients receiving definitive and postoperative IMRT. *Int J Radiat Oncol Biol Phys* 2002;53:1174–1184.

## 5.1. Tumors of the Tonsil

- T1 or T2 lesions can be treated with irradiation or surgery alone.
- T1, T2, and T3 tumors are treated with irradiation alone (60 to 75 Gy in 6 to 8 weeks, depending on stage); regional lymph nodes are treated with 50 Gy (subclinical disease) to 75 Gy, depending on nodal involvement (8,9,17). Interstitial brachytherapy has been used to deliver additional dose (25 to 30 Gy) to the primary tumor.[7]
- In T3 and T4 tumors, a combination of irradiation and surgery has been advocated because of the higher incidence of recurrences with either modality alone.[5,6,8] These lesions are treated with radical tonsillectomy with ipsilateral neck dissection followed by irradiation (50 to 60 Gy), depending on the status of the surgical margins and extent of cervical lymph node involvement.[9]

## 5.2. Tumors of Faucial Arch

- T1 lesions less than 1 cm in diameter are treated with wide surgical resection or irradiation alone (60 to 65 Gy in 6 to 7 weeks).[10–12]
- T2 tumors require more extensive surgical procedures, including partial resection of the mandible if there is bone involvement.[13] Because of the tendency of these tumors to extend to the midline, the site of lymph node metastasis is less predictable; therefore neck dissection should be done only in patients with palpable cervical lymph nodes.
- T2 tumors can also be treated with irradiation alone (65 to 70 Gy); irradiation has the advantage of treating subclinical disease in the neck (50 Gy total dose).[10,11,14–16]

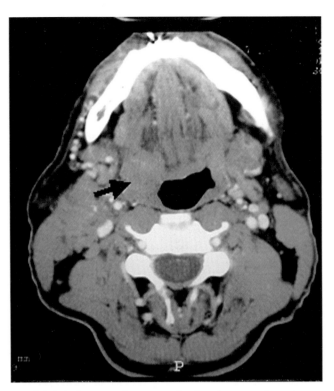

**FIGURE 8-4.** Computed tomography showing a tonsil carcinoma originating from right tonsil (*arrow*).

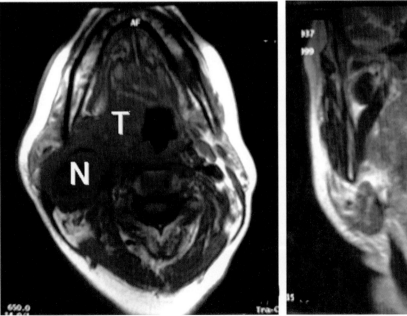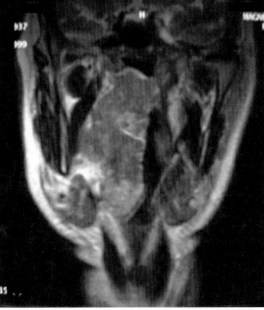

**FIGURE 8-5.** Axial and coronal MRI sections of a patient with a T3N2b tonsil squamous cell carcinoma. (T, tumor; N, metastatic lymph node.)

# Intensity Modulated Radiation Therapy for Head and Neck Cancer

## TABLE 8-2. INCIDENCE OF CONTRALATERAL OR BILATERAL NECK NODE METASTASES BY PRIMARY TUMOR SITE

| Tumor Site | cN+, Bilateral | cN+, Contralateral Only | cN–, pN+ Bilateral |
|---|---|---|---|
| Tonsil | 16% | 2% | — |

c, clinical; p, pathologic.
*Source:* Modified from Chao KSC, Wippold FJ, Ozyigit G, et al. Determination and delineation of nodal target volumes for head and neck cancer based on the patterns of failure in patients receiving definitive and postoperative IMRT. *Int J Radiat Oncol Biol Phys* 2002 *(in press).*

- Interstitial brachytherapy (20 to 30 Gy) in the primary tumor has been combined with external irradiation (50 Gy) (7,22).
- In more extensive lesions, preoperative or postoperative irradiation can be used in doses similar to those used in the tonsil.

## 5.3. Chemotherapy

- We prefer platinum-based chemotherapy given concurrently with radiation in locally advanced tonsillar carcinoma.
- Drugs of choice include cisplatin. Weekly carboplatinum and Taxol have been used in our institution since 1999 with good tumor response.
- Some reports describe complete response in 40% of patients given three cycles of chemotherapy before irradiation or surgery and an additional 30% partial response, for an overall response rate of 75% or higher. Disease-free survival has been prolonged by a few months, but after 3 years no enhancement of overall survival has been demonstrated.
- The potential benefit of adjuvant chemotherapy combined with irradiation or surgery in the treatment of these advanced lesions should be further evaluated.
- Agents that selectively enhance the effects of irradiation

## TABLE 8-4. DIAGNOSTIC WORK-UP FOR MALIGNANT TUMORS OF THE TONSIL AND FAUCIAL ARCH

General
  History, with emphasis on alcohol intake, smoking, tobacco chewing
  General physical examination

Head and neck examination
  Oral cavity, oropharynx (palpation is very important)
  Nasopharynx (mirror examination)
  Laryngopharynx (indirect laryngoscopy)
  Examination of the neck for lymph nodes
  Direct laryngoscopy
  Biopsy of tumor and any suspicious areas

Laboratory studies
  Complete blood count
  Blood chemistry profile
  Urinalysis

Radiographic studies
  Chest x-ray
  Plain radiographs of neck or mandible (as clinically indicated)
  Computed tomography (or magnetic resonance) scans
  Radionuclide bone scan (optional, as indicated)

Special studies (for malignant lymphoma)
  Immunologic typing of tumor
  Electron microscopy
  Special staging procedures

in the tumor are under investigation, such as hypoxic cell sensitizers, chemical modifiers, hyperthermia, and high linear energy transfer irradiation.

## 6. INTENSITY MODULATED RADIATION THERAPY IN TONSILLAR FOSSA AND FAUCIAL ARCH CARCINOMA

### 6.1. Target Volume Determination

- Target volume determination is an innovative modality that can be very useful in the treatment of oropharyngeal cancer.[17]

## TABLE 8-3. T- AND N-STAGE DISTRIBUTION OF TONSILLAR CARCINOMA PATIENTS AT INITIAL PRESENTATION

| Author | T1 | T2 | T3 | T4 | N0 | N1 | N2 | N3 |
|---|---|---|---|---|---|---|---|---|
| Galati et al.[20] | 24 | 34 | 37 | 12 | 51 | 25 | 20 | 11 |
| Withers et al.[21*] | 97 | 260 | 256 | 63 | 272 | 144 | 141 | 67 |
| O'Sullivan et al.[22] | 73 | 118 | 30 | 7 | 133 | 56 | 36 | 3 |
| Mendenhall et al.[23] | 56 | 150 | 126 | 68 | 137 | 56 | 170 | 37 |
| Kagei et al.[24] | 6 | 12 | 12 | 2 | 22 | 5 | 4 | 1 |
| Jackson et al.[25] | 43 | 94 | 85 | 28 | 101 | 54 | 7 | 16 |
| Gwozdz et al.[26] | 5 | 29 | 41 | 4 | 26 | 13 | 31 | 12 |
| Perez et al.[6] | 46 | 131 | 138 | 69 | 152 | 113 | 69 | 50 |
| Total | 350 (16%) | 828 (38%) | 725 (34%) | 253 (12%) | 894 (42%) | 579 (27%) | 478 (22%) | 197 (9%) |

*Data of nine institutions (Princess Margeret, Massachusetts, General, MD Anderson, Christie, Clatterbridge, University of Florida, Royal Marsden, Mt. Vernon, Portsmouth).

*Tonsillar Fossa and Faucial Arch* **105**

## TABLE 8-5. TNM CLASSIFICATION FOR CARCINOMA OF THE OROPHARYNX

*Primary Tumor (T)*

| | |
|---|---|
| TX | Primary tumor cannot be assessed |
| T0 | No evidence of primary tumor |
| Tis | Carcinoma *in situ* |
| T1 | Tumor <2 cm in greatest dimension |
| T2 | Tumor >2 cm but not >4 cm in greatest dimension |
| T3 | Tumor >4 cm in greatest dimension |
| T4 | Tumor invades adjacent structures (pterygoid muscle[s], mandible, hard palate, deep muscle of tongue, larynx) |

*Regional Lymph Nodes (N)*

| | |
|---|---|
| NX | Regional lymph nodes cannot be assessed |
| N0 | No regional lymph node metastasis |
| N1 | Metastasis in a single ipsilateral lymph node, <3 cm in greatest dimension |
| N2 | Metastasis in a single ipsilateral lymph node, >3 cm but not >6 cm in greatest dimension; in multiple ipsilateral lymph nodes, none >6 cm in greatest dimension; or in bilateral or contralateral lymph nodes, none >6 cm in greatest dimension |
| N2a | Metastasis in a single ipsilateral lymph node >3 cm but not >6 cm in greatest dimension |
| N2b | Metastasis in multiple ipsilateral lymph nodes, none >6 cm in greatest dimension |
| N2c | Metastasis in bilateral or contralateral lymph nodes, none >6 cm in greatest dimension |
| N3 | Metastasis in a lymph node >6 cm in greatest dimension |

*Distant Metastases (M)*

| | |
|---|---|
| MX | Presence of distant metastasis cannot be assessed |
| M0 | No distant metastasis |
| M1 | Distant metastasis |

*Stage Grouping*

| | | | |
|---|---|---|---|
| Stage 0 | Tis | N0 | M0 |
| Stage I | T1 | N0 | M0 |
| Stage II | T2 | N0 | M0 |
| Stage III | T3 | N0 | M0 |
| | T1 | N1 | M0 |
| | T2 | N1 | M0 |
| | T3 | N1 | M0 |
| Stage IV A | T4 | N0 or N1 | M0 |
| | Any T | N2 | M0 |
| Stage IV B | Any T | N3 | M0 |
| Stage IV C | Any T | Any N | M1 |

*Source:* Fleming ID, Cooper JS, Henson DE, et al., eds. *AJCC cancer staging manual*, 5th ed. Philadelphia: Lippincott-Raven, 1997:37–39, by permission.

## TABLE 8-6. CARCINOMA OF THE TONSIL: INITIAL LOCAL CONTROL ACCORDING TO T STAGES WITH IRRADIATION ALONE

| | Stage | | | | | | | |
|---|---|---|---|---|---|---|---|---|
| | T1 | | T2 | | T3 | | T4 | |
| Author | No. | % | No. | % | No. | % | No. | % |
| Amornmarn et al.[36] | 4/4 | 100 | 7/8 | 88 | 21/38 | 55 | 5/20 | 25 |
| Bataini et al.[4] | 32/36 | 89 | 78/93 | 84 | 111/173 | 64 | 77/163 | 47 |
| Dubois et al.[27] | 34/49 | 69 | 39/84 | 46 | 7/82 | 9 | — | — |
| Fayos et al.[28] | 8/10 | 80 | 36/47 | 77 | 12/31 | 39 | 4/14 | 29 |
| Lusinchi et al.[29] | 42/48 | 88 | 114/145 | 79 | — | — | — | — |
| Mantravadi et al.[30] | 3/3 | 100 | 16/21 | 76 | 20/61 | 33 | 1/9 | 11 |
| Mendenhall et al.[15] | 4/4 | 100 | 17/18 | 94 | 23/31 | 74 | 5/12 | 42 |
| Million et al.[16] | 11/13 | 85 | 18/23 | 78 | 6/13 | 46 | 1/4 | 25 |
| Mizono et al.[31] | 5/10 | 50 | 25/41 | 61 | 17/55 | 31 | 3/25 | 12 |
| Wong et al.[32] | 15/16 | 94 | 41/52 | 79 | 30/52 | 58 | 3/6 | 50 |
| Fein et al.[33] | 20/23 | 87 | 69/87 | 79 | 45/63 | 71 | 12/27 | 44 |
| Perez et al.[34] | 14/16 | 87 | 26/41 | 63 | 31/41 | 76 | 19/36 | 53 |
| Total | 192/233 | 82 | 486/660 | 74 | 223/640 | 35 | 130/316 | 41 |

Number of patients observed is in parentheses.

## TABLE 8-7. CARCINOMA OF THE TONSIL: LOCAL CONTROL ACCORDING TO T STAGES

| | | | Local Control Rates (%) | | | | |
| --- | --- | --- | --- | --- | --- | --- | --- |
| | Treatment | No. of Patients | T1 | T2 | T3 | T4 | Overall |
| Perez et al.[34] | Sx+RT | 230 | 80 | 71 | 65 | 58 | 68 |
| Foote et al.[8] | Sx+/–RT | 72 | 78 | 76 | 44 | — | 71 |
| Pernot et al.[35] | RT–Ir192 | 361 | 89 | 85 | 67 | — | 80 |
| Bataini et al.[4] | RT | 465 | 90 | 84 | 64 | 47 | 64 |
| Wong et al.[32] | RT | 150 | 94 | 81 | 67 | 63 | 75 |
| Perez et al.[34] | RT | 154 | 76 | 63 | 59 | 33 | 56 |
| Amornmarn et al.[36] | RT | 185 | 94 | 80 | 51 | 19 | 58 |
| Mendenhall et al.[15] | RT | 400 | 83 | 81 | 74 | 60 | 76 |

RT, radiotherapy; Sx, surgery.

## TABLE 8-8. TONSIL CARCINOMA: DISEASE-SPECIFIC SURVIVAL RATES

| | Treatment | No. of Patients | % with Stage IV Disease | 5-Year Cause-Specific Survival Rate |
| --- | --- | --- | --- | --- |
| Givens et al.[5] | Surgery + RT | 22 | 68 | 32 |
| Pernot et al.[35] | RT-Ir192 | 361 | 8 | 63 |
| Wong et al.[32] | RT | 150 | — | 70 |
| Gwozdz et al.[26] | RT | 83 | 53 | 71 |
| Garrett et al.[37] | RT | 372 | 54 | 54 |
| Amornmarn et al.[36] | RT | 185 | 46 | 42 |
| Mendenhall et al.[15] | RT | 400 | 56 | 70 |

## TABLE 8-9. TARGET VOLUME SPECIFICATION FOR DEFINITIVE AND POSTOPERATIVE IMRT IN TONSIL CANCER

| Target | Definitive IMRT | High-Risk Postoperative IMRT | Intermediate-Risk Postoperative IMRT |
| --- | --- | --- | --- |
| CTVI | Gross tumor and the adjacent soft tissue/nodal regions | Surgical bed with soft-tissue involvement or nodal region with extracapsular extension | Surgical bed without soft-tissue involvement or nodal region without capsular extension |
| CTV2 | Elective nodal regions (I, II, III, IV, V)* | Elective nodal regions (I, II, III, IV, V)* | Elective nodal regions (I, II, III, IV, V)* |

*Source:* Modified from Chao KSC, Wippold FJ, Ozyigit G, et al. Determination and delineation of nodal target volumes for head and neck cancer based on the patterns of failure in patients receiving definitive and postoperative IMRT. *Int J Radiat Oncol Biol Phys* 2002;53:1174–1184.
*N0 include level II, III, IV and retropharyngeal nodes. N1 include level Ib, II, III, IV and retropharyngeal nodes. N2–3 include level Ib, II, III, IV, V and retropharyngeal nodes.

## TABLE 8-10. SUGGESTED TARGET VOLUME DETERMINATION FOR TONSIL CARCINOMA IMRT

| Clinical Presentation | CTV1 | CTV2 |
| --- | --- | --- |
| T1–2 N0 | P | IN ± CN (I–IV, RPLN) |
| T3–4N+* | P + IN (I†–V, RPLN) | CN (II–IV, RPLN) |
| N2c | P + IN + CN (I†–V, RPLN) | |

*Source:* Modified from Chao KSC, Wippold FJ, Ozyigit G, et al. Determination and delineation of nodal target volumes for head and neck cancer based on the patterns of failure in patients receiving definitive and postoperative IMRT. *Int J Radiat Oncol Biol Phys* 2002;53:1174–1184.
CN, contralateral neck nodes; IN, ipsilateral neck nodes; P, gross tumor with margins for definition IMRT or surgical bed for postop IMRT; RPLN, retropharyngeal lymph nodes.
*N*= N1–3 except N2c.
†Ib only. Level Ia should be included when Ib node was involved.

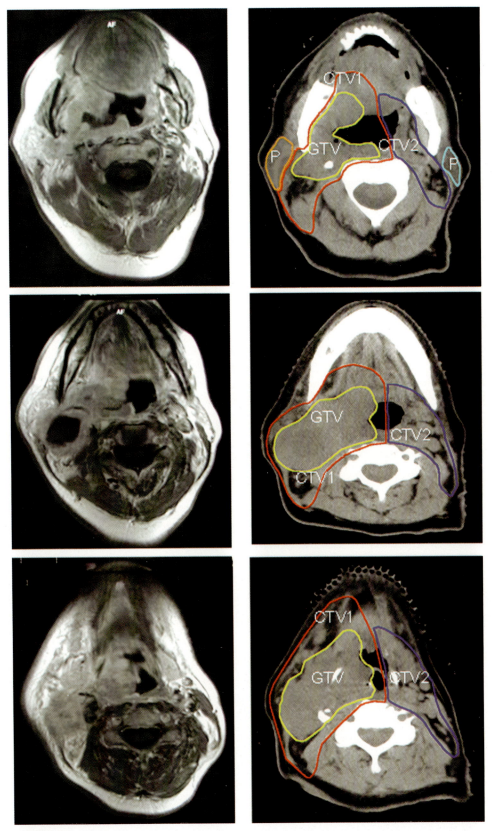

**FIGURE 8-6.** Clinical target volume (CTV) delineation of a T3N2b tonsil carcinoma patient receiving definitive IMRT. CTV, clinical target volume; CTV1, red line; CTV2, dark blue line; P, parotid gland; right parotid gland, rust line; left parotid gland, aqua line.

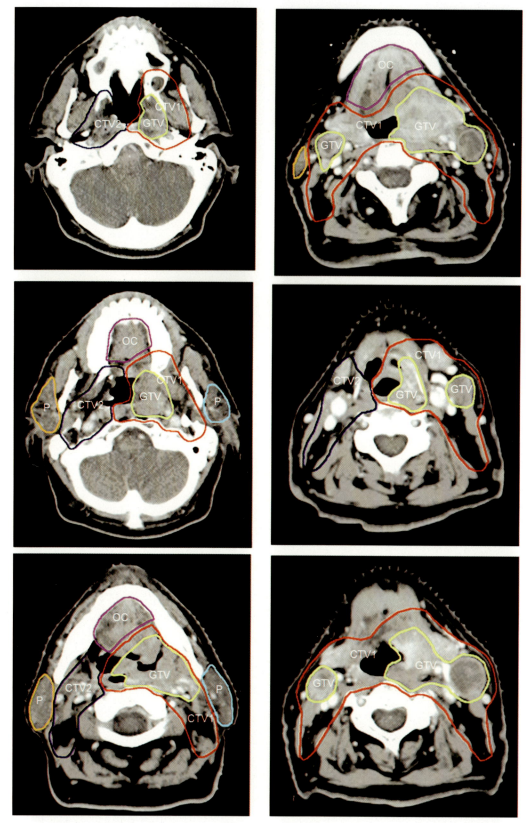

**FIGURE 8-7.** Clinical target volume (CTV) delineation of a T4N2c tonsil carcinoma patient receiving definitive IMRT. CTV1, red line; CTV2, dark blue line; P, parotid gland; right parotid gland, rust line; left parotid gland, aqua line; oral cavity (OC), magenta line.

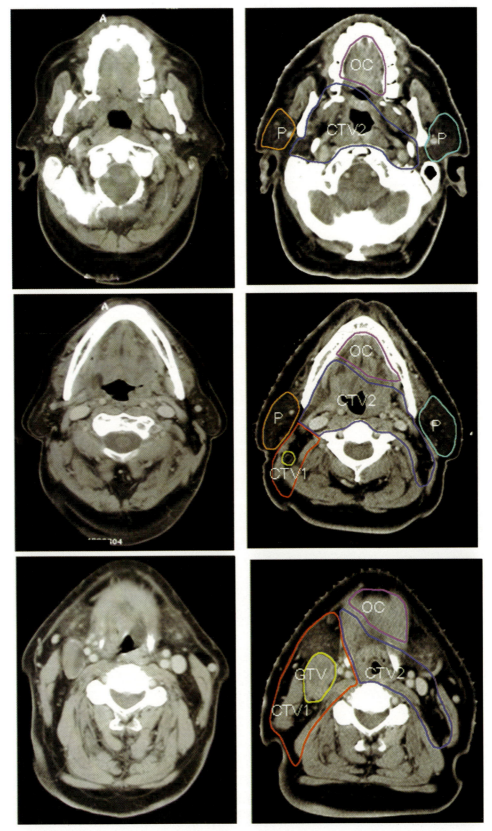

**FIGURE 8-8.** Clinical target volume (CTV) delineation of a T2N2b tonsil carcinoma patient receiving postoperative IMRT. CTV1, red line; CTV2, dark blue line; P, parotid gland; right parotid gland, rust line; left parotid gland, aqua line; oral cavity (OC), magenta line.

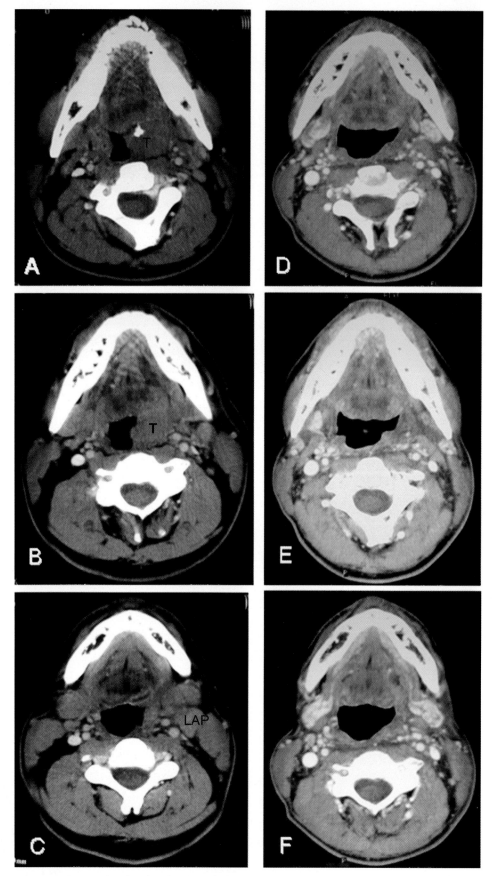

**FIGURE 8-9.** Pre-IMRT (**A–C**) and post-IMRT (**D–F**) CT sections of a patient with T2N2b tonsil carcinoma showing complete regression of the tumor after a total IMRT dose of 70 Gy (T, tumor; LAP, lymphadenopathy.)

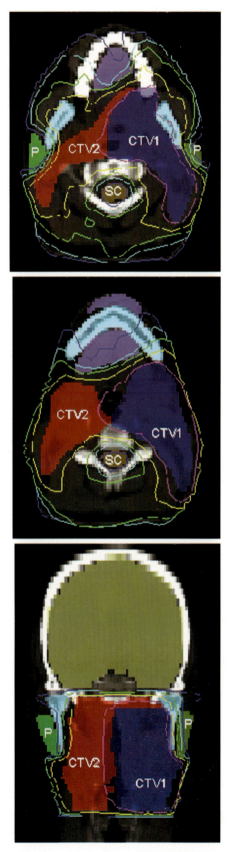

**FIGURE 8-10.** IMRT dose distribution of a patient with T2N2b definitive tonsillar carcinoma. CTV, clinical target volume; CTV1, dark blue area; CTV2, red area; P, parotid gland; SC, spinal cord. Pink line, 70 Gy; yellow line, 50 Gy; green line, 40 Gy; aqua line, 30 Gy; dark blue, 20 Gy.

- The primary tumor and palpable lymph nodes are treated to 70 Gy tumor dose, calculated to the 85% to 90% isodose.
- Daily dose is 2 Gy to CTV1.
- Nonpalpable lymph nodes simultaneously receive about 1.6 Gy daily to a total prescribed dose of 54 Gy.
- Gross tumor volume for tonsil carcinoma is the volume seen on CT or MRI.
- If chemotherapy was delivered before radiation, the targets should be outlined on the planning CT according to their prechemotherapy extent.
- Lymph node groups at risk in the tonsillar fossa region include the following:
  a. Submandibular nodes (surgical level I): all cases
  b. Upper deep jugular (junctional, parapharyngeal) nodes: all cases
  c. Subdigastric (jugulodigastric) nodes, midjugular, lower neck, and supraclavicular nodes (levels II through IV): all cases
  d. Posterior cervical nodes (level V): when level II/III involved
  e. Retropharyngeal nodes: all cases
- Table 8-9 summarizes the target volume specification for definitive and postoperative IMRT in tonsil cancer.
- Table 8-10 shows suggested target volume determination for tonsil carcinoma.

## 6.2. Target Volume Delineation

- Figure 8-6 shows CTV1 and CTV2 delineation in a patient with clinically T3N2bM0 squamous cell carcinoma of tonsil receiving definitive IMRT.
- Figure 8-7 shows CTV1 and CTV2 delineation in a patient with clinically T4N2cM0 squamous cell carcinoma of tonsil receiving definitive IMRT.
- Figure 8-8 shows CTV1 and CTV2 delineation in a patient with clinically T2N2b squamous cell carcinoma of tonsil receiving postoperative IMRT.

## 6.3. Normal Tissue Delineation

- See Chapter 5 for normal tissue delineation (Fig. 5-16).

## 6.4. Suggested Target and Normal Tissue Doses

- See Chapter 4 for suggested target and normal tissue doses (Table 4-9).

## 6.5. IMRT Treatment Results

- Following these guidelines, 42 tonsil carcinoma patients were treated with IMRT between February 1997 and December 2000 at Washington University. Twenty-two patients were treated postoperatively and 20 patients were treated with definitive IMRT. The T stages were 10 T1, 14 T2, eight T3, and 10 T4. The N stages were five N0, 12 N1, 23 N2, and two N3 (AJCC staging; 13 stage III and 29 stage IV). Median follow-up time was 23 months (9 to 51 months). We observed five locoregional recurrences; two of them were salvaged with surgery. Distant metastasis developed in four patients. Three patients died of either recurrent disease or distant metastasis; one patient died of intercurrent disease.
- Figure 8-9 shows pre- and posttreatment CT slices of a patient with T2N2bM0 tonsil cancer receiving definitive IMRT. Figure 8-10 shows IMRT dose distribution for the same patient.
- A G-tube was placed in eight patients during the course of IMRT. We observed no grade 3 or 4 late complications in our patients treated with IMRT. Five grade 2 and 16 grade 1 late xerostomia were observed. Trismus was seen in one patient after radiotherapy, and chronic serous otitis media developed in another patient as late sequelae. Decreased hearing was observed in three patients after IMRT.

## 7. SEQUELAE OF TREATMENT

- Xerostomia (moderate to severe) occurs in approximately 75% of patients treated with conventional beam arrangement. IMRT can significantly reduce this complication rate to 25%.[18]
- Oropharyngeal mucositis and moderate to severe dysphagia are the most common acute irradiation sequelae.
- Laryngeal edema, fibrosis, hearing loss, and trismus occasionally occur.
- The incidence of necrosis of the mandible depends on stage of tumor, irradiation dose delivered to the mandible, use of prophylactic dental care, trauma (including dental extractions), and irradiation technique, and is about 6% when the tumor is over or adjacent to the mandible and 0 when it is not.[2] Severe necrosis requiring mandibulectomy was reported in 6 of 88 patients (6.8%) with T1 and T2 carcinomas of the tonsillar fossa and 13 of 88 (14.8%) with T3 and T4 tumors[19]; the incidence of bone exposure was 29.5% and 45.4%, respectively. The incidence of osteonecrosis was higher with single homolateral fields, unilateral wedge filter arrangements, or a combination of external irradiation and interstitial implants.
- Carotid artery rupture occurs in up to 3% of patients treated with surgery for irradiation failure.

## REFERENCES

1. MacComb W, Fletcher G. *Cancer of the head and neck.* In: Baltimore: Williams & Wilkins, 1967:179–212.

2. Perez C. Tonsillar fossa and faucial arch. In: Brady L, editor. *Principles and practice of radiation oncology.* Philadelphia: Lippincott-Raven, 1998:1003–1032.

3. Byers R, Anderson B, Schwarz E, et al. Treatment of squamous carcinoma of the retromolar trigone. *Am J Clin Oncol (CCT)* 1984;7:647–652.

4. Bataini J, Asselain B, Jaulerry C, et al. A multivariate primary tumour control analysis in 465 patients treated by radical radiotherapy for cancer of the tonsillar region: clinical and treatment parameters as prognostic factors. *Radiother Oncol* 1989;14:265–277.

5. Givens CJ, Johns M, Cantrell R. Carcinoma of the tonsil: analysis of 162 cases. *Arch Otolaryngol* 1981;107:730–734.

6. Perez C, Patel M, Chao K, et al. Carcinoma of the tonsillar fossa: prognostic factors and long-term therapy outcome. *Int J Radiat Oncol Biol Phys* 1998;42:1077–1084.

7. Behar R, Martin P, Fee WJ, et al. Iridium-192 interstitial implant and external beam radiation therapy in the management of squamous cell carcinoma of the tonsil and soft palate. *Int J Radiat Oncol Biol Phys* 1994;28:221–227.

8. Foote R, Schild S, Thompson W, et al. Tonsil cancer: patterns of failure after surgery alone and surgery combined with postoperative radiation therapy. *Cancer* 1994;73:2638–2647.

9. Kramer S, Gelber R, Snow J, et al. Combined radiation therapy and surgery in the management of advanced head and neck cancer: final report of study 73-03 of the Radiation Therapy Oncology Group. *Head Neck Surg* 1987;10:19–30.

10. Horton D, Tran L, Greenberg P, et al. Primary radiation therapy in the treatment of squamous cell carcinoma of the soft palate. *Cancer* 1989;63:2442–2445.

11. Keus R, Pontvert D, Brunin F, et al. Results of irradiation in squamous cell carcinoma of the soft palate and uvula. *Radiother Oncol* 1988;11:311–317.

12. Lo K, Fletcher GH, Byers RM, et al. Results of irradiation in the squamous cell carcinomas of the anterior faucial pillar-retromolar trigone. *Int J Rad Oncol Biol Phys* 1987;113:969–974.

13. Leemans C, Engelbrecht W, Tiwari R, et al. Carcinoma of the soft palate and anterior tonsillar pillar. *Laryngoscope* 1984;104:1477–1481.

14. Barker J, Fletcher G. Time, dose, tumor volume relationships in megavoltage irradiation of squamous cell carcinomas of the RMT and AFP. *Int J Radiat Oncol Biol Phys* 1977;2:407–414.

15. Mendenhall W, Parsons J, Cassisi N, et al. Squamous cell carcinoma of the tonsillar area treated with radical irradiation. *Radiother Oncol* 1987;10:23–30.

16. Million R, Cassisi N, Mancuso A. Oropharynx. In: Cassisi N, ed. *Management of head and neck cancer: a multidisciplinary approach,* 2nd ed. Philadelphia: JB Lippincott, 1994:401–429.

17. Chao KSC, Low D, Perez CA, et al. Intensity modulated radiation therapy in head and neck cancers: the Mallinckrodt experience. *Int J Cancer* 2000;90:92–103.

18. Chao KSC, Deasy JO, Markman J, et al. A prospective study of salivary function sparing in patients with head and neck cancers receiving intensity-modulated or three-dimensional radiation therapy: initial results. *Int J Radiat Oncol Biol Phys* 2001;49:907–916.

19. Grant B, Fletcher G. Analysis of complications following megavoltage therapy for squamous cell carcinomas of the tonsillar area. *Am J Roentgenol* 1966;96:27–36.

20. Galati L, Myers E, Johnson J. Primary surgery as treatment for early squamous cell carcinoma of the tonsil. *Head Neck* 2000;22:294–296.

21. Withers H, Peters L, Taylor J, et al. Local control of carcinoma of the tonsil by radiation therapy: an analysis of patterns of fractionation in nine institutions. *Int J Radiat Oncol Biol Phys* 1995;33:549–562.

22. O'Sullivan B, Warde P, Grice B, et al. The benefits and pitfalls of ipsilateral radiotherapy in carcinoma of the tonsillar region. *Head Neck* 2001;51:332–343.

23. Mendenhall W, Amdur R, Stringer S, et al. Radiation therapy for squamous cell carcinoma of the tonsillar region: a preferred alternative to surgery? *J Clin Oncol* 2000;11:2219–2225.

24. Kagei K, Shirato H, Nishioka T, et al. Ipsilateral irradiation for carcinomas of tonsillar region and soft palate based on computed tomographic simulation. *Radiother Oncol* 2000;54:117–121.

25. Jackson S, Hay J, Flores A, et al. Cancer of the tonsil: the results of ipsilateral radiation treatment. *Radiother Oncol* 1999;51:123–128.

26. Gwozdz J, Morrison W, Garden A, et al. Concomitant boost radiotherapy for squamous carcinoma of the tonsillar fossa. *Int J Radiat Oncol Biol Phys* 1997;39:127–135.

27. Dubois J, Broquerie J, Delard R, et al. Analysis of the results of irradiation in the treatment of tonsillar region carcinomas. *Int J Radiat Oncol Biol Phys* 1983;9:1195–1203.

28. Fayos J, Lampe I. Radiation therapy of carcinoma of the tonsillar region. *Am J Roentgenol* 1971;111:85–94.

29. Lusinchi A, Wibault P, Marandas P, et al. Exclusive radiation therapy: the treatment of early tonsillar tumors. *Int J Radiat Oncol Biol Phys* 1989;17:273–277.

30. Mantravadi R, Liebner E, Ginde J. An analysis of factors in the successful management of cancer of the tonsillar region. *Cancer* 1978;41:1054–1058.

31. Mizono G, Diaz R, Fu K, et al. Carcinoma of the tonsillar region. *Laryngoscope* 1986;96:240–244.

32. Wong C, Ang K, Fletcher G, et al. Definitive radiotherapy for squamous cell carcinoma of the tonsillar fossa. *Int J Radiat Oncol Biol Phys* 1989;16:657–662.

33. Fein D, Lee W, Amos W, et al. Oropharyngeal carcinoma treated with radiotherapy: a 30-year experience. *Int J Radiat Oncol Biol Phys* 1996;34:289–296.

34. Perez C, Carmichael T, Devineni V, et al. Carcinoma of the tonsillar fossa—a nonrandomized comparison of irradiation alone or combined with surgery: long-term results. *Head Neck* 1991;13:282–290.

35. Pernot M, Malissard L, Hoffstetter S, et al. Influence of tumoral, radiobiological, and general factors on local control and survival of a series of 361 tumors of the velotonsillar area treated by exclusive irradiation (external beam irradiation-brachytherapy or brachytherapy alone. *Int J Radiat Oncol Biol Phys* 1994;30:1051–1057.

36. Amornmarn R, Prempree T, Jaiwatana J, et al. Radiation management of carcinoma of the tonsillar region. *Cancer* 1984;54:1293–1299.

37. Garrett P, Beale F, Cummings B, et al. Carcinoma of the tonsil: the effect of dose-time-volume factors on local control. *Int J Radiat Oncol Biol Phys* 1985;11:703–706.

# 9

# BASE OF THE TONGUE

**K.S. CLIFFORD CHAO**
**GOKHAN OZYIGIT**

## 1. ANATOMY

- The base of the tongue (BOT) is bounded anteriorly by the circumvallate papillae, laterally by the glossopharyngeal sulci and oropharyngeal walls, and inferiorly by the glossoepiglottic fossae or valleculae and the pharyngoepiglottic fold (Fig. 9-1).
- The vallecula is the transition zone between the base of tongue and the epiglottis, and is considered as part of the base of the tongue.
- The surface of the tongue is irregular because of submucosal lymphoid follicles, but the mucous membrane is smooth when compared with the dorsum of the oral tongue. The lymphoid tissue at the base of the tongue does not penetrate the intrinsic tongue muscles.
- The base of the tongue is almost parallel to the posterior pharyngeal wall. Its musculature is continuous with that of the oral tongue and the floor of the mouth anteriorly. The genioglossus fibers fan out in the tongue and finally interdigitate with the intrinsic tongue musculature (Fig. 9-2). The tongue base also is continuous with the preepiglottic space.[1]

## 2. NATURAL HISTORY

- Squamous cell carcinoma of the base of the tongue tends to have early, silent, and deep infiltration; therefore it is difficult to estimate the tumor extension by clinical examination. But tumors originating from the peripheral regions usually remain there.[1–3]
- Base-of-tongue cancers have little tendency to spread to the palatine tonsils, whereas tonsillar cancers tend to invade the base of the tongue.
- Vallecular lesions are often exophytic and invade along the mucosa to the lingual surface of the epiglottis, laterally along the pharyngoepiglottic fold, and then to the lateral pharyngeal wall and anterior wall of the pyriform sinus.
- The first-echelon nodes are the subdigastric (level II) nodes, then along the jugular chain to the midjugular and lower jugular nodes. If anterior extension into the oral tongue or massive upper neck disease is present, then

the submandibular lymph nodes may be involved. The posterior cervical lymph nodes are often involved, but submental spread is rare.
- Bilateral and contralateral lymphatic spread is common (Fig 9-3); retrograde spread to retropharyngeal lymph nodes has been reported, particularly in advanced lesions.[1–3]
- The deeply infiltrating nature of BOT cancers correlates with the high frequency of lymphatic metastases at presentation (80% of patients overall, with bilateral spread in 37% to 55%).[1–5]
- The incidence of clinically positive neck node at presentation is about 50% to 83% (Table 9-1).
- The incidence of pathologically positive neck node in clinical N0 neck is about 22% to 33%. Contralateral lymphatic metastasis at presentation is 37%. Table 9-2 shows the percentage of the incidence and distribution of metastatic disease in clinically negative and positive neck nodes in base-of-tongue cancers.

## 3. DIAGNOSIS AND STAGING SYSTEM

### 3.1. Signs and Symptoms

- The base of the tongue is visualized only by indirect mirror examination, so early diagnosis is rare. The earliest symptom is a mild sore throat. Many of the early lesions are asymptomatic and relatively silent. A subdigastric neck mass is frequently the first sign.
- Necrosis and internal bleeding may cause sudden enlargement and mild tenderness.
- Difficulty in swallowing, a nasal quality to the voice, and deep-seated ear pain occur with enlargement of the mass. Otalgia is associated with tumor involvement of retropharyngeal space.
- Hypoglossal nerve invasion is rare but causes unilateral paralysis and atrophy of the tongue if it occurs.

### 3.2. Physical Examination

- Early lesions are usually submucosal and relatively soft. Since the surface of the base of the tongue is irregular, it

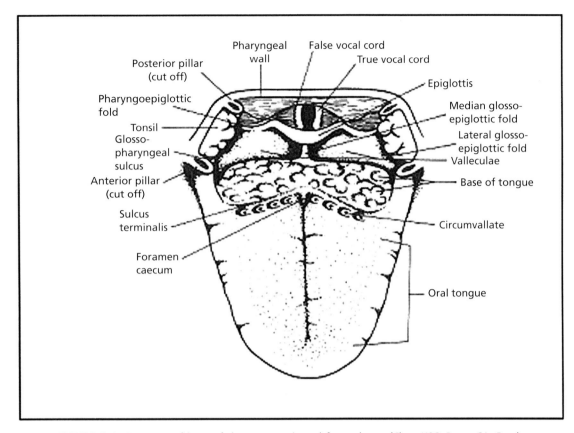

**FIGURE 9-1.** Anatomy of base of the tongue viewed from above. (Chao KSC, Perez CA, Brady LW, eds: *Radiation oncology: management decisions*. Philadelphia: Lippincott-Raven, 1999:245, by permission.)

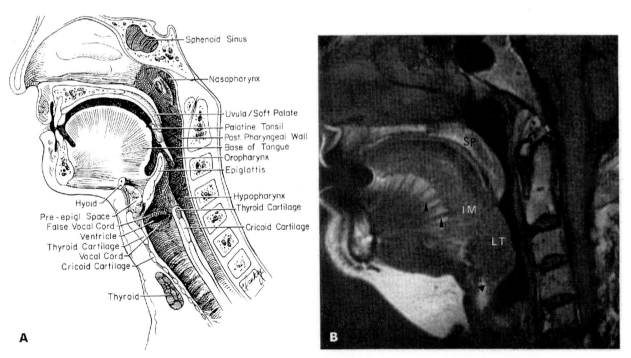

**FIGURE 9-2. A:** Sagittal section of the upper aerodigestive tract. **B:** Sagittal MRI. Lymphoid tissue at the tongue base (LT) does not penetrate the intrinsic tongue muscles (IM): it is limited to the surface. Genioglossus fibers fan out in the tongue (*arrowheads*) to finally interdigitate with the intrinsic tongue musculature. The tongue base is continuous with the preepiglottic space (*arrow*). Areas of high signal intensity within soft palate (SP) are due to its fatty content. (Million RR, Cassisi NJ, Mancuso AA. Oropharynx. In: Million RR, Cassisi NJ, eds. *Management of head and neck cancer: a multidisciplinary approach,* 2nd ed. Philadelphia: JB Lippincott, 1994:402, by permission.)

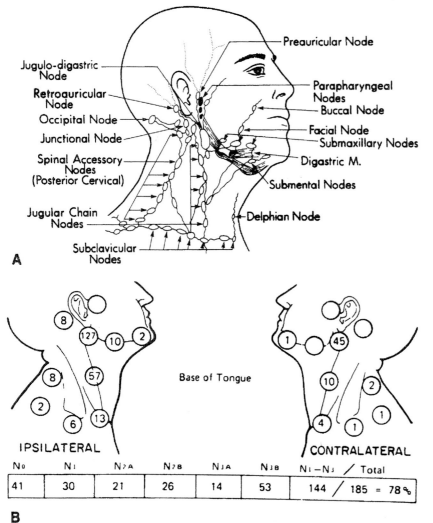

FIGURE 9-3. A: Lymphatics of head and neck. Both deep (*shaded*) parapharyngeal and superficial nodes (jugulodigastric) are commonly involved. (Chao KSC, Perez CA, Brady LW, eds: *Radiation oncology: management decisions.* Philadelphia: Lippincott-Raven, 1999: 246.) B: Distribution of nodal involvement at presentation of squamous cell carcinoma of base of the tongue. (Lindberg RD. Distribution of cervical lymph node metastases from squamous cell carcinoma of the upper respiratory and digestive tract. *Cancer* 1972;29:1446—1449, by permission.)

is very difficult to palpate the mass. The rigid or flexible endoscopes permit examination in some patients.
- Palpation through the lateral floor of the mouth can be helpful to detect anterior extension.
- Fullness in the soft tissue around the hyoid bone may be a sign of inferior penetration through the valleculae.
- Fixation of the tongue causes incomplete protrusion to the site that is fixed.

**TABLE 9-1. CLINICALLY DETECTED NODAL METASTASES (%) ON ADMISSION BY T STAGE (2,328 PATIENTS)**

|    | N0    | N1    | N2–3  |
|----|-------|-------|-------|
| T1 | 26–30 | 15–28 | 46–55 |
| T2 | 26–29 | 14–36 | 38–56 |
| T3 | 26–30 | 23    | 47–52 |
| T4 | 16–24 | 8–26  | 50–76 |

*Source:* Compiled from the data of the Curie Institute,[4] MSKCC,[5] MD Anderson.[3]

### 3.3. Imaging

- The main imaging tools of the oropharyngeal region are computed tomography (CT) and magnetic resonance imaging (MRI).
- CT is better for the lymph nodes and bone detail, so it is the preferred initial study. MRI is used adjunctively.
- Evaluation of the base of the tongue should include slices from the nasopharynx to the lower neck (Fig. 9-4). Axial sections are often sufficient; however, coronal sections may be needed when lesions invade the base of the skull. Sagittal MRI is necessary for detection of early preepiglottic space invasion.[6]
- CT and MRI sections of this region require injection of contrast media. Contiguous 3- to 4-mm slices should be used through the primary and the neck. It is important to keep the field of view small so that the pictures are magnified and spatial resolution is optimized. Evaluation of the base of the tongue must include a complete CT study of the cervical and retropharyngeal nodes (Fig. 9-5).[7]

**TABLE 9-2. INCIDENCE AND DISTRIBUTION OF METASTATIC DISEASE IN CLINICALLY NEGATIVE (N–)* AND POSITIVE (N+)† NECK NODES**

| | Pathologic Nodal Metastasis | | | | | | | | | | | |
|---|---|---|---|---|---|---|---|---|---|---|---|---|
| | Radiologically Enlarged Retropharyngeal Nodes | | Level I | | Level II | | Level III | | Level IV | | Level V | |
| Clinical presentation | N– | N+ | N– | N+ | N– | N+ | N– | N+ | N– | N+ | N– | N+ |
| Base of tongue | 0 | 6% | 4% | 19% | 30% | 89% | 22% | 22% | 7% | 10% | 0 | 18% |

*Sources:* Compiled from McLaughlin 1995,[21] Candela 1990,[22] Shah 1990,[23] Bataini 1985,[24] Byers 1988,[25] Lindberg 1972.[3]
*In patients who underwent bilateral neck dissection, 55% were found to have pathologic metastasis in both necks.
†Bilateral neck node metastasis was found in 37% of N+ patients at presentation.

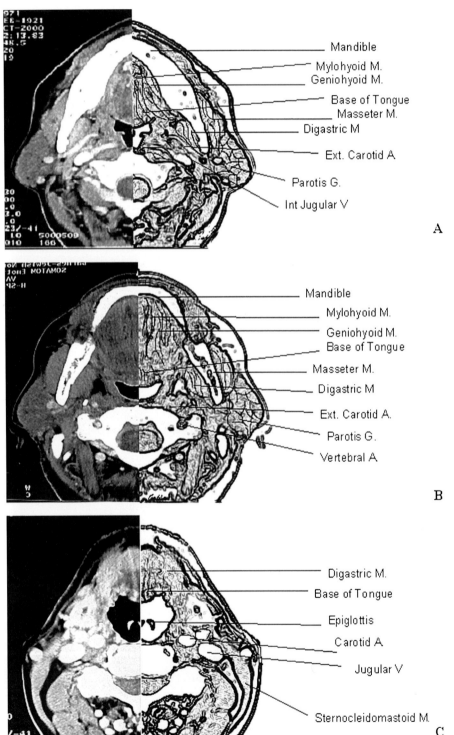

**FIGURE 9-4. A–C:** Anatomic line diagrams from the mid oropharynx to the level of the valleculae, including the base of tongue, to correlate with the accompanying CT images at the same level.

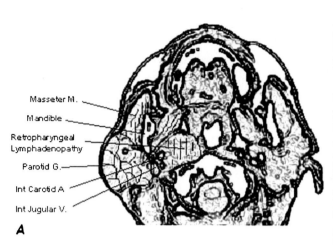 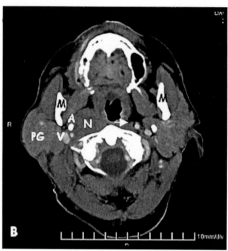

**FIGURE 9-5. A:** Anatomic relations of junctional and retropharyngeal lymph nodes. **B:** CT study shows an enlarged retropharyngeal lymph node (N). The node lies medial to the carotid artery (A), parotid gland (PG) and jugular vein (V). A more normal-sized retropharyngeal node (*arrow*) is present on the opposite side.

- CT and MRI are excellent at showing the deep structures surrounding the pharynx. The deep-tissue planes are generally symmetric, and obliteration of the deep fat spaces such as the parapharyngeal space or invasion of deep musculature is a sign of invasion. Such spread is frequently not expressed as signs and symptoms, or detected by physical examination. Lower in the oropharynx, the pharyngeal wall becomes tightly surrounded by musculature and the intervening fat planes are less visible, making diagnosis of invasion more difficult.[8]
- Lymphoid tissue is present throughout the oropharynx and is responsible for most of the variation seen in the surface contours on CT and MRI. Inexperienced interpreters may frequently misinterpret various bumps and bulges on the mucosal surfaces for tumors. These regions should be either ignored or used as prompts to look for adjacent deep infiltration as a sign of pathology. These surfaces are best evaluated by physical examination, not by CT or MRI. There are no findings that can distinguish lymphoid tissue and other benign mucosal lesions from cancer other than infiltration of the deeper structures.[9]
- Any tumor that is suspicious for deep infiltration should be studied primarily with CT. A significant portion of MRI studies in this area will be of low quality due to motion artifacts. MRI in general is preferred for the evaluation of the parapharyngeal space.[6–9]
- The relationship of tumor margins to both lingual neurovascular bundles can be anticipated on imaging with far greater precision than on physical examination. Occasionally, retrograde spread of tumor out of the tongue along the lingual neurovascular bundles to the external carotid artery is visible.
- Tumors in the region may also grow onto the styloid musculature. Inferior growth along the mylohyoid and hyoglossus muscles may bring the tumor to the insertion of these muscles on the hyoid bone, and there may be direct extension into the soft tissues of the suprahyoid and infrahyoid neck at that point. Occult spread from the base of the tongue to the preepiglottic space may also be visualized.[6–9]

### 3.4. Staging

- Table 9-3 shows the American Joint Committee on Cancer staging system for carcinoma of the oropharynx.

## 4. PROGNOSTIC FACTORS

- *Tumor size and extent:* Base-of-tongue cancers have a worse prognosis than those in the oral tongue because of greater size at diagnosis, more frequent spread to adjacent structures, and higher rate of lymphatic spread. However, stage for stage, they may have a prognosis similar to that of oral tongue cancers.[10]
- *Stage:* One of the most dominant prognostic factors is tumor stage.
- *Response to radiotherapy and the influence of complete regression at the end of irradiation:* Survival and local regional control are better for complete responders.
- *Histopathologic grade:* Poorly differentiated or undifferentiated carcinomas are shown to have better survival and local control rates.[4]
- *Others:* Other prognosticators include age (better survival over 45 years) and extension to both epilarynx and endolarynx (associated with poor survival).[4,10]

## 5. GENERAL MANAGEMENT

- Exophytic or surface tumors respond well to irradiation alone; ulcerative, endophytic cancers that are partly or completely fixed require surgery.[2,11,12]

## TABLE 9-3. TNM CLASSIFICATION FOR CARCINOMA OF THE OROPHARYNX

*Primary Tumor (T)*

| | |
|---|---|
| TX | Primary tumor cannot be assessed |
| T0 | No evidence of primary tumor |
| Tis | Carcinoma *in situ* |
| T1 | Tumor <2 cm in greatest dimension |
| T2 | Tumor >2 cm but not >4 cm in greatest dimension |
| T3 | Tumor >4 cm in greatest dimension |
| T4 | Tumor invades adjacent structures (pterygoid muscle[s], mandible, hard palate, deep muscle of tongue, larynx) |

*Regional Lymph Nodes (N)*

| | |
|---|---|
| NX | Regional lymph nodes cannot be assessed |
| N0 | No regional lymph node metastasis |
| N1 | Metastasis in a single ipsilateral lymph node, <3 cm in greatest dimension |
| N2 | Metastasis in a single ipsilateral lymph node, >3 cm but not >6 cm in greatest dimension; in multiple ipsilateral lymph nodes, none >6 cm in greatest dimension; or in bilateral or contralateral lymph nodes, none >6 cm in greatest dimension |
| N2a | Metastasis in a single ipsilateral lymph node >3 cm but not >6 cm in greatest dimension |
| N2b | Metastasis in multiple ipsilateral lymph nodes, none >6 cm in greatest dimension |
| N2c | Metastasis in bilateral or contralateral lymph nodes, none >6 cm in greatest dimension |
| N3 | Metastasis in a lymph node >6 cm in greatest dimension |

*Distant Metastases (M)*

| | |
|---|---|
| MX | Presence of distant metastasis cannot be assessed |
| M0 | No distant metastasis |
| M1 | Distant metastasis |

*Stage Grouping*

| | | | |
|---|---|---|---|
| Stage 0 | Tis | N0 | M0 |
| Stage I | T1 | N0 | M0 |
| Stage II | T2 | N0 | M0 |
| Stage III | T3 | N0 | M0 |
| | T1 | N1 | M0 |
| | T2 | N1 | M0 |
| | T3 | N1 | M0 |
| Stage IV A | T4 | N0 or N1 | M0 |
| | Any T | N2 | M0 |
| Stage IV B | Any T | N3 | M0 |
| Stage IV C | Any T | Any N | M1 |

*Source:* Fleming ID, Cooper JS, Henson DE, et al., eds. *AJCC cancer staging manual,* 5th ed. Philadelphia: Lippincott-Raven, 1997:37–39.

- Overall treatment results for base-of-tongue cancer, when all stages are considered, appear to be best for combinations of surgery and irradiation when compared with conventional irradiation alone.

### 5.1. Surgical Management

- Radical neck dissection yields information to determine the need for postoperative irradiation, which is recommended for patients with disease more extensive than stage N1 or with extracapsular extension.
- At Washington University in St. Louis, 47% of patients treated with combined surgery and preoperative irradiation had the mandible preserved.[13]
- Tumors of the lower base of the tongue that involve the valleculae and extend inferiorly to the supraglottic larynx and pyriform sinus may be controlled by partial glossectomy and subtotal supraglottic laryngectomy or partial laryngopharyngectomy with preservation of voice.[13,14]

- Prerequisites for a subtotal supraglottic laryngectomy include no gross involvement of the pharyngoepiglottic fold, preservation of one lingual artery, resection of less than 80% of the base of the tongue, pulmonary function suitable for supraglottic laryngectomy, and medical condition suitable for a major operation.
- Locoregional control is about 48% with surgery alone.[15]

### 5.2. Irradiation Alone

- Doses to the primary tumor and palpable lymph nodes range from 65 to 75 Gy delivered in 6.5 to 7.5 weeks. Doses for elective irradiation of subclinical, miroscopic lymphatic metastases should be at least 50 Gy.
- Small T1 and T2 base-of-tongue tumors without significant infiltration and surface or exophytic T2 and T3 lesions of the glossopharyngeal sulcus (glossopalatine sulcus) are controlled by high-dose radiation, with locoregional control of 70%.[11]

## TABLE 9-4. BASE OF TONGUE: LOCAL CONTROL RESULTS CORRELATED WITH T STAGE (IRRADIATION ALONE)

| | Local Control by T Stage | | | |
|---|---|---|---|---|
| | T1 | T2 | T3 | T4 |
| Puthawala et al.[26] | 2/2 (100%) | 14/16 (88%) | 30/40 (75%) | 8/12 (67%) |
| Crook et al.[11] | 11/13 (85%) | 25/35 (71%) | No data | No data |
| Lusinchi et al.[27] | 15/18 (83%) | 20/39 (51%) | 35/51 (69%) | No data |
| Spanos et al.[28] | 29/32 (91%) | 35/49 (71%) | 50/64 (78%) | 15/29 (52%) |
| Foote et al.[29] | 8/9 (89%) | 27/30 (90%) | 25/31 (81%) | 5/14 (36%) |
| Wang et al.[30] | 35/40 (89%) | 55/69 (79%) | 37/78 (48%) | 8/37 (21%) |
| Brunin et al.[4] | 27/29 (93%) | 35/56 (63%) | 42/95 (44%) | 8/36 (23%) |
| Harrison et al.[5] | 14/17 (87%) | 29/31 (93%) | 14/18 (82%) | 2/2 (100%) |
| Chao et al.[31] | 10/18 (55%) | 14/23 (61%) | 8/16 (50%) | 5/11 (45%) |
| Total | 151/178 (85%) | 254/348 (73%) | 241/393 (61%) | 51/141 (36%) |

- Large, unresectable base-of-tongue cancers that cross the midline, infiltrate, and fix the tongue are often irradiated palliatively to achieve as much tumor regression as possible.
- Local control results correlated with T and N stage, and disease-specific survival rates according to T and N stage in literature are summarized in Tables 9-4, 9-5, and 9-6, respectively.

### 5.3. Surgery and Irradiation

- Surgery combined with irradiation is best suited for larger tumors that extend beyond the base of the tongue or infiltrate and partially fix the tongue.
- Adjuvant irradiation should be routinely used for resectable T3 and T4 base-of-tongue cancers to reduce the likelihood of recurrence.[13]
- Bilateral fields covering the primary site and upper necks are necessary because of the significant primary tumor burden and high rate of contralateral and bilateral lymphatic spread.
- To eradicate residual microscopic disease, doses of 56 to 60 Gy (66 Gy for positive margins or extracapsular extension) may be delivered to the primary tumor bed and necks beginning 4 to 6 weeks after surgery.
- Locoregional control ranges from 57% to 84% with the combined approach (Table 9-7).

### 5.4. Chemotherapy

- In a metaanalysis of 63 trials (10,741 patients), locoregional treatment with chemotherapy yielded a pooled hazard ratio of death of 0.90 (95% CI 0.85 to 0.94, $p$ <.0001), corresponding to an absolute survival benefit of 4% at 2 and 5 years compared with patients receiving no chemotherapy. No significant benefit was associated with adjuvant or neoadjuvant chemotherapy. Chemotherapy given concomitantly to radiotherapy gave significant benefits.
- Newer drug combinations, usually containing cisplatin, have shown high complete-response rates in nonkeratinizing head and neck cancers and may improve results of treatment.[16–19]
- At Washington University, patients with locally advanced carcinoma of the oropharynx are treated with concomitant platinum-based chemo-IMRT. Regimens include cisplatin 21 days or weekly carboplatin plus Taxol.

## TABLE 9-5. BASE OF TONGUE: LOCAL CONTROL RESULTS CORRELATED WITH N STAGE (IRRADIATION ALONE)

| | Local Control by N Stage | | |
|---|---|---|---|
| | N0 | N1 | N2–3 |
| Brunin et al.[4] | 39/68 (57%) | 25/56 (46%) | 47/92 (51%) |
| Harrison et al.[5] | 6/10 (60%) | 21/24 (87%) | 31/32 (96%) |
| Wang et al.[30] | 53/75 (71%) | 23/42 (55%) | 59/107 (55%) |
| Chao et al.[31] | 21/23 (91%) | 7/10 (70%) | 24/35 (68%) |
| Total | 119/176 (64%) | 69/122 (68%) | 161/266 (61%) |

**TABLE 9-6. BASE OF TONGUE: DISEASE-SPECIFIC SURVIVAL RATES CORRELATED WITH T AND N STAGE (IRRADIATION ALONE)**

| | Massachusetts General Hospital (31) | | Institute Curie (4) | | Washington University (32) | |
|---|---|---|---|---|---|---|
| | DSS | No. of Pts | DSS | No. of Pts | DSS | No. of Pts |
| T1 | 78% | 40 | 60% | 29 | 18 | 61% |
| T2 | 76% | 69 | 42% | 56 | 23 | 65% |
| T3 | 40% | 78 | 29% | 95 | 16 | 39% |
| T4 | 16% | 37 | 20% | 36 | 11 | 42% |
| | | | | | | |
| N0 | 67% | 75 | 48% | 68 | 23 | 59% |
| N1 | 56% | 42 | 32% | 56 | 10 | 50% |
| N2–3 | 42% | 107 | 27% | 92 | 35 | 41% |

DSS, disease-specific survival; MIR, Mallinkrodt Institute of Radiology; Pts, patients.

## 6. INTENSITY MODULATED RADIATION THERAPY IN BASE-OF-TONGUE CARCINOMA

### 6.1. Target Volume Determination

- If chemotherapy was delivered before radiation, the targets should be outlined on the planning CT according to their prechemotherapy extent.
- Lymph node groups at risk in the base of the tongue include the following:
  a. Submandibular nodes (surgical level I): N+ cases
  b. Upper deep jugular (junctional, parapharyngeal) nodes: all cases (ipsilateral to the primary tumor)
  c. Subdigastric (jugulodigastric) nodes, midjugular, lower neck, and supraclavicular nodes (levels II through IV): all cases, bilaterally
  d. Posterior cervical nodes (level V): all cases, at the neck side where there is evidence of jugular nodal metastases
  e. Retropharyngeal nodes: all cases, if there is evidence of jugular nodal metastases
- Table 9-8 summarizes the target volume specification for definitive and postoperative IMRT in base-of-tongue cancer.
- Table 9-9 summarizes suggested target volume determination for base-of-tongue carcinoma.

### 6.2. Target Volume Delineation

- In patients receiving definitive IMRT, CTV1 encompasses gross tumor (primary and enlarged nodes) and the region adjacent to it but not directly involved. CTV2 includes primarily the prophylactically treated neck (Fig. 9-6).
- Figure 9-7 shows CTV1 and CTV2 delineation in a patient with clinically T4N2bM0 squamous cell carcinoma of BOT receiving definitive IMRT.
- In patients receiving postoperative IMRT, CTV1 encompasses residual tumor and the region adjacent to it but not directly involved by the tumor, the surgical bed with soft-tissue invasion by the tumor, or extracapsular extension by metastatic neck nodes. CTV2 includes primarily the prophylactically treated neck.
- Figure 9-8 shows CTV1 and CTV2 delineation in a patient with pathologic T2N0M0 squamous cell carcinoma of BOT receiving postoperative IMRT.

### 6.3. Normal Tissue Delineation

- Figure 5-16 shows normal tissue delineation is shown in.

### 6.4. Suggested Target and Normal Tissue Doses

- Table 4-9 shows the Washington University guideline for clinical target volume dose specification with biological

**TABLE 9-7. LOCOREGIONAL CONTROL AND DISEASE-SPECIFIC SURVIVAL RATES FOR POSTOPERATIVE RADIOTHERAPY SERIES**

| | Primary Site | Neck | Disease-Specific Survival |
|---|---|---|---|
| Kraus et al.[32] | 80% (50/63) | 82% (52/63) | 61% |
| Zelefsky et al.[33] | 84% (26/31) | 84% (26/31) | 64% |
| Goffinet et al.[34] | 64% (9/14) | 50% (7/14) | NA (6/14)* |
| Chao et al.[31] | 85% (79/93) | 89% (83/93) | 57% |
| Total | 82% (164/201) | 84% (168/201) | 57–64% |

*Out of 14 patients, six died as a result of disease.

**TABLE 9-8. TARGET VOLUME SPECIFICATION FOR DEFINITIVE AND POSTOPERATIVE IMRT IN BASE-OF-TONGUE CANCER**

| Target | Definitive IMRT | High-Risk Postoperative IMRT | Intermediate-Risk Postoperative IMRT |
|---|---|---|---|
| CTV1 | Soft-tissue and nodal regions adjacent to the gross tumor | Surgical bed with soft-tissue involvement or nodal region with extracapsular involvement | Surgical bed without soft-tissue involvement or nodal region without capsular extension |
| CTV2 | Elective nodal regions (I, II, III, IV, V)* | Elective nodal regions (I, II, III, IV, V)* | Elective nodal regions (I, II, III, IV, V)* |

*N0 includes levels II, III, IV and retropharyngeal nodes. N1 includes levels Ib, II, III, IV, and retropharyngeal nodes. N2–3 includes levels Ib, II, III, IV, V, and retropharyngeal nodes.

equivalent dose correction and normal tissue tolerance for IMRT.
- Figure 9-9 shows an example of IMRT dose distribution of a patient receiving postoperative IMRT for a T2N0 base-of-tongue cancer.

### 6.5. IMRT Treatment Results

- Following these guidelines, 15 base-of-tongue carcinoma patients were treated with IMRT between February 1997 and December 2000 at Washington University.[20] Seven patients were treated postoperatively and eight were treated with definitive IMRT. The T stages were two T1, five T2, two T3, and six T4. The N stages were one N0, one N1, 11 N2, and two N3 (AJCC staging; one stage I, one stage III, and 13 stage IV). Median follow-up time was 22 months (12 to 54 months). We observed two locoregional recurrences. One patient was salvaged with surgery; the other died of disease progression. No distant metastasis developed. A G-tube was placed in seven patients during the course of IMRT. We observed no grade 3 or 4 late complications in our patients treated with IMRT. Five grade 1 and three grade 2 xerostomia were observed, and hypothyroidism developed in one patient as a late sequela.

**TABLE 9-9. SUGGESTED TARGET VOLUME DETERMINATION FOR BASE-OF-TONGUE IMRT (35)**

| Clinical Presentation | CTV1 | CTV2 |
|---|---|---|
| T1–2 N0 | P | IN + CN (Ib–IV, RPLN) |
| T3–4N+* | P + IN (I†–IV, RPLN) | CN (I–V, RPLN) |
| N2c | P + IN + CN (I–V, RPLN) | |

Source: Modified from Chao KSC, Wippold FJ, Ozyigit G, et al. Determination and delineation of nodal target volumes for head and neck cancer based on the patterns of failure in patients receiving definitive and postoperative IMRT. *Int J Radiat Oncol Biol Phys* 2002;53:1174–1184.
CN, contralateral neck nodes; IN, ipsilateral neck nodes; P, gross tumor with margins for definition IMRT or surgical bed for postop IMRT; RPLN, retropharyngeal lymph nodes.
*N* = N1–3 except N2c.
†Level Ib only. Level Ia should be included when Ib node on oral tongue is involved.

## 7. SEQUELAE OF TREATMENT

- Moderate to severe xerostomia (RTOG grade 2 or above) occurs in approximately 75% of patients treated with conventional beam arrangement. In contrast, only approximately 25% of patients treated with IMRT developed moderate to severe xerostomia.
- Self-healing soft-tissue necrosis and bone exposure can be seen in patients treated with radiotherapy. But bone necrosis is very rare.
- The patient may lose weight due to dysphagia and require nutritional support. Hemorrhage is also rare.
- Hypoglossal nerve palsy is reported. Unilateral hypoglossal nerve palsy does not produce serious morbidity because the opposite site compensates rather well.
- Other infrequent complications include mild trismus and otitis media.
- Aspiration is unusual, even if the tip of epiglottis has been amputated by tumor.

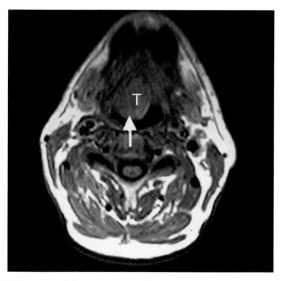

**FIGURE 9-6.** Axial MRI image of a patient with T2N0 base-of-tongue carcinoma (*white arrow*).

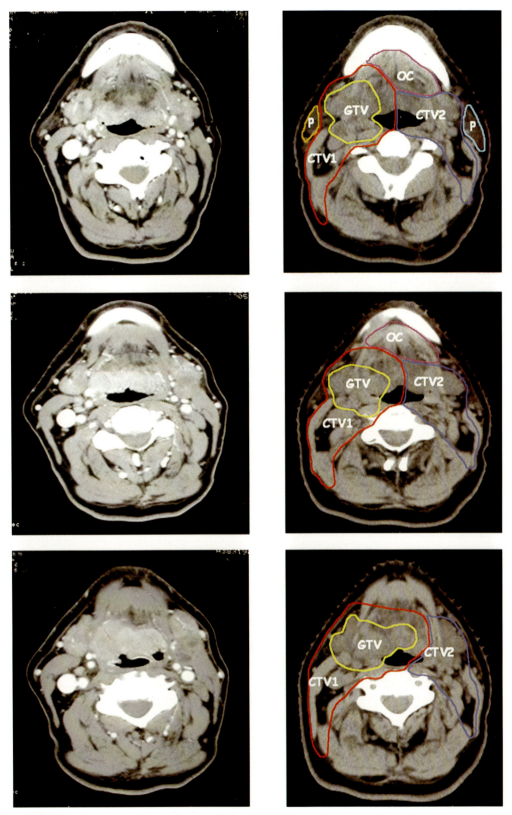

**FIGURE 9-7.** Clinical target volume (CTV) delineation in a patient with a T4N2bM0 squamous cell carcinoma of the base of tongue receiving definitive IMRT. Gross tumor volume (GTV), yellow line; CTV1, red line; CTV2, dark blue line; P, parotid gland; right parotid gland, rust line; left parotid gland, aqua line; oral cavity (OC), magenta line.

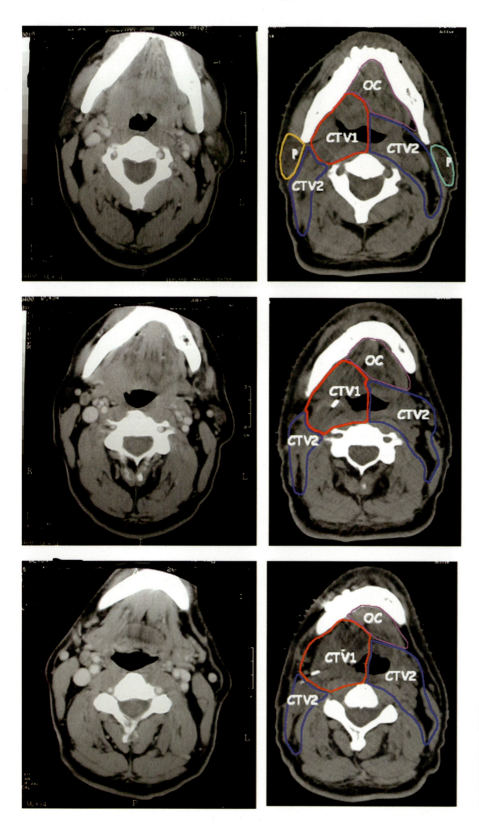

**FIGURE 9-8.** Clinical target volume (CTV) delineation in a patient with a T2N0M0 squamous cell carcinoma of the base of tongue receiving postoperative IMRT. Gross tumor volume (GTV), yellow line; CTV1, red line; CTV2, dark blue line; P, parotid gland; right parotid gland, rust line; left parotid gland, aqua line; oral cavity (OC), magenta line.

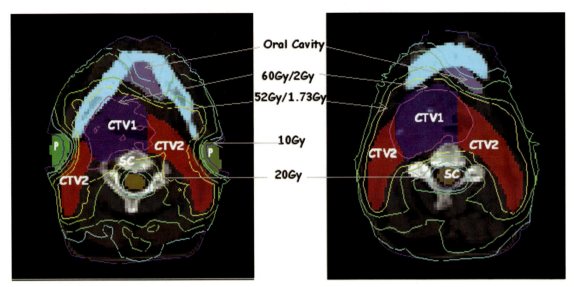

**FIGURE 9-9.** IMRT dose distribution of a T2N0 base-of-tongue cancer. CTV, clinical target volume; P, parotid gland; SC, spinal cord.

## REFERENCES

1. Shumrick D, Gluckman J. In Coto I, et al. *Cancer of the head and neck.* New York: Churchill Livingstone, 1981.
2. Fletcher G. *Textbook of radiotherapy,* 3rd ed. Philadelphia: Lea & Febiger, 1980:322.
3. Lindberg R. Distribution of cervical lymph node metastases from squamous cell carcinoma of the upper respiratory and digestive tracts. *Cancer* 1972;29:1447.
4. Brunin F, Mosseri V, Jaulerry C, et al. Cancer of the base of the tongue: past and future. *Head Neck* 1999;21:751–759.
5. Harrison L, Lee H, Pfister D, et al. Long-term results of primary radiotherapy with/without neck dissection for squamous cell cancer of the base of tongue. *Head Neck* 1998;20:668–673.
6. Mancuso A. Diagnostic imaging. In: Rice D, ed. *Otolaryngology: head and neck surgery.* Philadelphia: WB Saunders, 1992:18–27.
7. Mancuso A, Hanafee W. *Computed tomography and magnetic resonance imaging of the head and neck,* 2nd ed. Baltimore: Williams & Wilkins, 1985.
8. Mancuso A, Harnsberger H, Dillon W. *Workbook for MRI and CT of the head and neck,* 2nd ed. Baltimore: Williams & Wilkins, 1989.
9. Som P, Bergeron R. *Head and neck imaging.* St. Louis: Mosby Year Book, 1991.
10. Ildstad S, Bigelow M, Remensnyder J. Squamous cell carcinoma of the tongue: a comparison of the anterior two thirds of the tongue with its base. *Am J Surg* 1983;146:456–461.
11. Crook J, Mazeron J, Marinello J, et al. Combined external irradiation and interstitial implantation for T1 and T2 epidermoid carcinomas of base of the tongue: the Creteil experience (1971–1981). *Int J Radiat Oncol Biol Phys* 1989;15:105–114.
12. Parsons J, Million R, Cassisi N. Carcinoma of the base of tongue: results of radical irradiation with surgery reserved for irradiation failure. *Laryngoscope* 1982;92:689–696.
13. Thawley S, Simpson J, Marks J, et al. Preoperative irradiation and surgery for carcinoma of the base of tongue. *Ann Otol Rhinol Laryngol* 1983;92:485–490.
14. Rollo J, Rosenbom J, Thawley S, et al. Squamous cell carcinoma of the base of tongue: a clinicopathological study of 81 cases. *Cancer* 1992;69:2736–2743.
15. Foote R, Olsen K, Davis D, et al. Base of tongue carcinoma: patterns of failure and predictors of recurrence after surgery alone. *Head Neck* 1993;15:300–307.
16. Ervin TJ, Clark JR, Weichselbaum RR. Multidisciplinary treatment of advanced squamous carcinoma of the head and neck. *Semin Oncol* 1985;12:71–78.
17. Merlano M, Benasso M, Corvo A, et al. Five-year update of a randomized trial of alternating radiotherapy and chemotherapy compared with radiotherapy alone in treatment of unresectable squamous cell carcinoma of the head and neck. *J Natl Cancer Inst* 1996;88:583–589.
18. Pfister D, Harrison L, Strong E, et al. Organ function preservation in advanced oropharynx cancer: results with induction chemotherapy and radiation. *J Clin Oncol* 1995;13:671–680.
19. Slotman G, Doolittle C, Glicksman A. Preoperative combined chemotherapy and radiation therapy plus radical surgery in advanced head and neck cancer: five-year results with impressive complete response rates and high survival. *Cancer* 1992;69:2736–2743.
20. Chao K, Ozyigit G, Cengiz M, et al. Patterns of failure in patients receiving definitive and post-operative IMRT for head and neck cancer. *Int J Radiat Oncol Biol Phys* 2002 (in press).
21. McLaughlin MP, Mendenhall WM, Mancuso AA, et al. Retropharyngeal adenopathy as a predictor of outcome in squamous cell carcinoma of the head and neck. *Head Neck* 1995;17:190–198.
22. Candela F, Kothari K, Shah J. Patterns of cervical node metastasis from squamous carcinoma of the oropharynx and hypopharynx. *Head Neck* 1990;12:197–203.
23. Shah J, Candela F, Poddar A. The patterns of cervical lymph node metastases from squamous cell carcinoma of oral cavity. *Cancer* 1990;66:109–113.
24. Bataini JP, Bernier J, Brugere J, et al. Natural history of neck disease in patients with squamous cell carcinoma of the oropharynx and pharyngolarynx. *Radiother Oncol* 1985;3:245–255.
25. Byers R, Wolf P, Ballantyne A. Rationale for elective modified neck dissection. *Head Neck Surg* 1988;10:160–167.
26. Puthawala AA, Syed AM, Eads DL, et al. Limited external beam and interstitial 192 iridium irradiation in the treatment of carcinoma of the base of the tongue: a ten-year experience. *Int J Radiat Oncol Biol Phys* 1988;14:839–848.

27. Lusinchi A, Eskandari J, Haie J, et al. External irradiation plus brachytherapy boost in the base of tongue carcinoma (Abstract 13.). *Proceedings of the Second International Conference on Head and Neck Cancer,* vol. 51. Boston, MA, 1988.
28. Spanos W, Shukowsky L, Fletcher G. Time, dose, and tumor volume relationships in irradiation of squamous cell carcinomas of the base of the base of the tongue. *Cancer* 1976;37:2591–2599.
29. Foote R, Parsons J, Mendenhall W, et al. Is interstitial implantation essential for successful radiotherapeutic treatment of base of tongue carcinoma? *Int J Radiat Oncol Biol Phys* 1990;18:1293–1298.
30. Wang C. Carcinoma of the oropharynx. In: Wang C, ed. *Radiation therapy for head and neck neoplasms.* New York: Wiley-Liss, 1997.
31. Chao K, Majhail N, Huang C, et al. Intensity-modulated radiation therapy reduces late salivary toxicity without compromising tumor control in patients with oropharyngeal carcinoma: a comparison with conventional techniques. *Radiother Oncol* 2001;61:275–280.
32. Kraus D, Vastola A, Huvos A. Surgical management of squamous cell carcinoma of the base of the tongue. *Am J Surg* 1993;166:384–388.
33. Zelefsky M, Harrison L, Armstrong J. Long-term treatment results of post-operative radiation therapy for advanced oropharyngeal carcinoma: long term treatment results. *Cancer* 1992;70:2388–2395.
34. Goffinet D, Fee W, Wells J, et al. [192]Ir pharyngoepiglottic fold interstitial implants: the key to successful treatment of base tongue carcinoma by radiation therapy. *Cancer* 1985;55:941–948.

# 10

# HYPOPHARYNX

**GOKHAN OZYIGIT**
**K.S. CLIFFORD CHAO**

## 1. ANATOMY

- The hypopharynx is the most inferior portion of the pharynx from the level of the hyoid bone that is the base of the vallecula and pharyngoepiglottic folds to the beginning of the esophagus at the plane of the lower border of the cricoid cartilage (Fig. 10-1). It communicates the oropharynx with the esophageal inlet.
- The larynx indents the anterior wall of the hypopharynx to form a horseshoe-shaped hollow cavity. This creates a central aerodigestive passageway and two lateral fossae (i.e., the pyriform sinuses) (Fig. 10-2).
- The hypopharyngeal walls are composed of four layers of tissue: mucosa, fibrous fascia, muscular layer, and areolar coat. The epithelium of the pharyngeal mucous membrane is squamous and continuous with the nasopharyngeal epithelial membrane. There is no visible transitional zone between these two regions. The mucosal membrane, which is lined by ciliated pseudostratified columnar epithelium, is exposed to air. The surfaces that allow the transport of both food and air or food only are lined with stratified squamous epithelium. These differences have importance in the type and differentiation of malignancies in various parts of the pharynx.
- Beneath the mucous membrane of the posterior and lateral walls is the thin muscular layer. The muscular layer of the hypopharynx is composed of two paired constrictor muscles, the middle and the inferior constrictors. These muscles attach anteriorly to the hyoid bone and thyroid cartilage and fuse posteriorly with each other.
- Between the constrictor muscles and the prevertebral fascia that covers the longitudinal spinous muscles is a thin layer of loose areolar tissue, the retropharyngeal space. This is a potential space that may act as a conduit for tumor extension.
- The areolar layer contains the vessels, nerves, and lymphatics that lie lateral to the pharyngeal walls in a potential parapharyngeal space of loose connective tissue surrounded by the deep cervical and visceral fascia.
- Clinically, the hypopharynx is separated from the other parts of pharynx by certain anatomic landmarks (Fig. 10-1). The superior border arises anteriorly at the base of vallecula (inferior border of the hyoid bone) and proceeds laterally to the pharyngoepiglottic folds. The superior border is the plane connecting these points with the posterior pharyngeal wall at the level of the fourth cervical vertebra.
- The posterior and lateral hypopharyngeal walls are continuous with those of the oropharynx without certain anatomic separation. The lateral border of the epiglottis, the aryepiglottic folds, and lateral laryngeal wall makes the medial wall.
- The inferior constrictor muscle has two specialized divisions. The first is the cricopharyngeus muscle, which is composed of the lowermost fibers and the sphincteric guardian of the esophagus. The second part forms the cricothyroid muscle, which is the tensor of the vocal folds. This muscle inserts into the thyroid cartilage. The external branch of the superior laryngeal nerve innervates the cricothyroid muscle.
- The anterior border is the postcricoid region, which extends from the interarytenoid area and cricothyroid muscle. The inferior border is at the inferior edge of the pharyngeal aponeurosis and its cricopharyngeal ligament.
- The hypopharynx is also subdivided into three clinical regions: the pyriform sinus, the posterolateral pharynx, and the postcricoid region. The posterior border of the larynx forms the postcricoid region. The pyriform sinuses lie lateral to the larynx. The medial wall is formed by the aryepiglottic fold and the lateral laryngeal wall (cricothyroid muscle). The anterior and lateral walls are formed by the thyroid ala.
- The posterior wall is open and communicates with the hypopharyngeal lumen. The pyriform sinus apex lies below the level of the vocal cords and occasionally below the cricoid cartilage. So the tumors that extend to the pyriform sinus apex or postcricoid area are not amenable to voice conservational surgical procedures.
- The arterial supply of the hypopharynx is mainly from the ascending pharyngeal arteries, superior thyroid arteries, and branches from the lingual artery, all divisions from the external carotid system. A venous plexus

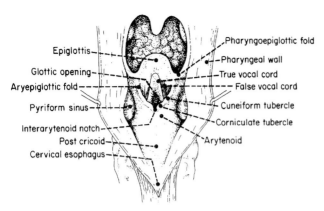

**FIGURE 10-1.** Hypopharynx. Posterior view showing the topography of the Pyriform sinus, pharyngeal wall, and postcricoid region. (Sobotta J. *Atlas of human anatomy,* vol. II. Munich: Urban & Schwarzenberg, 1983, by permission.)

drains the pharynx and communicates with the internal jugular vein.
- The lymphatics generally travel in cephalad direction, through the thyrohyoid membrane toward the upper deep cervical lymph nodes, to enter the jugulodigastric lymph nodes and the upper and middle jugular chain.
- There is also free communication with the spinal accessory lymph nodes and retropharyngeal lymph nodes; in this group the highest nodes (Rouviere) are at the skull base. This close proximity of the lymphatics to the mucosa partly explains the high incidence of early metastases.
- The lowest portions of the hypopharynx (the postcricoid region, pyriform apex, and inferior hypopharynx) drain into a lymphatic chain that follows the recurrent laryngeal nerve to the paratracheal, paraesophageal, and supraclavicular nodes.
- The motor neural supply of the hypopharyngeal muscles is from the pharyngeal plexus of nerves, which are motor-neural fibers from the glossopharyngeal (IX) and vagus (X) nerves.

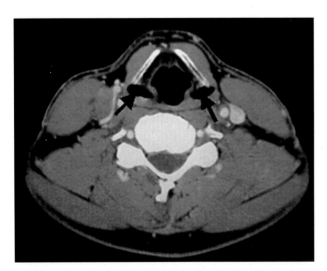

**FIGURE 10-2.** Axial CT section at the level of pyriform sinuses (*arrows*).

- The inferior hypopharynx is innervated by branches from the recurrent laryngeal nerve (X). Efferent pain fibers traveling with the internal branch of the superior laryngeal nerve through the auricular branch of the vagus (nerve of Arnold) to the ipsilateral ear cause pain, usually an ill-defined, dull ache in the superior-posterior wall of the external auditory canal or the posterior skin of the pinna.

## 2. NATURAL HISTORY

- In the United States, tumors occur in the following decremental frequency: pyriform fossa (>65%), postcricoid (20%), and hypopharyngeal wall (10% to 15%).[1]
- Medial wall pyriform fossa tumors, the most common group, may spread along the mucosal surface to involve the aryepiglottic folds (most common pattern). Sometimes they invade medially and deeply into the false vocal folds and larynx via the paraglottic space (Fig. 10-3). Involvement of the paraglottic space allows a lesion to behave as a transglottic carcinoma.[2]
- Cancers of the lateral wall and apex of the pyriform fossa commonly invade the thyroid cartilage and less frequently the cricoid cartilage.
- Once they penetrate the constrictor muscle, tumors can spread along the muscle and fascial planes to the base of the skull (the origin and suspension of the constrictor muscles) and along the neurovascular planes following the vagus, glossopharyngeal, and sympathetic nerves.
- Postcricoid area tumors commonly invade the cricoid cartilage, interarytenoid space, and posterior cricohyoid muscle to produce hoarseness.[3] Because of the tendency for early esophageal spread, some have suggested that these epiesophageal tumors are not hypopharyngeal in origin.[4]
- The abundant lymphatics of the hypopharynx, coupled with extensive primary disease at presentation, account for the high incidence of metastases to the regional lymph nodes (Table 10-1).
- The midcervical lymph nodes are most commonly involved. The incidence of metastases varies according to the site and origin in the hypopharynx (Tables 10-2 and 10-3, and Fig. 10-4).[5]
- Figure 10-5 shows the distribution of pathologically positive neck nodes after elective modified neck dissection. The contralateral subdigastric nodes are the most common site of harboring metastatic disease.
- Occult disease occurs irrespective of T stage in pyriform fossa tumors, with an incidence of 60% for T1 and T2 and 84% for T3 and T4 disease.[1]
- In 3,419 patients, the most common metastatic site was in level II (69%), and survival decreased as the level of metastases went from level II (39% survival) to the supraclavicular region (level IV, 21% survival).[6]
- Pathologically confirmed node metastases decreased survival by 26% to 28% (N0 versus N+), and size of nodal disease decreased survival by an additional 12% to 18%

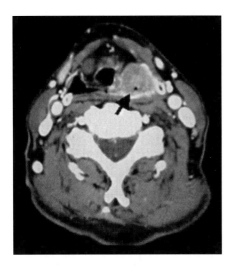 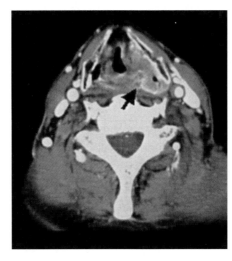

**FIGURE 10-3.** A T4N1 squamous cell carcinoma of the pyriform sinus (axial CT sections at two different levels).

(N1 versus N2 and N3).[7,8] There is a decremental survival rate with progressive nodal disease (N0, 57%; N1, 28%; N2, 6%; N3, 0) and a higher neck recurrence rate with progressively larger neck metastases (N0, 20%; N1, 37%; N2, 48%; N3, 83%).[9]
- Approximately 5% to 15% of presenting cases require an emergency tracheotomy.
- On rare occasions, direct tumor involvement or lymph node extension to the hypoglossal nerve may produce ipsilateral tongue paralysis.

## 3. DIAGNOSIS AND STAGING SYSTEM

### 3.1. Signs and Symptoms

- Early pharyngeal tumors generally produce a mild, nonspecific sore throat or vague discomfort on swallowing that persists for longer than 2 weeks.
- A major neurologic finding is referred pain to the ipsilateral ear, which is referred along the internal branch of the superior laryngeal nerve (sensory division to the larynx and hypopharynx) via the vagus nerve (X) to the auricular branch of the vagus nerve (Arnold's nerve).
- Dysphagia is produced by bulky tumors or by deep constrictor muscle invasion, prevertebral space invasion of the overlying strap muscles. This finding may be associated with salivary drooling, stiff neck, and a "hot potato"

**TABLE 10-1. CLINICALLY DETECTED NODAL METASTASES (%) ON ADMISSION BY T STAGE**

|    | N0 | N1 | N2–3 |
|----|----|----|------|
| T1 | 37 | 21 | 42   |
| T2 | 30 | 20 | 49   |
| T3 | 21 | 26 | 54   |
| T4 | 26 | 15 | 58   |

*Source:* Modified from Lindberg R. Distribution of cervical lymph node metastases from squamous cell carcinoma of the upper respiratory and digestive tracts. *Cancer* 1972;29:1446–1449.

voice. The last finding is due to laryngeal and especially base-of-tongue invasion.
- Advanced disease causes significant weight loss.
- Hoarseness by invasion of larynx, blood-streaked saliva, airway obstruction, halitosis, and nasal voice are other signs and symptoms that can be seen in hypopharyngeal cancers.

### 3.2. Physical Examination

- The initial history and physical examination should include indirect laryngoscopy and a flexible endoscopic examination under topical anesthesia. Posterior pharyngeal wall lesions may be missed during indirect laryngoscopy.
- Radiologic evaluation includes chest x-ray and computed tomography scan with contrast of the head and neck region, which is helpful in delineating cartilage and bone invasion by tumor, as well as extralaryngeal and paraglottic tumor invasion.
- In most cases, delineating the inferior border of the lesion and involvement of the esophageal inlet requires a barium swallow, including a video to evaluate the hypopharynx and cervical esophagus.

### 3.3. Imaging

- MRI can clearly distinguish the pharyngeal muscles from the mucosa and the lymphoid tissue lining the inner wall of the hypopharynx.
- The thickness of the posterior and lateral pharyngeal walls seen on MRI is usually less than 3 mm. If it reaches upper limits, it can be a sign of pathologic change.
- The pharyngeal constrictor muscles are relatively easy to distinguish from the mucosal lymphoid tissue on T2-weighted MRI.
- The penetration points of pharyngeal vessels are easily visible on CT and MRI. They are extremely important places, since they may provide early perineural and perivascular spread routes of tumor to the extrapharyngeal soft tissues.

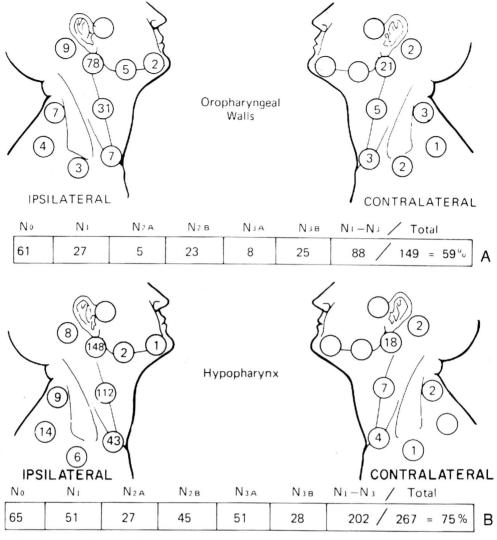

**FIGURE 10-4.** Nodal distribution of hypopharyngeal cancer on admission, MD Anderson Hospital. (Lindberg RD. Distribution of cervical lymph node metastases from squamous cell carcinoma of the upper respiratory and digestive tracts. *Cancer* 1972;29:1448, by permission.)

- The constrictor muscle fascia is normally not visible as a separate layer on either CT or MRI, but inflammatory or other invasive changes may cause the fascia to become pathologically visible.
- A small amount of fat is normally seen just lateral to the lateral pharyngeal wall in the deep neck in all patients. Similarly, prevertebral muscles are visible in all patients on axial CT or MRI; however, the prevertebral fascia is not normally visible. The potential retropharyngeal space is located between the constrictor fascia and the prevertebral fascia.

**TABLE 10-2. PERCENTAGE OF NODAL METASTASES (%) AS A FUNCTION OF LOCATION AND TUMOR SIZE[5]**

|  | T1 | T2 | T3 | T4 |
|---|---|---|---|---|
| Pyriform sinus | 38–91% | 67–83% | 69–80% | 60–98% |
| Pharyngeal wall | 33–70% | 31–79% | 47–85% | 70–82% |
| Postcricoid | 6% | 17% | 38% | 50% |

- The space lateral to the pharynx is referred as the parapharyngeal space above the level of hyoid bone.
- The retropharyngeal lymph nodes are located between the posterolateral corners of the pharynx and the carotid artery from the tip of the clivus to the C3 (hyoid) level.
- The degree of distention of the pyriform sinus seen on MRI or CT varies from side to side in any given individual and more greatly between patients, depending on their anatomy and the study technique. Any thickness on the surface of the pyriform sinus usually represents some type of pathology.
- Imaging particularly can show the deep anatomic relationships of the pyriform sinus apex. The mucosa of the pyriform sinus apex is always seen as a thin line that merges medially with the mucosa in the postcricoid region.
- The postcricoid region is easily visible as that zone posterior to the cricoid cartilage, where the constrictor muscle thickens to create the cricopharyngeus muscle. The lumen

**TABLE 10-3. INCIDENCE AND DISTRIBUTION OF METASTATIC DISEASE IN CLINICALLY NEGATIVE (N−)* AND POSITIVE (N+)† NECK NODES (IN PERCENTAGE)**

| | Pathological Nodal Metastasis | | | | | | | | | | | |
|---|---|---|---|---|---|---|---|---|---|---|---|---|
| | Radiologically Enlarged Retropharyngeal Nodes | | Level I | | Level II | | Level III | | Level IV | | Level V | |
| Clinical presentation | N− | N+ | N− | N+ | N− | N+ | N− | N+ | N− | N+ | N− | N+ |
| Pharyngeal walls | 16 | 21 | 0 | 11 | 9 | 84 | 18 | 72 | 0 | 40 | 0 | 20 |
| Pyriform sinus | 0 | 9 | 0 | 2 | 15 | 77 | 8 | 57 | 0 | 23 | 0 | 22 |

*Source:* Modified from Chao KSC, Wippold FJ, Ozyigit G, et al. Determination and delineation of nodal target volumes for head and neck cancer based on the patterns of failure in patients receiving definitive and postoperative IMRT. *Int J Radiat Oncol Biol Phys* 2002;53:1174–1184.
*In patients who underwent bilateral neck dissection, 38–56% were found to have pathologic metastasis in both necks.
†Bilateral neck node metastasis was found in 49% of N+ patients at presentation.

is usually not distended with air. Since the pharyngeal lumen is usually collapsed, the mucosa on enhanced CT or MRI is usually visible as parallel lines 1 mm or less in thickness, lying along the inner borders of cricopharyngeus muscle.

### 3.4. Staging

- Table 10-4 shows the American Joint Committee on Cancer staging system for carcinoma of the hypopharynx.

## 4. PROGNOSTIC FACTORS

- *Age:* Survival progressively declines with increasing age.
- *Gender:* Women have a significantly higher survival rate 3 to 20 years after therapy.
- *Surgical margin:* Pathologic findings in pyriform fossa tumors that adversely affect survival are positive surgical margins or tumor persistence in the irradiation field after initial definitive therapy.
- *Location:* Tumor location influences cure rates. The decremental frequency for survival with hypopharyngeal carcinomas at different sites is pyriform fossa, pharyngeal walls, and postcricoid region.[10] Aryepiglottic fold and medial wall pyriform fossa tumors are usually smaller and more localized, which leads to higher cure rates than with postcricoid and pharyngeal wall tumors. The poorest results are seen with pyriform apex, postcricoid, and two- or three-wall tumors.
- *Neck metastasis:* In pyriform fossa and aryepiglottic fold tumors, metastases reduce the cure rate by 28% and 26%, respectively (N0 > N+ by 26% to 28%). The presence of extracapsular tumor spread in the cervical lymph nodes

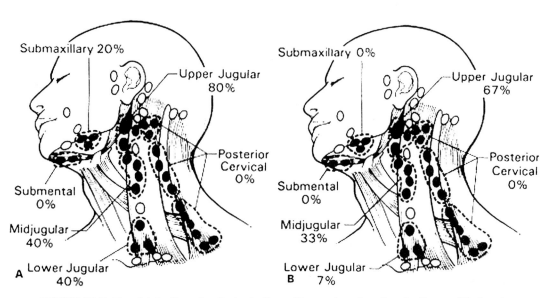

**FIGURE 10-5.** The distribution of pathologically positive neck nodes after elective modified neck dissection. **A:** Thirteen patients with pharyngeal wall cancer. **B:** Thirty-two patients with pyriform sinus carcinoma. (Byers RM, Wolf PF, Ballantyne AJ. Rationale for elective modified neck dissection. *Head Neck Surg* 1988;10:163–164.)

## TABLE 10-4. AMERICAN JOINT COMMITTEE STAGING SYSTEM FOR CANCERS OF THE HYPOPHARYNX

*Primary Tumor (T)*

| | |
|---|---|
| TX | Primary tumor cannot be assessed |
| T0 | No evidence of primary tumor |
| Tis | Carcinoma *in situ* |
| T1 | Tumor limited to one subsite of hypopharynx and <2 cm in greatest dimension |
| T2 | Tumor involves more than one subsite of hypopharynx or an adjacent site, or measures >2 cm but not >4 cm in greatest dimension without fixation of hemilarynx |
| T3 | Tumor measures >4 cm in greatest dimension or with fixation of hemilarynx |
| T4 | Tumor invades adjacent structures (e.g., thyroid/cricoid cartilage, carotid artery, soft tissues of neck, prevertebral fascia/muscles, thyroid, and/or esophagus) |

*Regional Lymph Nodes (N)*

| | |
|---|---|
| NX | Regional lymph nodes cannot be assessed |
| N0 | No regional lymph node metastasis |
| N1 | Metastasis in a single ipsilateral lymph node, <3 cm in greatest dimension |
| N2 | Metastasis in a single ipsilateral lymph node, >3 cm but not >6 cm in greatest dimension; or in multiple ipsilateral lymph nodes, none >6 cm in greatest dimension; or in bilateral or contralateral lymph nodes, none >6 cm in greatest dimension |
| N2a | Metastasis in a single ipsilateral lymph node, >3 cm but not >6 cm in greatest dimension |
| N2b | Metastasis in multiple ipsilateral lymph nodes, none >6 cm in greatest dimension |
| N2c | Metastasis in bilateral or contralateral lymph nodes, none >6 cm in greatest dimension |
| N3 | Metastasis in a lymph node >6 cm in greatest dimension |

*Distant Metastasis (M)*

| | |
|---|---|
| MX | Distant metastasis cannot be assessed |
| M0 | No distant metastasis |
| M1 | Distant metastasis |

*Stage Grouping*

| | | | |
|---|---|---|---|
| Stage 0 | Tis | N0 | M0 |
| Stage I | T1 | N0 | M0 |
| Stage II | T2 | N0 | M0 |
| Stage III | T3 | N0 | M0 |
| | T1 | N1 | M0 |
| | T2 | N1 | M0 |
| | T3 | N1 | M0 |
| Stage IVA | T4 | N0 or N1 | M0 |
| | Any T | N2 | M0 |
| Stage IVB | Any T | N3 | M0 |
| Stage IVC | Any T | Any N | M1 |

*Source:* Fleming ID, Cooper JS, Henson DE, et al., eds. *AJCC cancer staging manual,* 5th ed. Philadelphia: Lippincott-Raven Publishers, 1997:37–39.

and soft tissues of the neck is of paramount importance in survival.[11,12] The presence of neck metastases influences survival.

- *The size and number of neck node metastasis:* The size or number of metastases influences survival (higher for N1 than for N2 and N3) by an additional 12% to 18%.[7,8]
- *T stage:* T stage influences survival; most patients present with large tumors (82% are T3 or T4 pyriform sinus cancers).[13] In pyriform fossa tumors (T1 and T2 exceed T3 and T4 by 28%), there is a significant decrease in cure rates for T3 and T4 disease.[13]

## 5. GENERAL MANAGEMENT

- The best treatment for hypopharyngeal carcinoma achieves the highest locoregional control rate with the least functional damage.
- The functions that need to be preserved are respiration, deglutition, and phonation, if possible, with the least risk to the host and without the use of permanent prosthetic devices.
- Most T1N0 and selected T2N0 lesions can be treated equally well with curative irradiation or conservation surgery. Invasion of the larynx by a pyriform fossa tumor

## TABLE 10-5. PYRIFORM SINUS: LOCAL CONTROL RESULTS CORRELATED WITH T STAGE

| | No. of Patients | | Local Tumor Control | | |
| | | Therapy | T1–T2 | T4–T3 | Overall |
| --- | --- | --- | --- | --- | --- |
| Bataini et al.[19] | 434 | RT | 67% | 33% | 47% |
| Mendenhall et al.[20] | 50 | RT + ND | 74% | 26% | 49% |
| | 53 | S + RT | 4/6 | 72% | 25% |
| Mendenhall et al.[21] | 30 | RT (qd) | 80% | 1/5 | — |
| | 8 | RT (bid) | 3/4 | 1/4 | — |
| Mendenhall et al.[22] | 53 | RT + ND | 66% | 72% | 100% |
| Dubois et al.[23] | 209 | RT | 73% | 34% | 25% |
| | 154 | S ± RT | 43% | 33% | 35% |
| Wang et al.[3] | 28 | RT (qd) | 68% | 20% | 44% |
| | 54 | RT (bid) | 82% | 33% | 61% |
| El Badawi et al.[1] | 48 | RT | — | — | 75% |
| | 125 | RT + S | — | — | 89% |
| Vandenbrouck et al.[8] | 152 | RT | 77 | 49 | 45% |
| | 198 | S + RT | | | 80% |
| Marks et al.[24] | 137 | RT + S | — | — | 72% |

bid, twice daily; ND, neck dissection; qd, daily; RT, radiation therapy; S, surgery.

## TABLE 10-6. PHARYNGEAL WALL CANCER: LOCAL CONTROL RESULTS CORRELATED WITH T STAGE

| | No. of Patients | | Local Tumor Control (%) | | |
| | | Therapy | T1–T2 | T4–T3 | Overall |
| --- | --- | --- | --- | --- | --- |
| Meoz-Mendez[25] | 164 | RT | 91–73 | 61–37 | 60 |
| | 25 | S + RT | 5/5 | 75 | 45 |
| Wang[28] | 43 | RT (qd) | 55 | 36 | 47 |
| | 33 | RT (bid) | 74 | 44 | 64 |
| Mendenhall[26] | 49 | Rt qd ± Implant | 10/20 | 9/29 | 39 |
| | 13 | RT (bid) | 5/5 | 5/8 | 77 |
| Chang[27] | 44 | RT (qid) | 3/3–10/18 | 4/19–0/4 | |
| | 13 | RT (bid) | 1/1–1/2 | 5/7–2/3 | |

bid, twice daily; ND, neck dissection; qd, daily; RT, radiation therapy; S, surgery.

## TABLE 10-7. HYPOPHARYNGEAL CANCER: SURVIVAL RESULTS

| | No. of Patients | Therapy | T1 | T2 | T3 | T4 | Overall |
| --- | --- | --- | --- | --- | --- | --- | --- |
| | | | *Pyriform Sinus* | | | | |
| Bataini*[19] | 434 | RT | | 26% | | 17% | 19% |
| | 50 | RT + ND | | 60% | | 23% | 49% |
| Mendenhall*[20] | | | | | | | |
| | 53 | S + RT | | 43% | | 24% | 25% |
| Dubois†[23] | 209 | RT | | 11% | | 3% | 5% |
| | 154 | S ± RT | | 37% | | 30% | 33% |
| Spector*[7] | 128 | RT + S | 9/9 | 19/22 | 50/64 | 20/33 | 98/128(76.5%) |
| | 49 | S + RT | 5/5 | 7/9 | 13/19 | 7/16 | 32/49(65/3%) |
| | | | *Pharyngeal Wall* | | | | |
| Wang‡[28] | 43 | RT (qd) | 64% | 29% | 22% | 0% | 30% |

ND, neck dissection; qd, daily; RT, radiation therapy; S, surgery.
*5-year determinate survival.
†5-year overall survival.
5-year disease free survival.
‡3-year disease free survival.

### TABLE 10-8. TARGET VOLUME SPECIFICATION FOR DEFINITIVE AND POSTOPERATIVE IMRT IN HYPOPHARYNX CANCER

| Target | Definitive IMRT | High-Risk Postoperative IMRT | Intermediate-Risk Postoperative IMRT |
|---|---|---|---|
| CTV1 | Soft tissue and nodal regions adjacent to the GTV | Surgical bed with soft tissue involvement or nodal region with extracapsular involvement | Surgical bed without soft-tissue involvement or nodal region without capsular extension |
| CTV2 | Elective nodal regions (I, II, III, IV, V)* | Elective nodal regions (I, II, III, IV, V)* | Elective nodal regions (I, II, III, IV, V)* |

*Source:* Modified from Chao KSC, Wippold FJ, Ozyigit G, et al. Determination and delineation of nodal target volumes for head and neck cancer based on the patterns of failure in patients receiving definitive and postoperative IMRT. *Int J Radiat Oncol Biol Phys* 2002;53:1174–1184.
*N0 includes levels II, III, IV, and retropharyngeal nodes. N1 includes levels Ib, II, III, IV, and retropharyngeal nodes. N2–3 includes levels Ib, II, III, IV, V, and retropharyngeal nodes.

with vocal cord fixation predicts a poor outcome to curative irradiation.

- Larger lesions and neck metastases require combined surgical resection and adjuvant radiation therapy.[14]
- Tables 10-5 through 10-7 summarize treatment outcomes for hypopharyngeal cancer.

## 5.1. Surgical Management

- Contraindications for conservation surgery include the following: transglottic extension, cartilage invasion, vocal fold paralysis, pyriform apex invasion, postcricoid invasion, and extension beyond the laryngeal framework.
- In all cases, at a minimum, an ipsilateral neck dissection is performed (functional, modified, or radical resection), almost always followed by postoperative irradiation.
- Tumors of the aryepiglottic fold are resected with an extended subtotal supraglottic laryngectomy and neck dissection if they fulfill the resection criteria of no extension

### TABLE 10-9. SUGGESTED TARGET VOLUME DETERMINATION FOR HYPOPHARYNX IMRT

| Clinical Presentation | CTV1 | CTV2 |
|---|---|---|
| T1–2 N0 | P | IN + CN (II–IV) |
| T3–4N +* | P + IN (I†–IV, RPLN) | CN (II–IV) |
| N2c | P + IN + CN (I–V, RPLN) | |

*Source:* Modified from Chao KSC, Wippold FJ, Ozyigit G, et al. Determination and delineation of nodal target volumes for head and neck cancer based on the patterns of failure in patients receiving definitive and postoperative IMRT. *Int J Radiat Oncol Biol Phys* 2002 *(in press).*
CN, contralateral neck nodes; IN, ipsilateral neck nodes; P, gross tumor with margins for definition IMRT or surgical bed for postop IMRT; RPLN, retropharyngeal lymph nodes.
*N+ = N1–3 except N2c.
†Include Ib node when level II node involved.

beyond the larynx, transglottic extension, or vocal cord paralysis.

- Extension into the base of the tongue, epiglottis, and vallecula can be handled by extension of the operative field superiorly to resect these lesions and portions of the base of the tongue.
- Small lesions are amenable to partial laryngopharyngectomy and neck dissection if they are confined to the medial and anterior pyriform fossa walls or aryepiglottic folds, do not extend to the pyriform apex or beyond the larynx, show no postcricoid invasion or vocal cord (paralysis) or contralateral arytenoid involvement, and occur in patients who do not have pulmonary and cardiac disabilities.
- In patients who do not meet the criteria for conservation surgery, either a total laryngopharyngectomy or a total laryngectomy and partial pharyngectomy with reconstruction with neck dissection are performed.

## 5.2. Irradiation Alone

- Irradiation alone controls a substantial proportion of small surface lesions in the pyriform sinus. Of 25 T1 and T2 lesions of the pyriform sinus, 16 (64%) were controlled with irradiation alone (65 to 70 Gy in 7 to 8 weeks).[22]

## 5.3. Surgery and Irradiation

- Higher doses of adjuvant irradiation (60 to 66 Gy) are better delivered postoperatively than preoperatively because preoperative irradiation (usually 45 to 50 Gy in 4.5 to 5 weeks) retards healing of pharyngeal and cutaneous suture lines and may cause more complications than postoperative irradiation.[15]
- In pyriform fossa tumors, combined therapy had higher cure rates (71%) than surgery (53%) or irradiation (27%). In aryepiglottic fold tumors, combined therapy (68%) had

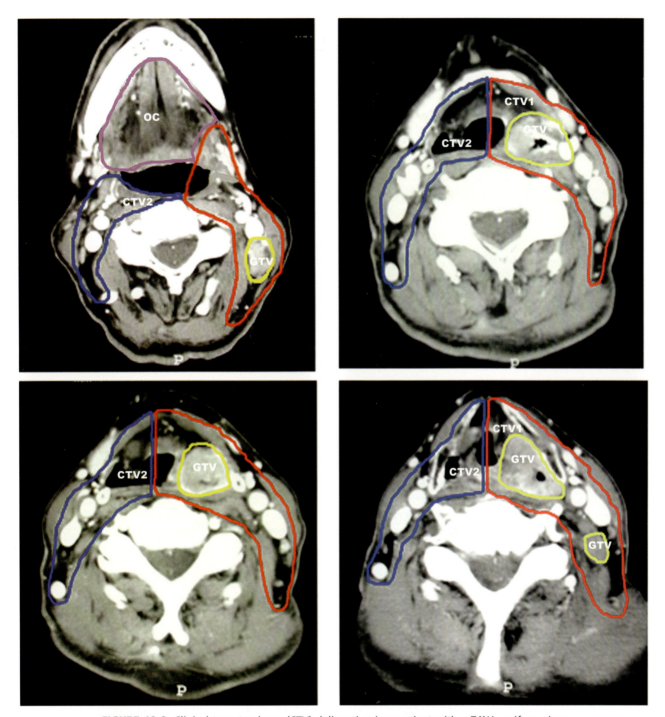

**FIGURE 10-6.** Clinical target volume (CTV) delineation in a patient with a T4N1 pyriform sinus cancer receiving definitive IMRT. CTV1, red line; CTV2, dark blue line; GTV, gross tumor volume (yellow line); OC, oral cavity (magenta line).

better disease-free results than surgery (61%) or irradiation (34%) at 5 years.[12]

## 5.4. Chemotherapy

- The European Organization for Research and Treatment of Cancer reported results of combined-modality therapy for head and neck cancer: 202 patients with operable, locally advanced squamous cell cancer of the pyriform sinus or the hypopharyngeal aspect of the aryepiglottic fold were randomly assigned to receive treatment with standard surgery and postoperative irradiation or induction chemotherapy (cisplatin and 5-fluorouracil).[16]

- Patients achieving a clinical complete response (CR) at the primary site after two or three cycles of chemotherapy received organ-sparing treatment with definitive irradiation

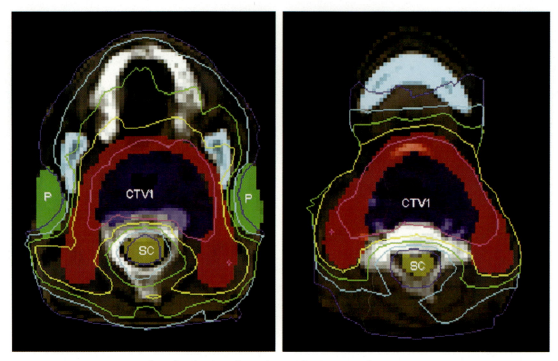

**FIGURE 10-7.** IMRT dose distribution of a patient with a T3N0 pyriform sinus carcinoma receiving postoperative IMRT. CTV, clinical target volume; CTV1, dark blue area; CTV2, red area; P, parotid gland; SC, spinal cord. pink line, 60 Gy; yellow line, 50 Gy; green line, 40 Gy; aqua line, 30 Gy; dark blue, 20 Gy.

(70 Gy), whereas those with less than a CR were treated surgically.

- At a median follow-up of 51 months (range, 3 to 106 months), the estimated survival outcomes for patients randomly assigned to receive induction chemotherapy or the surgery were 3-year overall survival of 57% versus 43%, 3-year disease-free survival of 43% versus 31%, and median survival of 44 versus 25 months.
- These differences reflected a trend for improved outcome from chemotherapy and meet the statistical criteria for survival equivalence for the two arms. The laryngeal preservation rate was estimated at 42%, considering only deaths from local disease as failure.

## 6. INTENSITY MODULATED RADIATION THERAPY IN HYPOPHARYNGEAL CARCINOMAS

### 6.1. Target Volume Determination

- If chemotherapy was delivered before radiation, the targets should be outlined on the planning CT according to their prechemotherapy extent.
- Lymph node groups at risk in the hypopharynx include the following:
  a. Submandibular nodes (surgical level I): N2c cases or when level II involved.
  b. Upper deep jugular (junctional, parapharyngeal) nodes: all cases
  c. Subdigastric (jugulodigastric) nodes, midjugular, lower neck, and supraclavicular nodes (levels II through IV): all cases, bilaterally
  d. Posterior cervical nodes (level V): all cases, when jugular node involved
  e. Retropharyngeal nodes: all cases, if there is evidence of jugular nodal metastases
- Table 10-8 summarizes the target volume specification for definitive and postoperative IMRT in hypopharynx cancer.
- Table 10-9 summarizes the suggested target volume determination for hypopharynx carcinoma.

### 6.2. Target Volume Delineation

- In patients receiving postoperative IMRT, CTV1 encompasses residual tumor and the region adjacent to it but not directly involved by the tumor, the surgical bed with soft-tissue invasion by the tumor, or extracapsular extension by metastatic neck nodes. CTV2 includes primarily the prophylactically treated neck.
- In patients receiving definitive IMRT, CTV1 encompasses gross tumor (primary and enlarged nodes) and the region adjacent to it but not directly involved. CTV2 includes primarily the prophylactically treated neck.

- Figure 10-6 shows CTV1 and CTV2 delineation in a patient with clinically T4N1M0 squamous cell carcinoma of pyriform sinus receiving definitive IMRT.

## 6.3. Normal Tissue Delineation

- See Chapter 5 (Fig. 5-16).

## 6.4. Suggested Target and Normal Tissue Doses

- Table 4-9 (Chapter 4) shows the Washington University guideline for clinical target volume dose specification with biologic equivalent dose correction and normal tissue tolerance for IMRT.

## 6.5. IMRT Treatment Results

- Following these guidelines, eight patients with hypopharyngeal carcinoma were treated with IMRT between February 1997 and December 2000 at Washington University.[17] Four patients were treated postoperatively and four were treated with definitive IMRT. The T stages were one T2, five T3, and two T4. The N stages were four N0, two N1, and two N2 (AJCC staging; one stage I, three stage III, and four stage IV). Median follow-up time was 21 months (range, 11 to 38 months). We observed two locoregional failures (both in the neck). All of them were salvaged with surgery. None of the patients developed distant metastasis. All but one patient are alive with no evidence of disease; the one patient died of intercurrent disease.
- Figure 10-7 provides an example of IMRT dose distribution of a patient receiving postoperative IMRT for a T3N0 pyriform sinus carcinoma.
- A G-tube was placed in two patients during the course of IMRT. We observed no grade 3 or 4 late complications in our patients treated with IMRT. Grade I xerostomia observed in one patient and trismus developed in another patient as late sequelae.

## 7. SEQUELAE OF TREATMENT

- The incidence of pharyngocutaneous fistulas after pharyngectomy is the same whether the pharynx has been irradiated before or not, but the time required to heal a preoperatively irradiated fistula is significantly greater than that for an unirradiated fistula.[15]
- Surgery-related mortality after low-dose preoperative irradiation and pharyngectomy for cancers of the pyriform sinus and pharyngeal wall ranges from 10% to 14%.[13]

## REFERENCES

1. El Badawi S, Goepfert H, Fletcher G, et al. Squamous cell carcinoma of the pyriform sinus. *Laryngoscope* 1982;92:357–364.
2. Richard J, Sancho-Garnier H, Saravane D, et al. Prognostic factors in cervical lymph node metastasis in upper respiratory and digestive tract carcinomas: study of 1713 cases during a 15-year period. *Laryngoscope* 1987;97:97–101.
3. Wang C, Schulz M, Miller D. Combined radiation therapy and surgery for carcinoma of the supraglottis and pyriform sinus. *Am J Surg* 1972;124:551–554.
4. Marks J, Kurnik B, Powers W, et al. Carcinoma of the pyriform sinus: an analysis of treatment results and patterns of failure. *Cancer* 1978;41:1008–1015.
5. McGavran M, Bauer W, Spjut H, et al. Carcinoma of the pyriform sinus. *Arch Otolaryngol* 1963;78:826.
6. Donald P, Hayes R, Dhaliwal R. Combined therapy for pyriform sinus cancer using postoperative irradiation. *Otol Head Neck Surg* 1980;88:738–744.
7. Spector J, Sessions D, Emami B, et al. Squamous cell carcinoma of the pyriform sinus: a nonrandomized comparison of therapeutic modalities and long-term results. *Laryngoscope* 1995;105:397–406.
8. Vandenbrouck C, Eschwege F, De la Rochefordiere A, et al. Squamous cell carcinoma of the pyriform sinus: retrospective study of 351 cases treated at the Institut Gustave-Roussy. *Head Neck Surg* 1987;10:4–13.
9. Lawrence WJ, Terz J, Rogers C, et al. Preoperative irradiation for head and neck cancer: a prospective study. *Cancer* 1974;33:318–323.
10. Farrington W, Weighill J, Jones P. Postcricoid carcinoma (a 10-year retrospective study). *J Laryngol Otol* 1986;100:79–84.
11. Brugere J, Mosseri V, Mamella G, et al. Nodal failures in patients with N0 N+ oral squamous cell carcinoma without capsular rupture. *Head Neck* 1996;18:133–137.
12. Spector J, Sessions D, Emami B, et al. Squamous cell carcinomas of the aryepiglottic fold: therapeutic results and long-term follow-up. *Laryngoscope* 1995;105:734–746.
13. Emami B, Spector J. Hypopharynx. In: Brady L, ed. *Principles and practice of radiation oncology,* 3rd ed. Philadelphia: Lippincott-Raven, 1998:1047–1068.
14. Sasaki T, Baker H, Yeager R. Aggressive surgical management of pyriform sinus carcinoma: a 15-year experience. *Am J Surg* 1986;151:590–592.
15. Cachin Y, Eschwege F. Combination of radiotherapy and surgery in the treatment of head and neck cancers. *Cancer Treat Rev* 1975;2:177–191.
16. McDonald T, DeSanto L, Weiland L. Supraglottic larynx and its pathology as studied by whole laryngeal sections. *Laryngoscope* 1976;86:635–648.
17. Chao K, Wippold F, Ozyigit G, et al. Determination and delineation of nodal target volumes for head and neck cancer based on the patterns of failure in patients receiving definitive and postoperative IMRT. *Int J Radiat Oncol Biol Phys* 2002;53:1174–1184.
18. Lindberg R. Distribution of cervical lymph node metastases from squamous cell carcinoma of the upper respiratory and digestive tracts. *Cancer* 1972;29:1446–1449.
19. Bataini P, Brugere J, Berniere J. Results of radical radiotherapeutic treatment of carcinoma of the pyriform sinus. *Int J Radiat Oncol Biol Phys* 1982;8:1277.
20. Mendenhall W, Parsons J, Cassisi N, et al. Squamous cell carcinoma of the pyriform sinus treated with surgery and/or radiotherapy. *Head Neck Surg* 1987;10:88–92.
21. Mendenhall W, Parsons J, Cassisi N, et al. Squamous cell

carcinoma of the pyriform sinus treated with radical radiation therapy. *Radiother Oncol* 1987;9:201.

22. Mendenhall W, Parsons J, Stringer S, et al. Radiotherapy alone or combined with neck dissection for T1–T2 carcinoma of the pyriform sinus: an alternative to conservation surgery. *Int J Radiat Oncol Biol Phys* 1993;27:1017–1027.

23. Dubois J, Guerrier B, Di Ruggiero J, et al. Cancer of the pyriform sinus: treatment by radiation therapy alone and after surgery. *Radiology* 1986;160:831–836.

24. Marks J, Sessions D. Hypopharynx. In: Brady L, ed. *Principles and practice of radiation oncology,* 2nd ed. Philadelphia: JB Lippincott, 1992.

25. Meoz-Mendez R, Fletcher G, Guillamondeque O. Analysis of the results of irradiation in the treatment of squamous cell carcinoma of the pharyngeal wall. *Int J Radiat Oncol Biol Phys* 1978;4:579.

26. Mendenhall W, Parsons J, Mancuso A, et al. Squamous cell carcinoma of the pharyngeal wall treated with irradiation. *Radiother Oncol* 1988;11:205–212.

27. Chang L, Stevens K, Moss W, et al. Squamous cell carcinoma of the pharyngeal walls treated with radiotherapy. *Int J Radiat Oncol Biol Phys* 1996;35:477–483.

28. Wang C. *Carcinoma of the hypopharynx,* 2nd ed. Chicago: Year Book Medical Publishers, 1990.

# 11

# LARYNX

**GOKHAN OZYIGIT**
**K.S. CLIFFORD CHAO**

## 1. ANATOMY

- The larynx is divided into the supraglottic (epiglottis, false vocal cords, ventricles, aryepiglottic folds, arytenoids), glottic (true vocal cords, anterior commissure), and subglottic (located below the vocal cords) regions (Figs. 11-1 and 11-2).[1]
- The lateral line of demarcation between the glottis and supraglottic larynx clinically is the apex of the ventricle. The demarcation between the glottis and subglottis is ill defined, but the subglottis is considered to begin 5 mm below the free margin of the vocal cord and to end at the inferior border of the cricoid cartilage and the beginning of the trachea (Fig. 11-3).
- The recurrent laryngeal nerve innervates the intrinsic muscles of the larynx. A branch of the superior laryngeal nerve supplies the cricothyroid muscle, an intrinsic muscle responsible for tensing the vocal cords (Fig.11-4). Isolated damage to this nerve causes a bowing of the true vocal cord, which continues to be mobile, but the voice may become hoarse.
- The supraglottic structures have a rich capillary lymphatic plexus. The trunks pass through the preepiglottic space and thyrohyoid membrane and terminate mainly in the subdigastric lymph nodes; a few drain to the middle internal jugular chain lymph nodes.
- There are essentially no capillary lymphatics of the true vocal cords. Lymphat c spread from glottic cancer occurs only if tumor extends to the supraglottic or subglottic areas.
- The subglottic area has relatively few capillary lymphatics. The lymphatic trunks pass through the cricothyroid membrane to the pretracheal (Delphian) lymph nodes in the region of the thyroid isthmus. The subglottic area also drains posteriorly through the cricotracheal membrane, with some trunks going to the paratracheal lymph nodes and others continuing to the inferior jugular chain.

## 2. NATURAL HISTORY

- Cancer of the larynx represents about 2% of the total cancer risk and is the most common head and neck cancer (skin excluded).
- The ratio of glottic to supraglottic carcinoma is approximately 3:1.
- Cancer of the larynx is strongly related to cigarette smoking. The risk of tobacco-related cancers of the upper alimentary and respiratory tracts declines among ex-smokers after 5 years and approaches the risk of nonsmokers after 10 years of abstention.[2]

### 2.1. Supraglottic Larynx

- Destructive suprahyoid epiglottic lesions tend to invade the vallecula and preepiglottic space, lateral pharyngeal walls, and the remainder of the supraglottic larynx.
- Infrahyoid epiglottic lesions grow circumferentially to involve the false cords, aryepiglottic folds, medial wall of the pyriform sinus, and the pharyngoepiglottic fold. Invasion of the anterior commissure and cords and anterior subglottic extension usually occurs only in advanced lesions.
- Extension of false cord tumors to the lower portion of the infrahyoid epiglottis and invasion of the preepiglottic space are common.
- It may be difficult to decide whether aryepiglottic fold/ arytenoid lesions started on the medial wall of the pyriform sinus or on the aryepiglottic fold. Advanced lesions invade the thyroid, epiglottic, and cricoid cartilages, and eventually invade the pyriform sinus and postcricoid area.

### 2.2. Glottic Larynx

- At diagnosis, about two-thirds of tumors are confined to the cords, usually one cord. The anterior portion of the cord is the most common site.

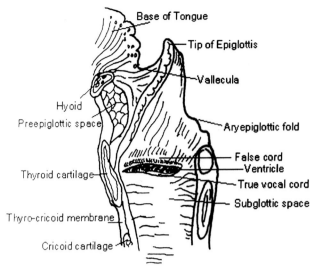

**FIGURE 11-1.** Sagittal section of the larynx. (Adapted from Sabotta J. In: Clemente CD, ed. *Anatomy: a regional atlas of the human body.* Philadelphia: Lea & Febiger, 1975. Copyright Urban & Schwarzenberg, Munich, 1975, by permission.)

- Subglottic extension may occur by simple mucosal surface growth, but it more commonly occurs by submucosal penetration beneath the conus elasticus; 1 cm of subglottic extension anteriorly or 4 to 5 mm of extension posteriorly brings the border of the tumor to the upper margin of the cricoid, exceeding the anatomic limits for conventional hemilaryngectomy.
- Advanced glottic lesions eventually penetrate through the thyroid cartilage or via the cricothyroid space to enter the neck, where they may invade the thyroid gland.

## 2.3. Lymphatic Spread

### 2.3.1. Supraglottic Carcinoma

- Disease spreads mainly to the subdigastric nodes.
- The incidence of clinically positive nodes is 55% at the time of diagnosis; 16% are bilateral (Fig. 11-5).[3]
- Table 11-1 summarizes the clinically detected nodal metastases (%) on admission by T stage for supraglottic laryngeal carcinoma.
- Elective neck dissection reveals pathologically positive nodes in 16% of cases. Observation of initially node-negative necks eventually identifies the appearance of positive nodes in 33% of cases (Table 11-2, Fig. 11-6).[4,5]
- Table 11-3 summarizes the incidence and distribution of metastatic disease in clinically negative (N−) and positive (N+) neck nodes for supraglottic laryngeal carcinoma patients.
- The risk of late-appearing contralateral lymph node metastasis is 37% if the ipsilateral neck is pathologically positive (Table 11-4).[6]

### 2.3.2. Glottic Carcinoma

- In carcinoma of the vocal cord, the incidence of clinically positive lymph nodes at diagnosis approaches zero for T1 lesions and 1.7% for T2 lesions; the incidence of neck metastases increases to 20% to 30% for T3 and T4 lesions (Fig. 11-7).[7]

## 3. DIAGNOSIS AND STAGING SYSTEM

### 3.1. Signs and Symptoms

- Hoarseness is the initial symptom of carcinomas arising on the true vocal cords. Advanced lesions of vocal cords may cause sore throat, ear pain, pain localized to thyroid cartilage, and airway obstruction.
- Hoarseness is not a prominent sign for supraglottic lesions. Mild pain in swallowing is the most frequent initial symptom. Pain is referred to the ear by vagus and auricular nerve of Arnold. Early epiglottic lesions may not give any signs or symptoms. A mass in the neck may be the first sign of supraglottic lesions. Weight loss, foul breath, dysphagia, and aspiration are late symptoms.

### 3.2. Physical Examination

- Rigid and flexible fiber-optic endoscopes are routinely used with laryngeal mirror examination.
- Determination of the mobility of the vocal cords may require multiple examinations.
- Ulceration of the infrahyoid epiglottis or fullness of the vallecula is an indirect sign of preepiglottic space invasion. Palpation of firm fullness above the thyroid notch with widening of the space between the hyoid and thyroid cartilages also may be a sign of preepiglottic space invasion.
- Tumor may penetrate the thyroid and be felt as a subcutaneous mass, suggesting the thyroid cartilage invasion.

### 3.3. Imaging

- The neck should be slightly hyperextended and the plane of section for laryngeal studies must be parallel to the true vocal cords with a slice thickness of no more than 3 to 4 mm. Occasionally, 1.5- to 2-mm slice thickness can be used for false vocal cord, true vocal cord and subglottic region, where 2- to 3-mm tumor extension might make a difference in treatment approach.
- Figure 11-8 shows the normal anatomy of the laryngeal region.
- T1 lesions of the true vocal cord usually required no imaging. Any tumor that is suspicious for deep invasion should be primarily studied with CT. MRI can be better for detection of cartilage invasion. The variation in ossification of the cartilages makes interpretation difficult. But in any

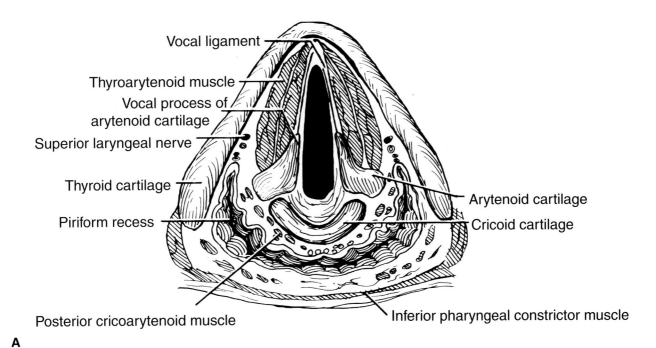

FIGURE 11-2. Cross section of larynx at the level of the vocal cords (A). Framework of the larynx (B). (Sabotta J. In: Clemente CD, ed. *Anatomy: a regional atlas of the human body.* Philadelphia: Lea & Febiger, 1975. Copyright Urban & Schwarzenberg, Munich, 1975, by permission.)

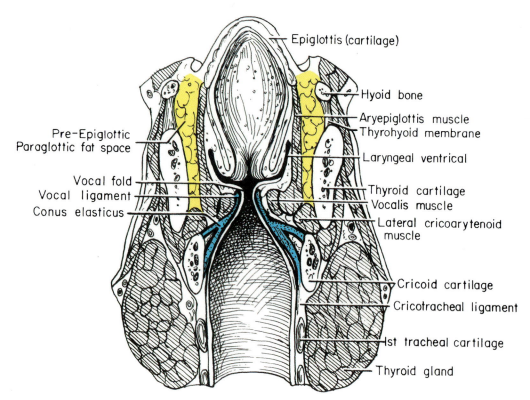

**FIGURE 11-3.** Coronal view of the larynx. (Sabotta J. In: Clemente CD, ed. *Anatomy: a regional atlas of the human body.* Philadelphia: Lea & Febiger, 1975. Copyright Urban & Schwarzenberg, Munich, 1975, by permission.)

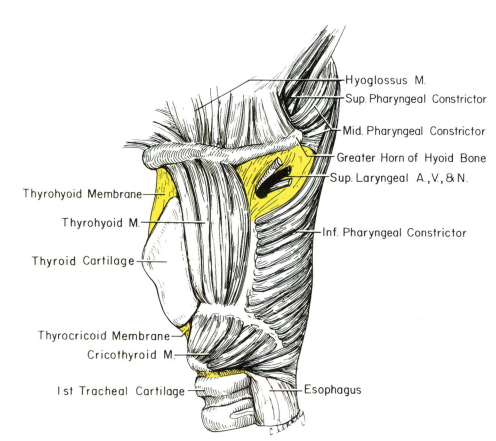

**FIGURE 11-4.** External view of the larynx. (Sabotta J. In: Clemente CD, ed. *Anatomy: a regional atlas of the human body.* Philadelphia: Lea & Febiger, 1975. Copyright Urban & Schwarzenberg, Munich, 1975, by permission.)

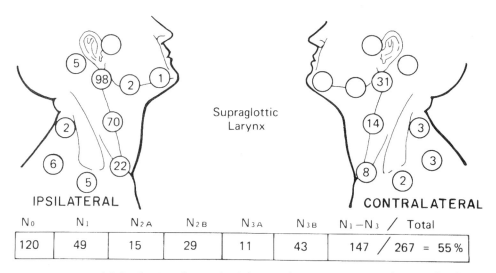

**FIGURE 11-5.** Nodal distribution of supraglottic laryngeal cancer patients on admission. (Lindberg RD. Distribution of cervical lymph node metastases from squamous cell carcinoma of the upper respiratory and digestive tracts. *Cancer* 1972;29:1449, by permission.)

case, both CT and MRI have limited capability in diagnosing subtle cartilage invasion.
- CT can distinguish extralaryngeal extension of the primary tumor from a lymph node mass and can define extension to the thyroid gland and other adjacent structures.
- CT is the preferred baseline examination for the detection of recurrence in the neck or postirradiation larynx.

## 3.4. Staging

- Table 11-5 shows the American Joint Committee on Cancer staging system for carcinoma of the hypopharynx.

## 4. PROGNOSTIC FACTORS

- *T stage:* T stage is the most important prognostic factor determining local control.
- *N stage:* N stage is an important prognostic factor for predicting the distant metastasis and survival.
- *Gender:* Female patients have generally better survival than male.

**TABLE 11-1. SUPRAGLOTTIC LARYNX: CLINICALLY DETECTED NODAL METASTASES (%) ON ADMISSION BY T STAGE**

|    | N0 | N1 | N2-3 |
|----|----|----|------|
| T1 | 61 | 10 | 29   |
| T2 | 58 | 16 | 26   |
| T3 | 36 | 25 | 40   |
| T4 | 41 | 18 | 41   |

*Source:* Compiled from the data of MD Anderson.[3]

## 5. GENERAL MANAGEMENT

- Table 11-6 summarizes the results of different treatment strategies used in laryngeal cancer.

### 5.1. Vocal Cord Carcinoma

#### 5.1.1. Carcinoma in Situ

- Stripping the cord may sometimes control carcinoma *in situ;* however, it is difficult to exclude the possibility of microinvasion in these specimens.
- Recurrence is frequent, and the cord may become thickened and the voice hoarse with repeated stripping.
- We recommend early radiation therapy because most patients with this diagnosis eventually receive this treatment, and earlier use of irradiation means a better chance of preserving a good voice.

#### 5.1.2. Early Vocal Cord Carcinoma

- In most centers, irradiation is the initial treatment for T1 and T2 lesions. Surgery is reserved for salvage after radiation therapy failure.[7-9]

**TABLE 11-2. ELECTIVE NODAL DISSECTION: INCIDENCE OF NODAL METASTASIS BY T CLASSIFICATION AND SITE IN LARYNX CANCER**

| Primary Site | Tx, T1, T2 | T3, T4 | Total |
|---|---|---|---|
| Supraglottic larynx | 31% | 25% | 26% |
| Glottic larynx | 21% | 14% | 16% |

*Source:* Modified from Byers et al. Rationale for elective modified neck dissection. *Head Neck Surg* 1988;10:165.

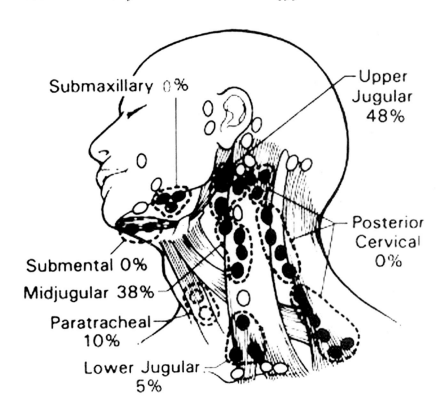

**FIGURE 11-6.** The distribution of pathologically positive neck nodes after elective modified neck dissection in 93 patients with supraglottic laryngeal carcinoma. (Byers RM, Wolf PF, Ballantyne AJ. Rationale for elective modified neck dissection. *Head Neck Surg* 1988;10:163–164, by permission.)

- The local control rate with definitive radiation therapy is about 90% for T1 lesions and 70% to 80% for T2 lesions.
- Although hemilaryngectomy or cordectomy produces comparable cure rates for selected T1 and T2 vocal cord lesions, irradiation is generally preferred.[10]

### 5.1.3. Moderately Advanced Vocal Cord Cancer

- Fixed-cord lesions (T3) can be subdivided into relatively favorable or unfavorable lesions.
- Patients with favorable T3 lesions have disease confined mostly to one side of the larynx, have a good airway, and are reliable for follow-up.
- Patients with unfavorable lesions usually have extensive bilateral disease with a compromised airway and are considered to be in the advanced group.

- Patients with favorable lesions are advised of the alternatives to irradiation with surgical salvage or immediate total laryngectomy.[11] They must be willing to return for follow-up examinations every 4 to 6 weeks for the first year, every 6 to 8 weeks for the second year, every 3 months for the third year, every 6 months for the fourth and fifth years, and annually thereafter.[6]

### 5.1.4. Advanced Vocal Cord Carcinoma

- The mainstay of treatment is total laryngectomy, with or without adjuvant irradiation.
- Indications for postoperative irradiation include close or positive margins, significant subglottic extension ($\geq 1$ cm), cartilage invasion, perineural invasion,

**TABLE 11-3. INCIDENCE AND DISTRIBUTION OF METASTATIC DISEASE IN CLINICALLY NEGATIVE (N−) AND POSITIVE (N+) NECK NODES (IN PERCENTAGE)**

| | Pathologic Nodal Metastasis ||||||||||||
| | Radiologically Enlarged Retropharyngeal Nodes || Level I || Level II || Level III || Level IV || Level V ||
| Clinical presentation | N− | N+ | N− | N+ | N− | N+ | N− | N+ | N− | N+ | N− | N+ |
|---|---|---|---|---|---|---|---|---|---|---|---|---|
| Supraglottic | 0 | 4 | 6 | 2 | 18 | 70 | 18 | 48 | 9 | 17 | 2 | 16 |
| Glottic | — | — | 0 | 9 | 21 | 42 | 29 | 71 | 7 | 24 | 7 | 2 |

*Source:* Modified from Chao KSC, Wippold FJ, Ozyigit G, et al. Determination and delineation of nodal target volumes for head and neck cancer based on the patterns of failure in patients receiving definitive and postoperative IMRT. *Int J Radiat Oncol Biol Phys* 2002;53:1174–1184.

**TABLE 11-4. INCIDENCE OF CONTRALATERAL OR BILATERAL NECK NODE METASTASES BY PRIMARY TUMOR SITE (IN PERCENTAGE)**†

| Tumor Site | cN+, Bilateral | cN+, Contralateral Only | cN−, pN+ Bilateral |
|---|---|---|---|
| Supraglottis | 39% | 2% | 26% |
| Glottis | — | — | 15% |

*Source:* Compiled from Northrop 1972; Bataini 1985; Byers 1988; Woolgar 1999; Buckley 2000.
c, clinical; p, pathologic.

extension of primary tumor into the soft tissues of the neck, multiple positive neck nodes, extracapsular extension, and control of subclinical disease in the opposite neck.[12–14]

### 5.1.5. Surgical Treatment

- One entire cord and as much as one-third of the opposite cord is the maximum cordal involvement suitable for hemilaryngectomy in men.
- Women have a smaller larynx, and usually only one vocal cord may be removed without compromising the airway.
- The maximum subglottic extension is 8 to 9 mm anteriorly and 5 mm posteriorly. These limits are necessary to preserve the integrity of the cricoid.
- Tumor extension to the epiglottis, false cord, or both arytenoids is a contraindication to hemilaryngectomy.

### 5.1.6. Treatment of Recurrence

- Radiation therapy failures may be salvaged by cordectomy, hemilaryngectomy, or total laryngectomy.
- Biller et al. reported a 78% salvage rate by hemilaryngectomy for 18 selected patients in whom irradiation failed.[15] Total laryngectomy was eventually required in two patients.
- The rate of salvage by irradiation for recurrences or new tumors that appear after initial treatment by hemilaryngectomy is about 50%.

## 5.2. Supraglottic Larynx Carcinoma

### 5.2.1. Early and Moderately Advanced Supraglottic Lesions

- Treatment of the primary lesion for the early group is by external-beam irradiation or supraglottic laryngectomy, with or without adjuvant irradiation.
- For early-stage primary lesions with advanced neck disease (N2b or N3), combined treatment is frequently necessary to control the neck disease.[14,16] In these cases, the primary lesion is usually treated by irradiation alone, with surgery added to treat the involved neck site(s). If the same patient were treated with supraglottic laryngectomy, neck dissection, and postoperative irradiation, the portals would unnecessarily cover the primary site and the neck.
- If a patient has early, resectable neck disease (N1 or N2a) and surgery is elected for the primary site, postoperative

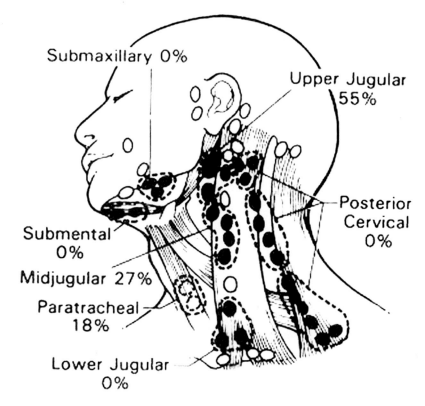

**FIGURE 11-7.** The distribution of pathologically positive neck nodes after elective modified neck dissection in 57 patients with glottic laryngeal carcinoma. (Byers RM, Wolf PF, Ballantyne AJ. Rationale for elective modified neck dissection. *Head Neck Surg* 1988;10:164, by permission.)

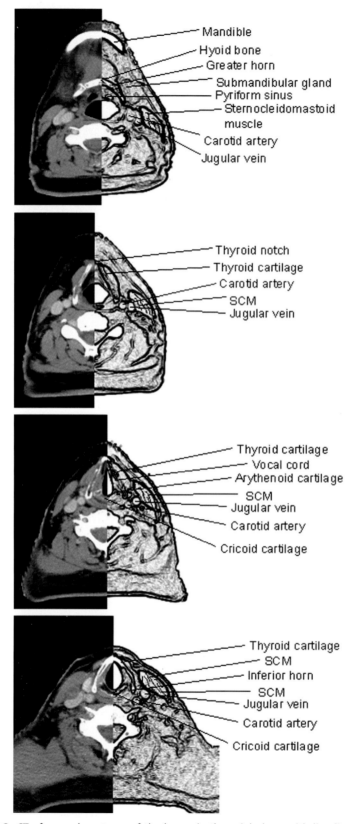

**FIGURE 11-8.** CT of normal anatomy of the larynx in the axial plane with linediagrams corresponding with anatomy seen in the same slice.

*Larynx* **147**

## TABLE 11-5. AJCC CLASSIFICATION FOR CARCINOMA OF THE LARYNX

*Primary Tumor (T)*

| | |
|---|---|
| TX | Primary tumor cannot be assessed |
| T0 | No evidence of primary tumor |
| Tis | Carcinoma *in situ* |

*Supraglottis*

| | |
|---|---|
| T1 | Tumor limited to one subsite of supraglottic with normal vocal cord mobility |
| T2 | Tumor invades mucosa of more than one adjacent subsite of supraglottic or glottis or region outside of supraglottis without fixation of the larynx |
| T3 | Tumor limited to larynx with vocal cord fixation and/or invades any of the following: postcricoid area, preepiglottic tissues |
| T4 | Tumor extends through the thyroid cartilage and/or extends into soft tissues of the neck, thyroid and/or esophagus |

*Glottis*

| | |
|---|---|
| T1 | Tumor limited to vocal cords (may involve anterior or posterior commissures) with normal mobility (T1a = Limited one vocal cord, T2a = Involves both vocal cord) |
| T2 | Tumor extends to supraglottis and/or subglottis, and/or impaired vocal cord mobility |
| T3 | Tumor limited to larynx with vocal cord fixation |
| T4 | Tumor extends through the thyroid cartilage, and/or extends into soft tissues of the neck, thyroid and/or esophagus |

*Regional Lymph Nodes (N)*

| | |
|---|---|
| NX | Regional lymph nodes cannot be assessed |
| N0 | No regional lymph node metastasis |
| N1 | Metastasis in a single ipsilateral lymph node, <3 cm in greatest dimension |
| N2 | Metastasis in a single ipsilateral lymph node, >3 cm but not >6 cm in greatest dimension; in multiple ipsilateral lymph nodes, none >6 cm in greatest dimension; or in bilateral or contralateral lymph nodes, none >6 cm in greatest dimension |
| N2a | Metastasis in a single ipsilateral lymph node >3 cm but not >6 cm in greatest dimension |
| N2b | Metastasis in multiple ipsilateral lymph nodes, none >6 cm in greatest dimension |
| N2c | Metastasis in bilateral or contralateral lymph nodes, none >6 cm in greatest dimension |
| N3 | Metastasis in a lymph node >6 cm in greatest dimension |

*Distant Metastases (M)*

| | |
|---|---|
| MX | Presence of distant metastasis cannot be assessed |
| M0 | No distant metastasis |
| M1 | Distant metastasis |

*Stage Grouping*

| | | | |
|---|---|---|---|
| Stage 0 | Tis | N0 | M0 |
| Stage I | T1 | N0 | M0 |
| Stage II | T2 | N0 | M0 |
| Stage III | T3 | N0 | M0 |
| | T1 | N1 | M0 |
| | T2 | N1 | M0 |
| | T3 | N1 | M0 |
| Stage IVA | T4 | N0 or N1 | M0 |
| | Any T | N2 | M0 |
| Stage IVB | Any T | N3 | M0 |
| Stage IVC | Any T | Any N | M1 |

From Fleming ID, Cooper JS, Henson DE, et al., eds. *AJCC cancer staging manual,* 5th ed. Philadelphia: Lippincott-Raven, 1997:45–46, by permission.

irradiation is added only because of unexpected findings (positive margins, multiple positive nodes, extracapsular extension).

### 5.2.2. Advanced Supraglottic Lesions

- The surgical alternative for these lesions is total laryngectomy.

- Selected advanced lesions, especially those that are mainly exophytic, may be treated by radiation therapy, with total laryngectomy reserved for irradiation failures.
- Borderline lesions are given a trial of irradiation (45 to 50 Gy). If the response is good, irradiation is continued for cure; if the response is unsatisfactory, radiation therapy is stopped, and total laryngectomy is performed 4 to 6 weeks later.

## TABLE 11-6. LARNYNGEAL STUDIES WITH SURGERY OR RADIOTHERAPY

| Author | No. of Patients | Site | Stage | Therapy | Outcome |
|---|---|---|---|---|---|
| Mittal et al.[23] | 98 | Glottic | T3–T4 | Surgery alone ± adjuvant RT | 75% LC, 50% OS |
| Yuen et al.[24] | 155 | Glottic | T3 | Surgery alone | 82% LC |
| Lundgren et al.[25] | 141 | Glottic | | RT alone | 51% OS |
| Meredith et al.[26] | 68 | Glottic | T3 | RT alone | 64% DSS |
| Razak et al.[27] | 128 | Glottic | T3–T4 | Total laryngectomy | 53% LC, 63% OS |
| Mendenhall et al.[28] | 65 | Glottic | | Surgery alone ± adjuvant RT | 75% LC, 71% DSS |
| Simpson et al.[29] | 38 | Glottic | T3N0 | RT alone | 57% OS |
| Simpson et al.[29] | 36 | Glottic | T3N0 | Laryngectomy | 52% OS |
| Foote et al.[30] | 81 | Glottic | T3 | Surgery alone | 74% LC, 78% DSS |
| Kligerman et al.[31] | 76 | Glottic | T3–T4N0 | Surgery alone ± adjuvant RT | 72% LC, 52% OS |
| Hao et al.[32] | 114 | Glottic | T3 | Total laryngectomy | 11% 2-year local recurrence rate |
| Bryant et al.[33] | 42 | Glottic | T3N0 | Surgery alone | 69% LC |
| Kowalski et al.[34] | 45 | Glottic | T3N0-1 | RT alone | 59% LC |
| Mendenhall et al.[35] | 75 | Glottic | T3 | RT alone | 63% LC, 78% DSS |
| Nyugen et al.[36] | 116 | Larynx | Stage III | Surgery and adjuvant RT | 76% LC, 68% OS |
| Parsons et al.[37] | 43 | Larynx | T4 | RT alone | 52% LC, 37% OS |
| Mancuso et al.[38] | 63 | Supraglottic | T1–T4 | RT alone | 69% LC |
| MacKenzie et al.[39] | 82 | Larynx | T2N+ | RT alone | 54% OS, 65% ultimate LC (T3–4) |

DSS, disease-specific survival; LC, local control; RT, Radiotherapy.

- Neoadjuvant chemotherapy followed by radiation therapy for responders is a reasonable alternative for selected patients.
- Supraglottic laryngectomy is voice-sparing surgery that can be used successfully for selected lesions involving the epiglottis, a single arytenoid, the aryepiglottic fold, or the false vocal cord.
- Extension of the tumor to the true vocal cord, anterior commissure, or both arytenoids; fixation of the vocal cord; or thyroid or cricoid cartilage invasion precludes supraglottic laryngectomy.
- Supraglottic laryngectomy may be extended to include the base of the tongue if one lingual artery is preserved.
- All patients have difficulty swallowing, with a tendency to aspirate immediately after surgery, but almost all learn to swallow again in a short time. Motivation and the amount of tissue removed are key factors in learning to swallow again.
- Preoperatively, adequate pulmonary reserve is evaluated by blood gas determinations, function tests, chest roentgenography, and a work test involving walking a patient up two flights of stairs to determine tolerance to pulmonary stress.
- Voice quality is generally normal after supraglottic laryngectomy.
- Radiation technique and dose are similar to those for glottic tumors; however, because of richer lymphatics in the supraglottic region, regional lymphatics must be treated in tumors greater than T2 size.[6]
- The addition of a neck dissection usually increases the risk of temporary lymphedema; however, it is preferable in terms of tumor control and complications to the higher doses of irradiation required to control large neck nodes.[16]

### 5.2.3. Postoperative Treatment

- Irradiation is added for close or positive margins, invasion of soft tissues of the neck, significant subglottic extension ($\geq 1$ cm), thyroid cartilage invasion, multiple positive nodes, and extracapsular extension.
- The postoperative irradiation dose as a function of known residual disease is as follows: negative margins, 60 Gy in 30 fractions; microscopically positive margins, 66 Gy in 33 fractions; and gross residual disease, 70 Gy in 35 fractions.
- If there is subglottic extension, the dose to the stoma is boosted with electrons (usually 10 to 14 MeV) for an additional 10 Gy in five fractions.

## 6. FUNCTIONAL PRESERVATION

### 6.1. Comparison of Surgery and Radiation Therapy

- The 659 patients with stage I (T1N0M0) glottic carcinoma treated with curative intent at Washington University in St. Louis were subdivided into four groups:[12] 90 patients received low-dose irradiation (mean dose, 58 Gy; range, 55 to 65 Gy; daily fractionation, 1.5 to 1.8 Gy).[17] One hundred four patients received high-dose irradiation (mean dose, 66.5 Gy; range, 65 to 70 Gy; daily fractionation, 2 to 2.25 Gy).[18] Four hundred four patients underwent conservation surgery[15]; 61 patients had endoscopic resection. T1A (85%) and T1B (15%) disease was equally distributed among the groups.

- No significant difference in the 5-year cause-specific survival rate was observed among the four therapeutic groups for T1 tumors ($p = .68$). Actuarial survival was significantly decreased in the low-dose radiation therapy group as compared with the other three therapeutic groups ($p = .04$). Initial local control was poorer for the endoscopic (77%) and low-dose irradiation (78%) groups than it was for the high-dose irradiation (89%) and conservation surgery (92%) groups ($p = .02$), but significant differences were not found for ultimate local control following salvage treatment. Unaided laryngeal voice preservation was similar for high-dose radiation therapy (89%), conservation surgery (93%), and endoscopic resection (90%), but significantly poorer for low-dose irradiation (80%; $p = .02$).[19]
- Among 134 patients with stage II glottic carcinomas treated with curative intent and function preservation, 47 patients were treated with low-dose radiation therapy (median dose, 58.5 Gy at 1.5- to 1.8-Gy daily fractions), 16 patients with high-dose irradiation (67.5 to 70 Gy) at higher daily fractionation doses (2 to 2.25 Gy), and 71 patients underwent conservation surgery. There were no statistical differences in local control, voice preservation, and 5-year actuarial and disease-specific cure rates between conservation surgery and high-dose irradiation ($p = .89$). Patients treated with low-dose irradiation had statistically lower local control, 5-year survival, and voice preservation ($p = .014$).[20]

## 6.2. Chemoradiotherapy for Laryngeal Preservation in Advanced Tumors

- A metaanalysis included patients with locally advanced laryngeal or hypopharyngeal carcinoma and compared radical surgery plus radiation therapy with a neoadjuvant combination of cisplatin and 5-fluorouracil followed by irradiation in responders or radical surgery plus radiation therapy in nonresponders. Six hundred two patients were identified, with a median follow-up of 5.7 years. The pooled hazard ratio (1.19, 0.97–1.46) showed a nonsignificant trend ($p .1$) in favor of the control group, corresponding to an absolute negative effect in the chemotherapy arm that reduced survival at 5 years by 6% (from 45% to 39%). Adjustment for nodal status (N0/N1–3) or tumor subsite (glottic or subglottic versus supraglottic versus hypopharynx) led to similar results. This metaanalysis suggests that, because of the nonsignificant negative effect of chemotherapy on the organ-preservation strategy, this procedure must remain investigational.[21]
- Table 11-7 summarizes the results of the several randomized larynx preservation trials.

## 7. INTENSITY MODULATED RADIATION THERAPY IN LARYNGEAL CARCINOMAS

### 7.1. Target Volume Determination

- If chemotherapy was delivered before radiation, the targets should be outlined on the planning CT according to their prechemotherapy extent.
- Lymph node groups at risk in the larynx include the following:
  a. Submandibular nodes (surgical level I): N2c cases, especially when level II node is involved
  b. Upper deep jugular (junctional, parapharyngeal) nodes: all cases (at the neck side ipsilateral to the primary tumor)
  c. Subdigastric (jugulodigastric) nodes, midjugular, lower neck, and supraclavicular nodes (levels II through IV): all cases, bilaterally
  d. Posterior cervical nodes (level V): all cases, at the neck side where there is evidence of jugular nodal metastases
  e. Retropharyngeal nodes: if there is evidence of metastasis
- Table 11-8 summarizes the target volume specification for definitive and postoperative IMRT in laryngeal cancer.

## TABLE 11-7. RANDOMIZED LARYNX PRESERVATION TRIALS

| Trial | No. of Patients | Site | Stage | Induction Chemotherapy | Local Treatments | Survival | Laryngeal Preservation |
|---|---|---|---|---|---|---|---|
| VALCSG | 332 | Larynx (37% G, 63% SG) | III, IV | 2–3 CF (98% CR, PR) | RT (if PR) ± salvage surgery | 52% | 31% |
| | | | | | Total laryngectomy + postop RT | 57% | |
| GETTEC | 68 | Larynx (41% G, 28% TG) | T3 | 2–3 CF (42% CR, PR) | RT (if PR) ± salvage surgery | 69% | 20% |
| | | | | | Total laryngectomy + postop RT | 84% | |
| EORTC | 202 | HP/Larynx (78% HP, 22% LE) | II–IV | 2–3 CF (54% CR, PR) | RT (if PR) ± salvage surgery | 57% | 42% |
| | | | | | Total laryngectomy + postop RT | 43% | |

CF, cisplatin + 5-fluorouracil; CR, complete response; EORTC, European Organization for Research and Treatment of Cancer; G, glottic; GETTEC, Groupe d'Etudes des Tumeurs de la Tete et du Cou; HP, hypopharynx; PR, partial response; SG, supraglottic; TG, transglottic; VALCSG, Veterans Administration Laryngeal Cancer Study Group.

## TABLE 11-8. TARGET VOLUME SPECIFICATION FOR DEFINITIVE AND POSTOPERATIVE IMRT IN LARYNX CANCER

| Target | Definitive IMRT | High-Risk Postoperative IMRT | Intermediate-Risk Postoperative IMRT |
|---|---|---|---|
| CTV1 | Soft-tissue and nodal regions adjacent to the GTV | Surgical bed with soft-tissue involvement or nodal region with extracapsular involvement | Surgical bed without soft-tissue involvement or nodal region without capsular extension |
| CTV2 | Elective nodal regions* | Elective nodal regions* | Elective nodal regions* |

*Source:* Modified from Chao KSC, Wippold FJ, Ozyigit G, et al. Determination and delineation of nodal target volumes for head and neck cancer based on the patterns of failure in patients receiving definitive and postoperative IMRT. *Int J Radiat Oncol Biol Phys* 2002;53:1174–1184.
*See Table 11-10.

- Table 11-9 summarizes the suggested target volume determination for laryngeal carcinoma.

## 7.2. Target Volume Delineation

- In patients receiving postoperative IMRT, CTV1 encompasses residual tumor and the region adjacent to it but not directly involved by the tumor, the surgical bed with soft-tissue invasion by the tumor, or extracapsular extension by metastatic neck nodes. CTV2 includes primarily the prophylactically treated neck.
- In patients receiving definitive IMRT, CTV1 encompasses gross tumor (primary and enlarged nodes) and the region adjacent to it but not directly involved. CTV2 includes primarily the prophylactically treated neck.
- Figure 11-9 shows CTV1 and CTV2 delineation in a patient with pathologic T2N2bM0 squamous cell carcinoma of larynx receiving postoperative IMRT.
- Figure 11-10 shows CTV1 and CTV2 delineation in a patient with pathologic T2N0 squamous cell carcinoma of a glottic larynx receiving definitive IMRT.

## 7.3. Normal Tissue Delineation

- Figure 5-16 shows normal tissue delineation.

## TABLE 11-9. SUGGESTED TARGET VOLUME DETERMINATION FOR LARYNX IMRT

| Tumor Site | Clinical Presentation | CTV1 | CTV2 |
|---|---|---|---|
| Larynx[†] | T1–2N0 | P | IN + CN (II–IV) |
| | T3–4N+* | P + IN (II–IV) | CN (II–IV) |
| | N2c | P + IN + CN (I–V) | |

*Source:* Modified from Chao KSC, Wippold FJ, Ozyigit G, et al. Determination and delineation of nodal target volumes for head and neck cancer based on the patterns of failure in patients receiving definitive and postoperative IMRT. *Int J Radiat Oncol Biol Phys* 2002 *(in press).*
BOT, base of tongue; CN, contralateral neck nodes (level); FOM, floor of mouth; IN, ipsilateral neck nodes (level); P, gross tumor with margins for definition IMRT or surgical bed for post-op IMRT; RMT, retromolar trigone; RPNL, retropharyngeal lymph nodes.
*N+ = N1–3 except N2c.
[†]T1–2 carcinoma of the true vocal cord excluded.

## 7.4. Suggested Target and Normal Tissue Doses

- Table 4-9 gives the Washington University guideline for clinical target volume dose specification with biologic equivalent dose correction and normal tissue tolerance for IMRT.

## 7.5. IMRT Treatment Results

- Following these guidelines, seven supraglottic larynx carcinoma patients were treated with IMRT between February 1997 and December 2000 at Washington University. All patients were treated with postoperative IMRT. The T stages were two T2, three T3, and two T4. The N stages were three N0, one N1, and three N2 (AJCC staging; two stage III, and five stage IV). Median follow-up time was 22 months (range, 14 to 26 months). We observed one locoregional recurrence. This patient subsequently developed distant metastasis and died of disease. We observed no additional distant metastasis. All other patients are alive with no evidence of disease, except one who died of intercurrent disease.
- Figure 11-11 shows an example of IMRT dose distribution of a patient receiving postoperative IMRT for a T3N2b laryngeal cancer.
- A G-tube was placed in three patients during the course of IMRT. We observed no grade 3 or 4 late complications in our patients treated with IMRT. Grade 1 xerostomia was observed in three patients and grade 2 xerostomia occurred in one patient as late sequelae.

## 8. SEQUELAE OF TREATMENT

## 8.1. Surgical Sequelae

- Postoperative complications and sequelae of hemilaryngectomy include chondritis, wound slough, inadequate glottic closure, and anterior commissure webs.[22]
- Complications associated with supraglottic laryngectomy and total laryngectomy for supraglottic carcinomas include fistula (8%), carotid artery exposure or blowout

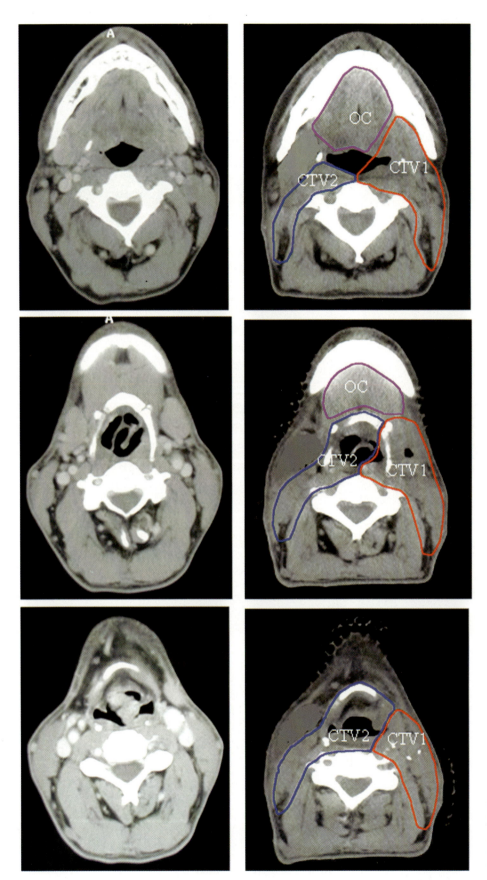

**FIGURE 11-9.** Clinical target volume (CTV) delineation in a patient with a T2N2b supraglottic larynx carcinoma receiving postoperative IMRT. CTV1, red line; CTV2, dark blue line; OC, oral cavity (magenta line).

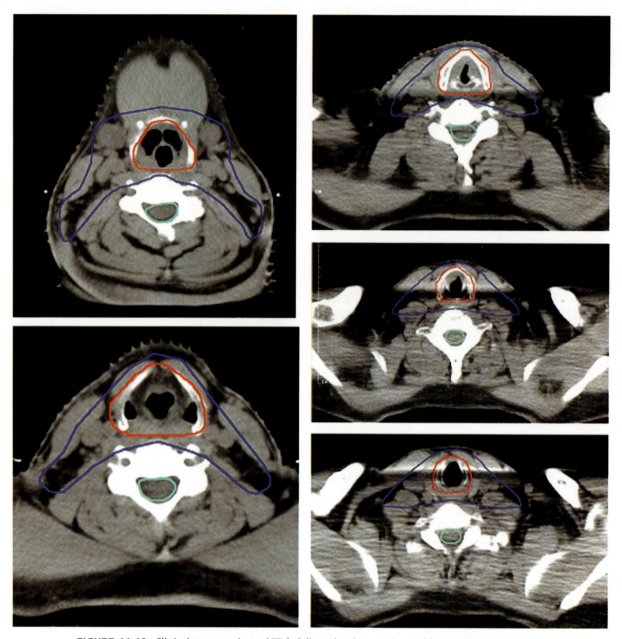

**FIGURE 11-10.** Clinical target volume (CTV) delineation in a patient with a T2N0 glottic larynx cancer receiving definitive IMRT. CTV1, red line; CTV2, dark blue line; Spinal cord, green line.

(3% to 5%), infection or wound sloughing (3% to 7%), and fatal complications (3%).[22]vspace*-2.5pt

### 8.2. Radiation Therapy Sequelae

- During the first 2 to 3 weeks, the voice may improve as the tumor regresses, but it generally becomes hoarse again because of radiation-induced changes, even though the tumor continues to regress.
- The voice begins to improve approximately 3 weeks after completion of treatment, usually reaching a plateau in 2 to 3 months.
- Edema of the larynx is the most common sequela after irradiation for glottic or supraglottic lesions. It may be accentuated by radical neck dissection and may require 6 to 12 months to subside.
- Soft-tissue necrosis leading to chondritis occurs in fewer than 1% of patients, usually in those who continue to smoke.
- Corticosteroids such as dexamethasone have been used to reduce radiation-induced edema after recurrence has been ruled out by biopsy. If ulceration and pain occur, administration of an antibiotic, such as tetracycline, may help.

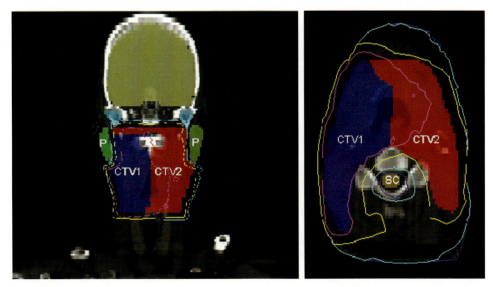

**FIGURE 11-11.** IMRT dose distribution of a patient with T3N2b supraglottic laryngeal carcinoma receiving postoperative IMRT. CTV, clinical target volume; CTV1, dark blue area; CTV2, red area; P, parotid gland; SC, spinal cord. Pink line, 66 Gy; yellow line, 50 Gy; aqua line, 30 Gy; dark blue, 20 Gy.

- It is unusual for patients to require a tracheotomy before irradiation, unless severe lymphedema develops at the time of direct laryngoscopy and biopsy. In patients who have recovered from direct laryngoscopy and biopsy without obstruction, a tracheotomy has rarely been required during a fractionated course of irradiation.
- Patients treated twice a day with 1.2-Gy fractions (continuous-course technique) to total doses of 74 to 76.8 Gy usually have more brisk acute reactions than those treated once a day with 2-Gy fractions.[6] Approximately 10% treated with twice-a-day irradiation require nasogastric feeding tubes because of difficulty in swallowing.

## REFERENCES

1. Clemente CD. *Anatomy: a regional atlas of the human body.* Philadelphia: Lea & Febiger, 1975.
2. Wynder EL. The epidemiology of cancers of the upper alimentary and upper respiratory tracts. *Laryngoscope* 1978;88[Suppl 8]: 50–51.
3. Lindberg R. Distribution of cervical lymph node metastases from squamous cell carcinoma of the upper respiratory and digestive tracts. *Cancer* 1972;29:1446–1449.
4. Fletcher GH. Elective irradiation of subclinical disease in cancers of the head and neck. *Cancer* 1972;29:1450–1454.
5. Ogura JH, Biller HF, Wette R. Elective neck dissection for pharyngeal and laryngeal cancers: an evaluation. *Ann Otol Rhinol Laryngol* 1971;80:646–651.
6. Mendenhall WM, Parsons JT, Mancuso AA, et al. Larynx. In: Brady LW, ed. *Principles and practice of radiation oncology,* 3rd ed. Philadelphia: Lippincott-Raven, 1998:1069–1093.
7. Mendenhall W, Parsons J, Stringer S, et al. T1–T2 vocal cord carcinomas: a basic for comparing the results of the radiotherapy and surgery. *Head Neck Surg* 1988;10:373–377.
8. Fein DA, Mendenhall WM, Parsons JT, et al. T1–T2 squamous cell carcinoma of the glottic larynx treated with radiotherapy: a multivariate analysis of variables potentially influencing local control. *Int J Radiat Oncol Biol Phys* 1993;25:605–611.
9. Mendenhall WM, Parsons JT, Stringer SP, et al. Management of Tis, T1, and T2 squamous cell carcinoma of the glottic larynx. *Am J Otolaryngol* 1994;15:250–257.
10. O'Sullivan B, Mackillop W, Gilbert R, et al. Controversies in the management of laryngeal cancer: results of an international survey of patterns of care. *Radiother Oncol* 1994;31:23–32.
11. Parsons JT, Mendenhall WM, Mancuso AA, et al. Twice-a-day radiotherapy for T3 squamous cell carcinoma of the glottic larynx. *Head Neck* 1989;11:123–128.
12. Amdur RJ, Parsons JT, Mendenhall WM, et al. Postoperative irradiation for squamous cell carcinoma of the head and neck: an analysis of treatment results and complications. *Int J Radiat Oncol Biol Phys* 1989;16:25–36.
13. Huang DT, Johnson CR, Schmidt-Ullrich R, et al. Postoperative radiotherapy in head and neck carcinoma with extracapsular lymph node extension and/or positive resection margins: a comparative study. *Int J Radiat Oncol Biol Phys* 1992;23:737–742.
14. Mendenhall WM, Parsons JT, Buatti JM, et al. Advances in radiotherapy for head and neck cancer. *Semin Surg Oncol* 1995;11:256–264.
15. Biller HF, Barnhill FR, Jr., Ogura JH, et al. Hemilaryngectomy following radiation failure for carcinoma of the vocal cords. *Laryngoscope* 1968;80:249–253.
16. Mendenhall WM, Parsons JT. Squamous cell carcinoma of the head and neck treated with irradiation: management of the neck. *Semin Radiat Oncol* 1992;2:163–170.
17. Beahrs OH, Henson DE, Hutter RVP, et al. *Manual for staging of cancer,* 4th ed. Philadelphia: JB Lippincott, 1992.
18. Archer CR, Yeager VL, Herbold DR. Improved diagnostic accuracy in laryngeal cancer using a new classification based on computed tomography. *Cancer* 1984;53:44–57.
19. Spector JG, Sessions DG, Chao KS, et al. Stage I (T1 N0 M0) squamous cell carcinoma of the laryngeal glottis: therapeutic results and voice preservation. *Head Neck* 1999;21:707–717.

20. Spector JG, Sessions DG, Chao KS, et al. Management of stage II (T2N0M0) glottic carcinoma by radiotherapy and conservation surgery. *Head Neck* 1999;21:116–123.

21. Pignon J, Bourhis J, Domenge C, et al. Chemotherapy added to locoregional treatment for head and neck squamous-cell carcinoma: three meta-analyses of updated individual data. *Lancet* 2000;18:949–955.

22. Gall AM, Sessions DG, Ogura JH. Complications following surgery for cancer of the larynx and hypopharynx. *Cancer* 1977;39:624–631.

23. Mittal B, Marks JE, Ogura JH. Transglottic carcinoma. *Cancer* 1984;53:151–161.

24. Yuen A, Medina JE, Goepfert H, et al. Management of stage T3 and T4 glottic carcinomas. *Am J Surgery* 1984;148:467–472.

25. Lundgren JA, Gilbert RW, van Nostrand AW, et al. T3N0M0 glottic carcinoma: a failure analysis. *Clin Otolaryngol* 1988;13:455–465.

26. Meredith AP, Randall CJ, Shaw HJ. Advanced laryngeal cancer: a management perspective. *J Laryngol Otol* 1987;101:1046–1054.

27. Razack MS, Maipang T, Sako K, et al. Management of advanced glottic carcinomas. *Am J Surg* 1989;158:318–320.

28. Mendenhall WM, Parsons JT, Stringer SP, et al. Stage T3 squamous cell carcinoma of the glottic larynx: a comparison of laryngectomy and irradiation. *Int J Radiat Oncol Biol Phys* 1992;23:725–732.

29. Simpson D, Robertson AG, Lamont D. A comparison of radiotherapy and surgery as primary treatment in the management of T3 N0 M0 glottic tumours. *J Laryngol Otol* 1993;107:912–915.

30. Foote RL, Olsen KD, Buskirk SJ, et al. Laryngectomy alone for T3 glottic cancer. *Head Neck* 1994;16:406–412.

31. Kligerman J, Olivatto LO, Lima RA, et al. Elective neck dissection in the treatment of T3/T4 N0 squamous cell carcinoma of the larynx. *Am J Surg* 1995;170:436–439.

32. Hao SP, Myers EN, Johnson JT. T3 glottic carcinoma revisited: transglottic vs pure glottic carcinoma. *Arch Otolaryngol Head Neck Surg* 1995;121:166–170.

33. Bryant GP, Poulsen MG, Tripcony L, et al. Treatment decisions in T3N0M0 glottic carcinoma. *Int J Radiat Oncol Biol Phys* 1995;31:285–293.

34. Kowalski LP, Batista MB, Santos CR, et al. Prognostic factors in T3, N0-1 glottic and transglottic carcinoma: a multifactorial study of 221 cases treated by surgery or radiotherapy. *Arch Otolaryngol Head Neck Surg* 1996;122:77–82.

35. Mendenhall WM, Parsons JT, Mancuso AA, et al. Definitive radiotherapy for T3 squamous cell carcinoma of the glottic larynx. *J Clin Oncol* 1997;15:2394–2402.

36. Nguyen TD, Malissard L, Theobald S, et al. Advanced carcinoma of the larynx: results of surgery and radiotherapy without induction chemotherapy (1980–1985): a multivariate analysis. *Int J Radiat Oncol Biol Phys* 1996;36:1013–1018.

37. Parsons JT, Mendenhall WM, Stringer SP, et al. T4 laryngeal carcinoma: radiotherapy alone with surgery reserved for salvage. *Int J Radiat Oncol Biol Phys* 1998;40:549–552.

38. Mancuso AA, Mukherji SK, Schmalfuss I, et al. Preradiotherapy computed tomography as a predictor of local control in supraglottic carcinoma. *J Clin Oncol* 1999;17:631–637.

39. MacKenzie RG, Franssen E, Balogh JM, et al. Comparing treatment outcomes of radiotherapy and surgery in locally advanced carcinoma of the larynx: a comparison limited to patients eligible for surgery. *Int J Radiat Biol* 2000;47:64–74.

# 12

# NECK NODE METASTASIS OF UNKNOWN PRIMARY

**GOKHAN OZYIGIT**
**K.S. CLIFFORD CHAO**

## 1. INTRODUCTION

- Neck node metastasis of unknown primary makes up 1% to 2% of head and neck malignancies. Jugulodigastric and mid-jugular lymph nodes are the most frequent sites.[1]
- The possible site of origin can be estimated from the histology of the neck node. But the biopsy often reveals a poorly differentiated neoplasm. Lymphoma should be excluded by proper immunohistochemical staining.
- Figure 12-1 shows the site of presentation and the nodal distribution for 69 unknown primary carcinoma patients. A solitary upper jugular chain is the most common site, since most head and neck cancer spreads first to this area. This metastasis site is very uncommon for tumors below the clavicle.[1]
- The mass between the angle of the mandible and the tip of the mastoid suggests origin in the nasopharynx, oropharynx, parotid, and occasionally malignant melanoma or other skin cancer.
- The oral cavity, larynx, and hypopharynx should be included as likely sites for the mass in the subdigastric region.
- Bilateral upper neck nodes usually originate from nasopharynx, base of tongue, soft palate, supraglottic larynx, and pyriform sinus.
- A solitary submandibular mass suggests a primary site of origin in the oral cavity, lip, nasal vestibule, or a primary submandibular salivary gland tumor. A solitary submental node is rare.
- A mass in the mid-neck region suggests a primary site from the larynx, hypopharynx, or less commonly, the thyroid, cervical esophagus, or tumor originating below the clavicle.
- The solitary lower neck mass is commonly metastatic from the chest or abdomen. A solitary spinal accessory mass suggests a nasopharyngeal site. Squamous cell carcinoma in the parotid lymph nodes is always from a skin cancer or parotid gland origin.

## 2. DIAGNOSIS AND STAGING SYSTEM

- Physical examination and assessment under anesthesia conducted by an experienced otolaryngologist detect primary site in more than 50% of patients with cervical lymph node metastasis.[1,2] In the absence of physical or radiographic suspicion, panendoscopy with biopsies yield a 17% detection rate.[3]
- Mendenhall et al. reported that the sites of primary tumor found through this process were at the tonsillar fossa and base of the tongue in 82% of patients. Repeat panendoscopy did not appear to increase the detection rate.[3]

### 2.1. Imaging

- Repeated examinations and contrast-enhanced CT or MRI scans are essential to finding primary lesion. CT or MRI to look for a possible primary site follows a diagnosis of squamous cell carcinoma. If the biopsy is not definitive, CT or MRI may redirect the work-up.
- The CT or MRI examination should be done with at least 3-mm sections from the nasopharynx to the entire neck. MRI is used as a supplement for focused evaluation of suspicious regions but not necessarily positive on CT or when CT is normal.
- With negative routine clinical examination and CT, positron emission tomography detects 5% to 25% of patients, whereas ipsilateral tonsillectomy discovered carcinoma in about 25% of patients.[1] Laser-induced fluorescence imaging with panendoscopy and directed biopsies showed encouraging results but needs further investigation. Positron emission tomography has an overall staging accuracy of 69%.[1]

### 2.2. Staging

- Table 12-1 shows the American Joint Committee on Cancer staging system for carcinoma of the unknown primary.

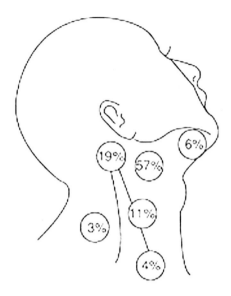

**FIGURE 12-1.** Site of presentation in unknown primary head and neck cancer treated for cure—69 cases (University of Florida data). (Million RR, Cassisi NJ, Mancuso AA. The unknown primary. In: Million RR, Cassisi NJ, *Management of head and neck cancer: a multidisciplinary approach,* 2nd ed. Philadelphia: JB Lippincott, 1994:312, by permission.)

## 3. GENERAL MANAGEMENT

### 3.1. Surgical Management

- Data of surgery alone revealed a median nodal recurrence rate of around 34% and a 5-year overall survival rate of approximately 66%.[4–7] The crude mucosal carcinoma emergence rate was about 25% (30 of 121 patients). These data suggested that selected patients, especially those with pathologic N1 disease with no extracapsular extension, can be treated adequately with surgery alone.[6]

### 3.2. Irradiation Alone

- Grau et al. reported a group of 213 patients treated with radiation alone. The 5-year actuarial mucosal carcinoma emergence rate was 16%, nodal relapse rate was 50%, and survival rate was 37%. But it should be noted that radiation-alone series have more unfavorable prognostic factors.[4]

### 3.3. Surgery and Irradiation

- Colletier et al. reported a series of 136 patients who received radiotherapy after nodal excision or neck dissection. The mucosal carcinoma emergence rate was 10%,

**TABLE 12-1. AMERICAN JOINT COMMITTEE STAGING SYSTEM FOR CANCERS OF THE UNKNOWN PRIMARY**[*]

| | *Primary Tumor (T)* |
|---|---|
| TX | Primary tumor cannot be assessed |
| | *Regional Lymph Nodes (N)* |
| NX | Regional lymph nodes cannot be assessed |
| N0 | No regional lymph node metastasis |
| N1 | Metastasis in a single ipsilateral lymph node, <3 cm in greatest dimension |
| N2 | Metastasis in a single ipsilateral lymph node, >3 cm but not >6 cm in greatest dimension; or in multiple ipsilateral lymph nodes, none >6 cm in greatest dimension; or in bilateral or contralateral lymph nodes, none >6 cm in greatest dimension |
| N2a | Metastasis in a single ipsilateral lymph node, >3 cm but not >6 cm in greatest dimension |
| N2b | Metastasis in multiple ipsilateral lymph nodes, none >6 cm in greatest dimension |
| N2c | Metastasis in bilateral or contralateral lymph nodes, none >6 cm in greatest dimension |
| N3 | Metastasis in a lymph node >6 cm in greatest dimension |
| | *Distant Metastasis (M)* |
| MX | Distant metastasis cannot be assessed |
| M0 | No distant metastasis |
| M1 | Distant metastasis |

*Source:* From Fleming ID, Cooper JS, Henson DE, et al., eds. *AJCC cancer staging manual,* 5th ed. Philadelphia: Lippincott-Raven Publishers, 1997:31–39; with permission.
[*]There is no Roman numeral classification of AJCC for neck node metastasis of unknown primary cancer.

the nodal failure rate was 9%, and the 5-year overall survival rate was 60%. The data from six earlier series are consistent with these findings.[8]

### 3.4. Radiotherapy to Ipsilateral Neck

- Weir et al. compared 85 patients treated with involved nodal regions with 59 patients irradiated to bilateral neck and putative primary sites. Mucosal primary tumors emerged in 7% of patients receiving involved nodal field irradiation compared with 1.7% in those with the second group. In multivariant analysis, no difference in survival or cause-specific survival was found between these groups.[9]
- Similarly, Marcial-Vega et al. did not show a significant difference of portal volume on mucosal emergence rate and 5-year overall survival in a study of 80 patients.[10]
- In the series of Grau et al., 26 patients received ipsilateral neck radiation. In multivariant analysis, there was no significant difference in the rates of mucosal emergence, nodal failure, disease-specific survival, and overall survival compared with bilateral neck radiation. However, combining all relapses above the clavicle unilateral neck radiation had a relative risk of 1.9 ($p = .05$) compared with bilateral neck radiation.[4]
- Table 12-2 summarizes the results of comprehensive and limited radiotherapy.

## TABLE 12-2. RESULTS OF COMPREHENSIVE AND LIMITED RADIOTHERAPY*

| | Unilateral Radiotherapy (Range) | Comprehensive Radiotherapy (Range) |
|---|---|---|
| Medial Mucosal emergence rate | 8% (5–44) | 9.5% (2–13) |
| Median neck relapse rate | 51.5% (31–63) | 19% (8–49) |
| Median distant metastasis rate | 38% | 19% (11–23) |
| Median 5-year overall survival rate | 36.5% (22–41) | 50% (34–63) |

*Source:* Modified from Nieder et al. Cervical lymph node metastases from occult squamous cell carcinoma: cut down a tree to get an apple? *Int Radiat Oncol Biol Phys* 2001;50,731.
*Comprehensive = Irradiation of bilateral neck nodes plus the pharyngeal axis; limited = Ipsilateral cervical irradiation.

## 3.5. Chemotherapy

- No data exist to support the benefit of chemotherapy.

## 4. INTENSITY MODULATED RADIATION THERAPY IN NECK NODE METASTASIS OF UNKNOWN PRIMARY CARCINOMAS

### 4.1. Target Volume Determination

- Table 12-3 summarizes the target volume specification for postoperative IMRT in unknown primary cancer.
- Table 12-4 summarizes suggested target volume determination for unknown primary carcinoma.

### 4.2. Target Volume Delineation

- In patients receiving postoperative IMRT, CTV1 encompasses residual tumor and the region adjacent to it but not directly involved by the tumor, the surgical bed with soft-tissue invasion by the tumor, or extracapsular extension

## TABLE 12-3. TARGET VOLUME SPECIFICATION FOR POSTOPERATIVE IMRT IN UNKNOWN PRIMARY CANCER

| Target | High-Risk Postoperative IMRT | Intermediate-Risk Postoperative IMRT |
|---|---|---|
| CTV1 | Surgical bed of nodal region with extracapsular involvement | Surgical bed of nodal region without capsular extension |
| CTV2 | Elective nodal regions (I, II, III, IV, V)* | Elective nodal regions (I, II, III, IV, V)* |

*N0 include levels II, III, IV, and retropharyngeal nodes. N1 include levels Ib, II, III, IV, and retropharyngeal nodes. N2–3 include levels Ib, II, III, IV, V, and retropharyngeal nodes.

## TABLE 12-4. SUGGESTED TARGET VOLUME DETERMINATION FOR UNKNOWN PRIMARY CARCINOMA IMRT

| Tumor Site | Clinical Presentation | CTV1 | CTV2 |
|---|---|---|---|
| Unknown primary | TXN+* N2c | IN (I–V) IN + CN (I–V) | CN (I–V) ± M ± M |

CN, contralateral neck nodes; IN, ipsilateral neck nodes; ±M, treating mucosal area at physician's discretion.
*N+, N1–3 except N2c.

by metastatic neck nodes. CTV2 includes primarily the prophylactically treated neck.

- Figure 12-2 shows CTV1 and CTV2 delineation in a patient with a medically inoperable TXN2M0 squamous cell carcinoma of unknown primary receiving definitive IMRT.

### 4.3. Normal Tissue Delineation

- Figure 5-16 shows normal tissue delineation.

### 4.4. Suggested Target and Normal Tissue Doses

- Table 4-9 shows the Washington University guideline for clinical target volume dose specification with biologic equivalent dose correction and normal tissue tolerance for IMRT.

### 4.5. IMRT Treatment Results

- Following these guidelines, nine patients with unknown primary carcinoma were treated with IMRT between February 1997 and December 2000 at Washington University. The N stages were N1 in one, N2 in seven, and N3 in one. Median follow-up time was 34 months (range, 10 to 55 months). We observed one locoregional recurrence, and none of the patients developed lung metastasis. All patients are alive except for one who died of recurrent disease.
- A G-tube was placed in one patient during the course of IMRT. We observed no grade 3 or 4 late complications in our patients treated with IMRT. Grade 1 xerostomia was observed in five patients, and grade 2 xerostomia developed in one patient as a late sequela.

## 5. COMPLICATIONS

- The main radiation therapy complication is marked xerostomia. Bone exposure is a rare complication after radiotherapy. Lympedema of the neck occurs more often in patients who underwent neck dissection.

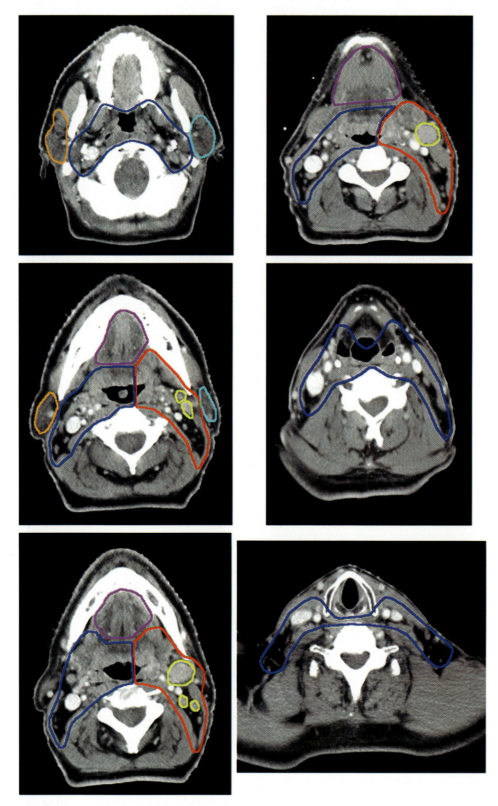

**FIGURE 12-2.** Clinical target volume (CTV) delineation in a patient with TXN2b squamous cell carcinoma of unknown primary receiving definitive IMRT. CTV1, red line; CTV2, dark blue line; oral cavity, magenta line; gross tumor volume, yellow line; left parotid gland, aqua line; right parotid gland, rust line.)

## REFERENCES

1. Nieder C, Gregoire V, Ang K. Cervical lymph node metastases from occult squamous cell carcinoma: cut down a tree to get an apple? *Int J Rad Oncol Biol Phys* 2001;50:727–733.
2. Jones A, Cook J, Phillips D, et al. Squamous carcinoma presenting as an enlarged cervical lymph node. *Cancer* 1993;72:1756–1761.
3. Mendenhall W, Mancuso A, Parsons J, et al. Diagnostic evaluation of squamous cell carcinoma metastatic to cervical lymph nodes from an unknown head and neck primary site. *Head and Neck* 1998;20:739–744.
4. Grau C, Johansen L, Jakobsen J, et al. Cervical lymph node metastases from unknown primary tumours: results from a national survey by the Danish Society for Head and Neck Oncology. *Radiother Oncol* 2000;55:121–129.
5. Coker D, Casterline P, Chamber R, et al. Metastases to lymph nodes of the head and neck from an unknown primary site. *Am J Surg* 1977;134:517–522.
6. Coster J, Foote R, Olsen K, et al. Cervical nodal metastasis of squamous cell carcinoma of unknown origin: indications for withholding radiation therapy. *Int J Radiat Oncol Biol Phys* 1992;23:743–749.
7. Wang R, Goepfert H, Barber A, et al. Unknown primary squamous cell carcinoma metastatic to the neck. *Head Neck Surg* 1990;116:1388–1393.
8. Colletier P, Garden A, Morrison W, et al. Postoperative radiation for squamous cell carcinoma metastatic to cervical lymph nodes from an unknown primary site: outcomes and patterns of failure. *Head Neck* 1998;20:674–681.
9. Weir L, Keane T, Cummings B, et al. Radiation treatment of cervical lymph node metastases from an unknown primary: an analysis of outcome by treatment volume and other prognostic factors. *Radiother Oncol* 1995;35:206–211.
10. Marcial-Vega V, Cardenes H, Perez C, et al. Cervical metastases from unknown primaries: radiotherapeutic management and appearance of subsequent primaries. *Int J Radiat Oncol Biol Phys* 1990;19:919–928.

# 13

# MANAGEMENT OF ACUTE AND LATE EFFECTS OF RADIATION THERAPY IN HEAD AND NECK CANCERS

## GOKHAN OZYIGIT

## 1. INTRODUCTION

- Rapid advances in radiation oncology, biology, and physics have led to the accumulation of information on the interactions of radiation with other therapeutic modalities (chemotherapy, biologic-response modifiers) and have had an impact on the understanding of normal tissue toxicities.
- During the treatment of malignant diseases unavoidable toxicities to normal cells may be produced. The mucosal lining of the upper respiratory and gastrointestinal tracts is a prime target for radiotherapy-related toxicity due to its rapid cell turnover rate. The oral cavity is highly sensitive to direct and indirect toxic effects of radiation therapy. This risk is caused by multiple factors such as a diverse and complex microflora, trauma to oral tissues during normal oral function like swallowing foods, and high cellular turnover rates for the lining mucosa.
- The most common oral complications related to radiation therapy are mucositis, infection, salivary gland dysfunction, taste dysfunction, and pain. These complications can lead to secondary complications such as dehydration, dysgeusia, and malnutrition.
- Radiation of the head and neck can irreversibly injure oral mucosa, vasculature, muscle, and bone. This can result in xerostomia, rampant dental caries, trismus, soft-tissue necrosis, and osteoradionecrosis.
- Severe oral toxicities can compromise delivery of optimal radiation therapy protocols. For example, dose reduction or treatment schedule modifications may be necessary to allow for resolution of oral lesions. In cases of severe oral morbidity, the patient may no longer be able to continue cancer therapy; treatment is then usually discontinued. These disruptions in dosing due to oral complications can thus directly affect patients' survival.
- Management of oral complications of cancer therapy includes identification of high-risk populations, patient education, initiation of pretreatment interventions, and timely management of lesions. Assessment of oral status and stabilization of oral disease before cancer therapy are critical to overall patient care. This care should be both preventive and therapeutic, as indicated to minimize risk for oral and associated systemic complications.

- Radiation doses customarily deemed safe may no longer be so because, when combined with another modality, these doses can lead to severe late effects in different vital organs. Previously defined radiation tolerance doses ($TD_{5/5}$ and $TD_{50/5}$) remain as valuable guides, but their applicability has changed.
- Emphasis is now placed on the volume of the organ irradiated, in addition to the dose, and a new construct relating global (whole organ) and focal (partial volume) injury as a function of the dose–volume histogram is presented.
- Mathematical models such as the nominal standard dose, time–dose factor, and cumulative radiation effect have been supplanted by the linear-quadratic equation using the $\alpha/\beta$ ratio and its clinical applicability to normal tissue complication probability estimates.
- Tables 13-1 and 13-2 summarize previously defined whole- and partial-organ tolerance.

## 2. ETIOPATHOGENESIS

- Oral complications associated with cancer chemotherapy and radiation result from complex interactions among multiple factors. The most prominent contributors are direct lethal and sublethal damage to oral tissues, attenuation of immune and other protective systems, and interference with normal healing.
- Elimination of preexisting dental/periapical, periodontal, and mucosal infections; institution of comprehensive oral hygiene protocols during therapy; and reduction of other factors that may compromise oral mucosal integrity (e.g., physical trauma to oral tissues), however, can reduce frequency and severity of oral complications in cancer patients.

## TABLE 13-1. TOLERANCE DOSES (TD$_{5/5}$–TD$_{50/5}$) TO WHOLE-ORGAN IRRADIATION

| Organ | Single Dose (Gy) | Organ | Fractionated Dose (Gy) |
|---|---|---|---|
| Brain | 15–25 | Brain | 60–70 |
| Eye (lens) | 2–10 | Eye (lens) | 6–12 |
| Skin | 15–20 | Skin | 30–40 |
| Spinal cord | 15–20 | Spinal cord | 50–60 |
| VCTS | 10–20 | VCTS | 50–60 |
| Mucosa | 5–20 | Mucosa | 65–77 |
| Peripheral nerve | 15–20 | Peripheral nerve | 65–77 |
| Muscle | >30 | Muscle | >70 |
| Bone and cartilage | >30 | Bone and cartilage | >70 |
| | | Thyroid | 30–40 |

*Source:* Modified from Rubin P. The law and order of radiation sensitivity, absolute vs. relative. In: Vaeth JM, Meyer JL, eds. *Radiation tolerance of normal tissues: frontiers of radiation therapy and oncology*, vol. 23. Basel: S. Karger, 1989:7–40.
VCTS, vasculoconnective tissue systems.

- Complications can be acute (developing during therapy) or chronic (developing months to years after therapy). Radiation protocols typically not only cause acute oral toxicities but induce permanent tissue damage that results in life-long risk for the patient.

- Head and neck irradiation not only can cause ulcerative oral mucositis clinically similar to that caused by high-dose chemotherapy, but also can induce damage that results in permanent dysfunction of vasculature, connective tissue, salivary glands, muscle, and bone.

- Loss of bone vitality occurs secondary to both injuries to osteocytes, osteoblasts, and osteoclasts as well as from a relative hypoxia due to reduction in vascular supply. These changes can lead to soft-tissue necrosis and osteoradionecrosis (ORN) that result in bone exposure, secondary infection, and severe pain.

- Unlike chemotherapy, however, radiation damage is anatomically site-specific; toxicity is localized to irradiated tissue volumes. Degree of damage depends on treatment regimen-related factors, including type of radiation used, total dose administered, and field size/fractionation.

- Radiation-induced damage also differs from chemotherapy-induced changes in that irradiated tissue tends to manifest permanent damage that places the patient at continual risk for oral sequelae. The oral tissues are thus more easily damaged by subsequent toxic drug or radiation exposure, and normal physiologic repair mechanisms are compromised as a result of permanent cellular damage.

## 3. MANAGEMENT BEFORE CANCER THERAPY

- Severity of oral complications in cancer patients can be reduced significantly when oral care is initiated before treatment. Primary preventive measures, such as appropriate nutritional intake, effective oral hygiene practices, and early detection of oral lesions, are important pretreatment interventions.

- The involvement of a dental team experienced with oral oncology may reduce the risk of oral complications either via direct examination of the patient or in consultation with the community-based dentist. The evaluation should be done as early as possible before treatment. The examination allows the dentist to determine the status of the oral cavity before cancer therapy and to initiate necessary interventions that may reduce oral complications during and after that therapy.

## TABLE 13-2. NORMAL TISSUE TOLERANCE TO THERAPEUTIC IRRADIATION

| Organ | TD$_{5/5}$ Volume | | | TD$_{50/5}$ Volume | | | Selected Endpoint |
|---|---|---|---|---|---|---|---|
| | 1/3 | 2/3 | 3/3 | 1/3 | 2/3 | 3/3 | |
| Brain infarction | 60 | 50 | 45 | 75 | 65 | 60 | Necrosis |
| Brainstem infarction | 60 | 53 | 50 | — | — | 65 | Necrosis |
| Spinal cord | 5 cm | 10 cm | 20 cm | 5 cm | 10 cm | 20 cm | Myelitis necrosis |
| | 50 | 50 | 47 | 70 | 70 | — | |

*Source:* Modified from Emami B, Lyman J, Brown A, et al. Tolerance of normal tissue to therapeutic irradiation. *Int J Radiat Oncol Biol Phys* 1991;21:109–122.

# 4. SITE EFFECTS AND MANAGEMENT DURING AND AFTER CANCER THERAPY

## 4.1. Oral Hygiene

- Routine systematic oral hygiene is important for reducing incidence and severity of oral sequelae of cancer therapy. The patient must be informed of the rationale for the oral hygiene program as well as of the potential side effects of cancer chemotherapy and radiation therapy. Effective oral hygiene is important throughout cancer treatment, with emphasis on oral hygiene before that treatment.

- Considerable variation exists across institutions relative to specific nonmedicated approaches to baseline oral care, given limited published evidence. Most nonmedicated oral care protocols utilize topical, frequent (every 4 to 6 hours) rinsing with 0.9% saline. Additional interventions include dental brushing with toothpaste, dental flossing, ice chips, and sodium bicarbonate rinses. Patients utilizing removable dental prostheses or orthodontic appliances have the risk of mucosal injury or infection.

- Dental brushing and flossing represent simple, cost-effective approaches to bacterial dental plaque control.

- Periodontal infection causes the risk of oral bleeding; healthy tissues should not bleed. Discontinuing dental brushing and flossing can increase the risk of gingival bleeding, oral infection, and bacteremia. Therefore reducing the risk for gingival bleeding and eliminating gingival infection before therapy and promoting oral health daily by removing bacterial plaque with gentle debridement via a soft or ultrasoft toothbrush during therapy reduce infection.

- Mechanical plaque control not only promotes gingival health, but also may decrease risk of exacerbation of oral mucositis secondary to microbial colonization of damaged mucosal surfaces.

- Oral rinsing with water or saline while brushing will further aid in removal of dental plaque dislodged by brushing. Rinses containing alcohol should be avoided. Since the flavoring agents in toothpaste can irritate oral soft tissues, toothpaste with relatively neutral taste should be considered.

- Patients skilled at flossing without traumatizing gingival tissues may continue flossing throughout the administration of chemotherapy. Flossing allows for removal of dental bacterial plaque and thus promotes gingival health.

- The oral cavity should be cleaned after meals. If xerostomia is present, plaque and food debris may accumulate secondarily to reduce salivary function, and more frequent hygiene may be necessary.

- It is important to prevent dryness of the lips to reduce risk for tissue injury. Mouth breathing and/or xerostomia secondary to anticholinergic medications used for nausea management can induce the condition. Lip care products containing petroleum-based oils and waxes can be useful.

Lanolin-based creams and ointments, however, may be more effective in protecting against trauma.

- Patients should receive a comprehensive oral evaluation several weeks before initiation of radiation. This timing provides an appropriate interval for tissue healing in the event that invasive oral procedures (including dental extractions, dental scaling/polishing, and endodontic therapy) are necessary. These interventions are principally directed to reducing risk of soft-tissue necrosis and osteoradionecrosis. The likelihood of these lesions occurring after radiation increases over the patient's lifetime.

- Most patients with smoking-related cancer appear motivated to quit smoking once cancer is diagnosed.

- Candidiasis is the most common clinical infection of the oropharynx in irradiated patients. Patients receiving head and neck radiation are frequently colonized with candida, as demonstrated by an increase in quantitative counts and rates for clinical infection. Candidiasis may exacerbate the symptoms of oropharyngeal mucositis.

- Treatment of oral candidiasis in the radiation patient has primarily utilized topical antifungals such as nystatin and clotrimazole. Compliance can be compromised secondary to oral mucositis, nausea, pain, and difficulty in dissolving nystatin pastilles and clotrimazole troches. Use of systemic antifungals, including ketoconazole and fluconazole, to treat oral candidiasis has proved effective and may have advantages over topical agents for patients experiencing mucositis.

- Bacterial infections may also occur early in the course of head/neck radiation and should be treated with antibiotics appropriately targeted to culture and sensitivity data.

- Late oral complications of radiation therapy are chiefly a result of chronic injury to vasculature, salivary glands, mucosa, connective tissue, and bone. Types and severity of these changes are directly related to radiation dosimetry, including total dose, fraction size, and duration of treatment.

- Mucosal changes include epithelial atrophy, reduced vascularization, and submucosal fibrosis. These changes lead to an atrophic, friable barrier. Fibrosis involving muscle, dermis, and temporomandibular joint results in compromised oral function.

- Salivary tissue changes include loss of acinar cells, alteration in duct epithelium, fibrosis, and fatty degeneration. Compromised vascularization and remodeling capacity of bone leads to risk for osteoradionecrosis.

- The risk of dental caries increases secondary to a number of factors, including shifts to a cariogenic flora, reduced concentrations of salivary antimicrobial proteins, and loss of mineralizing components. Treatment strategies must be directed to each component of the caries process. Optimal oral hygiene must be maintained. Xerostomia should be managed whenever possible via salivary substitutes or replacements. Resistance to caries can be enhanced via use of topical fluorides and/or remineralizing agents.

- Increased colonization with *Streptococcus mutans* and *Lactobacillus* species increases the risk of caries. Cultural data can be useful in defining the level of risk in relation to colonization patterns. Topical fluorides or chlorhexidine rinses may lead to reduced levels of *Streptococcus mutans* but not to those of *Lactobacillus* species. Because of adverse drug interactions, fluoride and chlorhexidine dosing should be separated by several hours.
- Remineralizing agents that are high in calcium phosphate and fluoride have demonstrated salutary *in vitro* and clinical effects. Delivering the drug via customized vinyl carriers may enhance the intervention. This approach extends the contact time of active drug with tooth structure, which leads to increased uptake into enamel.
- Necrosis and secondary infection of previously irradiated tissue are serious complications for patients who have undergone radiation for head and neck tumors. Acute effects typically involve oral mucosa. Chronic changes involving bone and mucosa are a result of the process of vascular inflammation and scarring that in turn result in hypovascular, hypocellular, and hypoxic changes. Infection secondary to tissue injury and osteoradionecrosis confounds the process.

## 4.2. Osteoradionecrosis

- The unilateral vascular supply to each half of the mandible results in osteoradionecrosis most frequently involving mandible versus maxilla. Presenting clinical features include pain, diminished or complete loss of sensation, fistula, and infection. Pathologic fracture can occur, as the compromised bone cannot repair itself at the involved sites. Risk for tissue necrosis is in part related to trauma or oral infection; however, idiopathic cases can also occur.
- Patients who develop osteoradionecrosis should be comprehensively managed, including eliminating trauma, avoiding removable dental prostheses if the denture-bearing area is within the necrosis field, ensuring adequate nutritional intake, and discontinuing use of tobacco and alcohol. Topical antibiotics (e.g., tetracycline) or antiseptics (e.g., chlorhexidine) may contribute to wound resolution. Wherever possible, the exposed bone with mucosa should be covered. Analgesics for pain control are often effective. Local resection of bone sequestrae may be possible.
- Hyperbaric oxygen therapy (HBO) is generally recommended for management of osteoradionecrosis in that it increases oxygenation of irradiated tissue, promotes angiogenesis, and enhances osteoblast repopulation and fibroblast function. HBO is usually prescribed as 20 to 30 dives at 100% oxygen and 2 to 2.5 atmospheres of pressure. If surgery is needed, 10 dives of postsurgical HBO are recommended. Unfortunately, HBO technology is not always accessible to patients who might benefit from it.

- Partial mandibulectomy may be necessary in severe cases of osteoradionecrosis. The mandible can be reconstructed to provide continuity for esthetics and function. A multidisciplinary cancer team that includes oncologists, oncology nurses, maxillofacial prosthodontists, general dentists, hygienists, and physical therapists is appropriate for managing these patients.
- Musculoskeletal syndromes may develop secondary to radiation and surgery. Lesions include soft-tissue fibrosis, surgically induced mandibular discontinuity, and parafunctional habits associated with emotional stress caused by cancer and its treatment. Patients can be instructed in physical therapy interventions, including mandibular stretching exercises as well as use of prosthetic aids designed to reduce severity of fibrosis. It is important that these approaches be instituted before trismus develops. If clinically significant changes develop, several approaches—including stabilization of occlusion, trigger point injection, and other pain management strategies, muscle relaxants, and/or tricyclic medications—can be considered.

## 4.3. Xerostomia

- Saliva is necessary for the normal execution of oral functions such as taste, swallowing, and speech. Unstimulated whole salivary flow rates of less than 0.1 mL/min are considered indicative of xerostomia (normal salivary flow rate = 0.3 to 0.5 mL/min). Xerostomia produces the following changes in the mouth that collectively cause patient discomfort and increase risk for oral lesions:
  - ☐ Salivary viscosity increases, with resultant impaired lubrication of oral tissues.
  - ☐ Buffering capacity is compromised, with increased risk for dental caries. Oral flora becomes more pathogenic. Plaque levels accumulate because of the patient's difficulty in maintaining oral hygiene. Acid production after sugar exposure results in further demineralization of the teeth and leads to dental decay.
- Xerostomia is caused by a marked reduction in salivary gland secretion.[1] Symptoms and signs of xerostomia include dryness, burning sensation of the tongue, fissures at lip commissures, atrophy of dorsal tongue surface, difficulty in wearing dentures, and increased thirst.
- Xerostomia results from inflammatory and degenerative effects of ionizing radiation on salivary gland parenchyma, especially serous acinar cells. Salivary flow decreases within 1 week after starting radiation treatment and diminishes progressively with continued treatment. The degree of dysfunction is related to the radiation dose and volume of glandular tissue in the radiation field. Parotid glands may be more susceptible to radiation effects than submandibular, sublingual, and other minor salivary glandular tissues. Salivary gland tissues that have been excluded from the radiation portal may become hyperplastic, partially

compensating for the nonfunctional glands at other oral sites.

- The mean dose thresholds for both unstimulated and stimulated parotid saliva flow rates to reduce to <25% of pretreatment level were 24 and 26 Gy, respectively.[1] Chao et al. reported that the saliva flow rate reduced exponentially and independently for each gland at the rate of approximately 4% per Gy of the mean parotid dose.[2] This implies that approximately 50% or more of the baseline saliva flow can be retained if both parotid glands receive a mean dose of less than 16 Gy. If both parotid glands receive a mean dose of 32 Gy, the reduction of stimulated saliva will be approximately 25% of the pretreatment value. The reduction of stimulated and unstimulated whole saliva flow did alter patients' subjective xerostomia/eating/speaking functions, and preserving saliva function translated into a better quality of life.
- Xerostomia alters the mouth's buffering capacity and mechanical cleansing ability, thereby contributing to dental caries and progressive periodontal disease. Development of dental caries also is accelerated in the presence of xerostomia due to reduction in delivery to the dentition of antimicrobial proteins normally contained in saliva.
- Patients who experience xerostomia must maintain excellent oral hygiene to minimize risk for oral lesions. Periodontal disease can be accelerated and caries can become rampant unless preventive measures are instituted. Multiple preventive strategies should be considered (Table 13-3).
- Management of xerostomia also includes use of saliva substitutes or sialagogues. Saliva substitutes or artificial saliva preparations (oral rinses containing hydroxyethyl-, hydroxypropyl-, or carboxymethylcellulose) are palliative agents that relieve the discomfort of xerostomia by temporarily wetting the oral mucosa. Sialagogues pharmacologically stimulate saliva production from intact salivary glandular tissues.

- Pilocarpine is approved by the U.S. Food and Drug Administration for use as a sialogogue (5-mg tablets of pilocarpine hydrochloride). Treatment is initiated at 5 mg orally, three times daily; the dose is then titrated to achieve optimal clinical response and minimize adverse effects. The most common adverse effect at clinically useful doses of pilocarpine is hyperhidrosis (excessive sweating).
- Amifostine (Ethyl) is approved for prevention of xerostomia and off-label use for reduction of mucositis. In a phase III study of conventional radiation therapy with or without amifostine, amifostine significantly reduced acute and late xerostomia. Using Radiation Therapy Oncology Group (RTOG) criteria, the incidence of grade 2 or higher acute xerostomia reduced from 78% to 51% ($p < 0.001$), and the incidence of late xerostomia reduced from 57% to 34% ($p = 0.0019$). The local regional control was not compromised.[16]

## 4.4. Dysphagia

- Dysphagia can be a prominent symptom in chemotherapy or head/neck radiation patients. Etiology is likely associated with several factors, including direct neurotoxicity to taste buds, xerostomia, infection, and psychologic conditioning.
- A total fractionated radiation dose of more than 3,000 Gy reduces acuity of sweet, sour, bitter, and salt tastes. Damage to the microvilli and outer surface of the taste cells has been proposed as the principal mechanism for loss of the sense of taste. In many cases, taste acuity returns in 2 or 3 months after cessation of radiation. However, many other patients develop permanent hypogeusia. Zinc supplementation (zinc sulfate 220 mg, twice a day) has been reported to be useful in some patients; the overall benefit of this treatment remains unclear.
- Loss of appetite can also occur in cancer patients concurrent with mucositis, xerostomia, taste loss, dysphagia, nausea, and vomiting. Quality of life is compromised as eating becomes more problematic.
- Oral pain upon eating may lead to selection of foods that do not aggravate the oral tissues, often at the expense of adequate nutrition. Modifying the texture and consistency of the diet, adding between-meal snacks to increase protein and caloric intake, and administering vitamin, mineral, and caloric supplements can minimize nutritional deficiencies.

## TABLE 13-3. MANAGEMENT OF THE XEROSTOMIC PATIENT

| Plaque removal | Tooth brushing<br>Flossing<br>Other oral hygiene aids |
|---|---|
| Remineralization | Topical high-concentration fluorides<br>Children: topical and systemic<br>Adults: topical<br>Remineralizing solutions |
| Antimicrobials | Chlorhexidine solutions (rinses)<br>Providone iodine oral rinses<br>Tetracycline oral rinses |
| Sialogogues | Pilocarpine<br>Bethanechol<br>Antholetrithione (Sialor TM) |

*Source:* Modified from: Schubert MM, Peterson DE, Lloid ME. Oral complications. In: Thomas ED, Blume KG, Forman SJ, eds. *Hematopoietic cell transplantation,* 2nd ed., Malden, Mass: Blackwell Science, 1999;751–763.
*Note:* Prescription strength fluorides should be used. Nonprescription fluoride preparations are inadequate in the face of moderate to high dental caries risk. If drinking water does not have adequate fluoride content to prevent dental decay, then oral fluoride (i.e., drops, vitamins, etc.) should be provided.

- Nutritional counseling may be required during and following therapy; maintenance of appropriate caloric and nutrient intake should be emphasized. Nasogastric feeding tubes or percutaneous esophageal gastrostomy may be required when swallowing is significantly impaired.
- Total parenteral nutrition represents a means to provide adequate nutrition but is generally reserved for patients who cannot eat due to mucositis or nausea, as opposed to dysgeusia alone.
- When cancer therapy-associated mucositis has resolved, nutritional counseling must consider long-term complications, including xerostomia, increased caries risk, altered ability to masticate, and dysphagia. Consideration must thus be given to taste, texture, moisture, calories, and nutrient content.
- Cancer patients undergoing high-dose chemotherapy and/or radiation can experience fatigue related to either disease or its treatment. These processes can produce sleep deprivation or metabolic disorders, which collectively contribute to compromised oral status. For example, the fatigued patient will likely have impaired compliance with mouth care protocols designed to otherwise minimize risk of mucosal ulceration, infection, and pain. In addition, biochemical abnormalities are likely involved in many patients. The psychosocial component can also play a major role, with depression contributing to the overall status.

## 5. OTHER ORGAN-SPECIFIC LATE EFFECTS OF HEAD AND NECK RADIATION THERAPY

### 5.1. Brain

- *Clinical detection:* Headache, somnolence, intellectual deficits, functional neurologic losses, and memory alterations may occur during, shortly after, or most often as a delayed effect at 6 months.
- *Time course of events:* Brain necrosis and gliosis require 6 to 12 months to develop.
- *Dose/time/volume:* Generally, doses of 50 Gy to whole brain in 1.8- to 2-Gy fractions are well tolerated; in children the threshold doses are 30 to 35 Gy.[3] $TD_5$ in adults for necrosis is $\geq$50 Gy (54 Gy).[4] A threshold dose of 57.6 Gy was noted by Leibel and Sheline using 1.8- to 2-Gy fractions.[5] With focal areas, the $TD_{50}$ is between 70 and 80 Gy, as evidenced by a recent Radiation Therapy Oncology Group study.[6]
- *Chemical/biologic modifiers:* Concomitant use of carmustine (BCNU) is well tolerated, but immediate subsequent use of methotrexate intrathecally or intravenously is of concern.
- *Radiologic imaging:* On magnetic resonance (MR) imaging, four stages have been described, from early whitening in the periventricular region to a diffuse coalescence of white and gray matter into an intense signal region and loss of structure.[7]
- *Differential diagnosis:* Positron emission tomography scans indicate hypometabolic zones for necrosis and hypermetabolic zones for tumor.
- *Pathologic diagnosis:* Establishing diagnosis is indicated only if tumor recurrence or progression is suspected. Alterations in vasculature and loss of myelination due to oligodendrocytic death are well documented.
- *Management:* This is often symptomatic treatment with analgesics and antiseizure medications, such as phenytoin (Dilantin) and barbiturates, but as headaches and neurologic deficits increase, high-dose corticosteroids are used.
- *Follow-up:* The patient is seen every day or week until relief is obtained, and then at 1- to 3-month intervals.

### 5.2. Spinal Cord

- *Clinical detection:* Paresthesias (tingling sensation, shooting pain, Lhermitte's sign), numbness, motor weakness, and loss of sphincter control may progress through Brown-Séquard's syndrome to total paraparesis and paraplegia.
- *Time course of events:* Clinically, Lhermitte's syndrome occurs 2 to 4 months after irradiation and persists or returns at 6 to 9 months. Paresis, numbness, and altered sphincter control appearing at 6 to 12 months with progression compose the classic onset of radiation-induced spinal cord transection.[8]
- *Dose/time/volume:* The most widely observed dose limit for the spinal cord is 45 Gy in 22 to 25 fractions. Marcus and Million found 45 Gy conventionally fractionated is on the flat part of the dose–response curve and yields an incidence of myelopathy of less than 0.2%.[9] $TD_5$ level is probably 57 to 61 Gy; $TD_{50}$ is 68 to 73 Gy. No volume effect has been shown. Shortening the interval from 24 hours to 6 to 8 hours reduces spinal cord tolerance by 10% to 15%.
- *Chemical/biologic modifiers:* Intrathecal and intravenous use of concomitant methotrexate, cisplatin (CDDP), and etoposide (VP-16) are neurotoxic.
- *Radiologic imaging:* MR imaging may show cord swelling or atrophy, decreased intensity on T1-weighted images, or increased intensity on T2-weighted images.[10]
- *Differential diagnosis:* Epidural metastasis or compression secondary to vertebral metastases must be excluded.
- *Pathologic diagnosis:* This is not possible until postmortem.
- *Management:* Currently, corticosteroids are prescribed using an intensive intravenous schedule, as with multiple sclerosis patients: methylprednisolone (Solu-Medrol) 1,000 mg IV for 3 to 5 days; then the dose is tapered to stabilize progress.

## 5.3. Cornea, Lacrimal Gland, and Lens

- *Clinical detection:* Mild keratitis may present as a foreign-body sensation, discomfort, or tearing. Damage to the lacrimal gland with resultant dry eye may lead to severe keratitis sicca, corneal ulceration, and perforation of the globe. Cataract may form after irradiation to the lens.
- *Time course of events:* Twenty-four hours following radiation, the conjunctiva and other periocular tissues were edematous and diffusely infiltrated by neutrophils. Vascular changes consisted of dilated blood vessels and hypertrophy of the endothelium, but the meibomian glands and goblet cells were normal at this time.
- *Dose/time/volume:* Keratitis, edema, and corneal ulcers can occur after 30 Gy when large fractions (10 Gy) are used, but the tolerance is higher (approximately 50 Gy) when conventional fractionation is used. The lacrimal glands have TD 5/50 at 50 to 60 Gy. A dose of more than 60 Gy will result in keratoconjunctivitis sicca and lead to permanent loss of secretions. The transient eyelid effects of eyelash loss, erythema, and conjunctivitis are noted at 30 to 40 Gy, but permanent lash loss is associated with doses of more than 50 Gy with conventional fractionation. Small doses (2 to 3 Gy), particularly when delivered in a single session, may lead to cataract formation. According to Merriam and Focht, fractionated radiation doses exceeding 12 Gy may cause cataracts.[11] When single-dose (8 to 10 Gy) TBI was used, cataracts developed in 80% of survivors. The incidence of cataracts fell to 10% when fractionated TBI (2 Gy/fraction) was given to an even higher total dose (12 to 14 Gy).
- *Chemical/biologic modifiers:* Little information in this aspect.
- *Management:* Management of keratitis and dry eyes consists of aggressive lubrication, patching, and antibiotic drops as necessary. Surgery is the treatment of choice for cataract should it occur.
- *Follow-up:* Once detected, radiation injury needs careful scrutiny.

## 5.4. Retina and Optic Tract

- *Clinical detection:* Radiation retinopathy may produce floaters, visual distortion, and decreased visual acuity. Microaneurysms, telangiectasis, macular edema, and retinal hemorrhages are common.
- *Time course of events:* Radiation retinopathy may occur in a few months. Symptoms for optic tract injury may take 5 to 10 years to develop.
- *Dose/time/volume:* Radiation retinopathy is rare at 45 Gy after conventional fractions of irradiation. Nakissa et al. reported that all patients who received more than 45 Gy to the posterior pole had recognizable changes.[12] However, most of these did not affect vision. Decreased visual acuity occurred only in patients receiving more than 65 Gy. Half of patients displayed some changes at 60 Gy, and 85% to 90% showed changes at 80 Gy. Parsons et al. reported no optic nerve injury in patients receiving less than 59 Gy ($\leq$1.9 Gy/day).[13] However, the 15-year actuarial incidence of optic nerve injury reached 11% for doses above 60 Gy ($\leq$1.9 Gy/day). When daily fraction size increased to 2.1 to 2.2 Gy/fraction, Jiang et al. observed a 5- and 10-year complication rate of 34%.[14] The dose to the optic apparatus during stereotactic radiosurgery should be under 8 Gy, because Tishler et al. reported that four of 17 patients (24%) receiving greater than 8 Gy to any part of the optic apparatus developed visual complications, compared with none in 35 who received less than 8 Gy ($p = .009$).[15]
- *Chemical/biologic modifiers:* Chemotherapy increases the toxic effects of radiation to the eye.
- *Management:* No effective treatment. Prevention is critical.
- *Follow-up:* Once detected, radiation injury needs careful scrutiny.

## REFERENCES

1. Eisbruch A, Ten-Haken RK, Kim HM, et al. Dose, volume, and function relationships in parotid salivary glands following conformal and intensity-modulated irradiation of head and neck cancer. *Int J Radiat Oncol Biol Phys* 1999;45:577–587.
2. Chao KSC, Deasy JO, Markman J, et al. A prospective study of salivary function sparing in patients with head and neck cancers receiving intensity-modulated or three-dimensional radiation therapy: initial results. *Int J Radiat Oncol Biol Phys* 2001;49:907–916.
3. Constine LS. Tumors in children: cure with preservation of function and aesthetics. In: Wilson JF, ed. *Syllabus: a categorical course in radiation therapy.* Oak Brook, IL: Radiological Society of North America, 1988:75–91.
4. Marks JE, Baglan RJ, Prassad SC, et al. Cerebral radionecrosis: incidence and risk in relation to dose, time, fractionation and volume. *Int J Radiat Oncol Biol Phys* 1981;7:243–252.
5. Leibel SA, Sheline GE. Tolerance of the brain and spinal cord to conventional irradiation. In: Gutin PH, Leibel SA, Sheline GE, eds. *Radiation injury to the nervous system.* New York: Raven Press, 1991:239–256.
6. Murray KG, Nelson DF, Scott C, et al. Quality-adjusted survival analysis of malignant glioma patients treated with twice-daily radiation and carmustine: a report of Radiation Therapy Oncology Group (RTOG) 83-02. *Int J Radiat Oncol Biol Phys* 1995;31:453–459.
7. Constine LS, Konski A, Ekholm S, et al. Adverse effects of brain irradiation correlated with MR and CT imaging. *Int J Radiat Oncol Biol Phys* 1988;15:319–330.
8. Rubin P, Casarett GW. *Clinical radiation pathology,* vols. I and II. Philadelphia: WB Saunders, 1968.
9. Marcus RB, Million RR. The incidence of myelitis after irradiation of the cervical spinal cord. *Int J Radiat Oncol Biol Phys* 1990;19:3–8.

10. Wang PY, Shen WC, Jan JS. Magnetic resonance imaging in radiation myelopathy. *Am J Neuroradiol* 1992;13:1049–1055.
11. Merriam GR Jr., Focht EF. A clinical study of radiation cataracts and the relationship to dose. *Am J Roentgenol, Rad Ther Nuc Med* 1957;77:759–785.
12. Nakissa N, Rubin P. Strohl R, et al. Ocular and orbital complications following radiation therapy of paranasal sinus malignancies and review of literature. *Cancer* 1983;51:980–986.
13. Parsons JT, Bova FJ, Fitzgerald CR, et al. Radiation optic neuropathy after megavoltage external-beam irradiation: analysis of time-dose factors. *Int J Radiat Oncol Biol Phys* 1994;30:755–763.
14. Jiang GL, Tucker SL, Guttenberger R, et al. Radiation-induced injury to the visual pathway. *Radiother Oncol* 1994;30:17–25.
15. Waldron JN, Laperriere NJ, Jaakkimainen L, et al. Spinal cord ependydmomas: a retrospective analysis of 59 cases. *Int J Radiat Oncol Biol Phys* 1993;27:215–221.
16. Brizel DM, Wasserman TH, Henke M, et al. Phase III randomized trial of ami fostive as a radioprotector in head and neck cancer. *J Clin Oncol* 2000;18:3339–3345.

# INDEX

Note: Page numbers followed by *f* indicate figures; page numbers followed by *t* indicate tables.

## A

Abdomen, as primary site, 155
Aerodigestic pathway, 30–31, 127
Age, as prognostic factor, 102, 131
AJCC. *See* American Joint Committee on Cancer
Alveolar ridge of the maxilla, 41*t*, 85
American Academy of Otolaryngology-Head and Neck Surgery, 1, 26*f*, 38
American Joint Committee on Cancer (AJCC), *See* TNM staging

Analgesics
Anatomy
base of tongue
base of tongue
faucial arch
hypopharynx
larynx, 1
lymphatics
lymph node
nasopharynx, 72, 71*f*
neck, 20–21, 22*f*, 23*ft*, 40*f*
oral cavity, 85, 85*f*, 117–118, 117*f*
paranasal sinuses and nasal cavity, 50, 51–55*f*
paraphyngeal spaces, 101*f*
tonsillar fossa, 100, 102*f*
Antibiotics, 152, 162, 163, 164*t*, 166
Antifungal medication, 162
Antiseizure medication, 165
Artifacts, 2, 5, 6, 10, 19, 118
Aspiration, 122, 140, 148
Attenuation-corrected images (AC), 31

## B

Barbiturates, 165
Barium contrast, 129
Base and fog, at zero dose, 5
Base of skull, 19, 21, 69*t*, 70*f*, 72*f*, 74*f*
Base of tongue (BOT)
anatomy, 114, 115*f*
general management, 118–120, 120*t*, 121*t*, 122*ft*, 123–125*f*
imaging, 116, 117*f*, 118, 118*f*
IMRT, 121–122, 122*ft*, 123–125*f*
incidence of metastasis, 41*t*, 42*ft*
invasion with tonsil or faucial arch cancer, 102
local control results, irradiation alone, 120*t*, 121*t*
natural history of cancer, 114, 115*ft*, 116*ft*
physical examination, 114, 116
sequelae of IMRT treatment, 122
survival rate, 121*t*
TNM staging, 116*t*, 119*t*

Beam angle, 4
Beam characteristics, 1, 3, 5
BED. *See* Biologic equivalent dose
Bilateral lymph node involvement, 42*t*, 76, 104*t*, 155
Biologic equivalent dose (BED), 47*t*
Biopsy, 18, 155
Bone
exposure, 112, 122, 161, 163
floor of the mouth, 94
paranasal sinuses and nasal cavity, 50, 51*f*
toxic effects of radiation, 161, 162, 163
Bone marrow, 27
BOT. *See* Base of tongue
Brain, effects of radiation therapy, 165
Buccal mucosa
anatomy, 85
general management, 92–93, 93*t*
incidence of metastasis, 40, 42*f*, 86
natural history of cancer, 87
signs and symptoms, 88
survival rate, 93*t*

## C

Calcifications, 19, 19*f*, 24
Calibration, 4, 5, 10, 11
Carboplatin, 104, 120
Cartilage
collapse, 27
cricoid, 40*f*, 127, 128, 128*f*, 140*f*, 141*f*, 142*f*
of the hypopharynx, 127
of the larynx, 139, 141*f*, 142*f*
of the paranasal sinuses and nasal cavity, 50, 51*f*
Cerebral aneurysm clips, 19
Chemotherapy
base of tongue cancer, 120
hypopharyngeal cancer, 135–136
laryngeal cancer, 147, 149, 149*t*
nasopharyngeal cancer, 77, 78*t*, 81
tonsillar fossa cancer, 104, 112
toxic side effects, 161, 164–165, 166
Chest, as primary site, 155
Children, hypopituitarism, 83
Cisplatin, 104, 120, 149*t*
Clinical target volume. *See* Target volume
Clusters. *See* Lymph nodes, clusters
Commissioning tests, IMRT TPS, 11
Complications. *See* Sequelae of IMRT treatment
Computed tomography (CT)
base of tongue, 116, 117*f*, 118, 118*f*
CT/PET hybrid machines, 34–35
floor of the mouth, 89, 91
hypopharynx, 129–131

image fusion with PET, 32, 33–36*f*, 34–36
imaging, 18
larynx, 140, 146*f*
lip, 88
nasopharynx, 72–73, 74*f*
neck node metastasis of unknown primary, 155
oral tongue, 91
overview, 18–28
paranasal sinuses and nasal cavity, 56, 57*f*, 58
retromolar trigone, 91
tonsillar fossa, 103*f*
*vs.* MRI, 18–19, 19*f*
*vs.* PET, 31–32, 31*t*, 32*t*, 33–34*f*
Contraindications, 19, 134
Contralateral lymph node involvement, 42*t*, 86, 88*t*, 104*t*, 114
Contrast media, 18, 19, 129
Copper ATSM (Cu-ATSM), 30, 35*f*
Corticosteroids, 152, 165
Couch, 3, 4, 12, 15
Cranial nerves, 72, 73*t*, 76, 82
Cricoid cartilage, 40*f*, 127, 128, 128*f*, 140*f*, 141*f*, 142*f*
Critical structures, 1, 11
Cross-sectional imaging, basics, 18–20
CT. *See* Computed tomography
CTV. *See* Target volume
Cysts, 18

## D

Data analysis as source of discrepancy, 10
Deep cervical fascia, 20, 20*f*
Densitometer, 5, 6*f*, 10
Dental care, 112, 160–162, 164*t*
Dental prostheses, 163
Dental side effects, 83, 96, 160, 161, 162–163, 164
Dermal toxicity, 27, 44, 45–46*f*, 48, 83
Dexamethasone, 152
Diabetes, 31
Diagnostic work-ups, 74*t*, 104*t*
Diazepam, 31
Diet, 164–165
Digitally reconstructed radiographs (DRR), 14*f*
Distance-to-agreement test (DTA), 8
Distribution of dose. *See* Dose distribution
DMLC. *See* Dynamic multileaf collimation
Dose
calculation algorithms, 1, 2
cumulative effects, 160
errors, 11, 12, 13*f*, 15
measurement as source of discrepancy, 8
modeling, 160
multiple simultaneous, 1–2

**170** *Index*

Dose (*Cont.*)
  nominal standard, 160
  relationship with optical density, 5, 6*f*
  threshold for side effects, 160, 163, 164,
    165, 166
  tolerance, 160, 161*t*
Dose delivery, temporal, 2
Dose distribution
  base of tongue, 122, 125*f*
  conformality, 1
  evaluation, 6–8, 9*f*
  gradient, 1, 4, 5, 7, 8, 15
  hypopharynx, 136*f*
  with ionization chamber, 4
  isodose to test localization, 12*f*
  larynx, 153*f*
  nasopharynx, 82
  oral cavity, 96, 99*f*
  oral tongue, 111*f*
  paranasal sinuses and nasal cavity, 61, 66*f*
  positioning, 1, 7–8
  reference, 9*f*
  sampling, 4
  shifted *vs.* unshifted to test localization
    effects, 12, 13*f*, 14*f*
  verification, 15
Dose prescription for cancer
  base of tongue, 119, 120
  buccal mucosa, 93
  floor of the mouth, 95
  hypopharynx, 134, 136
  larynx, 148–149, 152
  lip, 92
  oral tongue, 94
  paranasal sinuses and nasal cavity, 49*t*, 61
  and target delineation for nodal volumes,
    38–48
  tonsillar fossa and faucial arch, 103
  Washington University guidelines, 47–48,
    47*t*
Dose-volume histogram (DVH), 12, 13*f*, 15,
  48
Dosimeter, 15
Dosimetry, 2, 4–10, 7*f*, 11
DTA. *See* Distance-to-agreement test
DVH. *See* Dose-volume histogram
Dynamic multileaf collimation (DMLC), 2–3,
  11
Dysphagia, 112, 122, 129, 164–165

**E**

Ear, 40, 42*f*, 72, 122
Edema, 112, 148, 152, 157, 166
Epidemiological factors, 76, 102
Epiglottis, 27, 140*f*, 145
Esophagus, as primary site, 155
Etiopathogenesis, 160–161
European Organization for Research and
  Treatment of Cancer (EORTC), 135,
  149*t*
Extracapsular extension (ECE)
  with base of tongue cancer, 119, 121
  ± differentiation, 44, 46*f*
  with hypopharyngeal cancer, 136
  incidence, 47*t*
  with laryngeal cancer, 148
Eye, 58, 61, 83, 166

**F**

Failure of treatment. *See* Recurrent tumors
False-positive rate, PET, 32
False vocal cords, 18, 27, 139, 140*f*, 145
Fasting, 30, 31

Fat, 18, 19*f*, 20*f*, 27*f*
Faucial arch, 100, 102, 102*f*, 103–104
FDG. *See* $^{18}$F-Fluorodeoxyglucose
Feeding, 122, 152, 165
Fiber-optics, 71–72
Fibrosis, posttherapy, 18, 27, 83, 112, 162, 163
Field characteristics, 2, 10, 11
Film. *See* Portal film; Radiographic film
Filters, 3–4
Fistula, 96, 137
Floor of the mouth (FOM)
  anatomy, 85, 86*f*
  general management, 94–95, 95*t*
  imaging, 18, 19, 89, 91
  incidence of metastasis, 41*t*, 42*t*, 86, 88*t*
  natural history of cancer, 87
  signs and symptoms, 87
  survival, 95*t*
Fluoride, 162, 163, 164*t*
$^{18}$F-Fluorodeoxyglucose (FDG), 30, 31
5-Fluorouracil, 104, 149, 149*t*
FOM. *See* Floor of the mouth
Foramina of the base of the skull, 69*t*, 70*f*

**G**

Gadolinium-enhanced images, 18, 19, 19*f*, 20
Gallium-67, 30
Gastrointestinal tract, 160
Gender, as a prognostic factor, 131, 143
Gene therapy, 36
Gingiva, 85, 87, 93
Glossectomy, 119
Glottic larynx
  anatomy, 139
  carcinoma, 140, 144*t*, 145*ft*, 147*t*
  incidence of metastasis, 41*t*, 42*t*
Glucose, FDG as analog, 30, 31

**H**

HBO. *See* Hyperbaric oxygen therapy
Hearing, decreased, 72, 83, 112
Hemorrhage, 28, 122, 166
Heterogeneity corrections, 11
High linear transfer irradiation, 104
Histology, 31, 76, 155
Hoarseness, 129, 139, 140
Hyperbaric oxygen therapy (HBO), 163
Hyperthermia, 104
Hypoglossal nerves, 114, 122
Hypopharynx
  anatomy, 127–128, 128*f*
  general management, 132, 133–134*t*
  imaging, 129–131
  IMRT, 135*f*, 136–137, 136*f*
  incidence of metastasis, 41*t*
  natural history of cancer, 128–129, 129*ft*,
    130*ft*, 131*ft*
  physical examination, 129
  as primary site, 155
  prognostic factors, 131–132
  sequelae of IMRT treatment, 137
  signs and symptoms, 129
  survival rate, 133*t*
  TNM staging, 132, 132*t*
Hypopituitarism, 83
Hypoxia, loss of bone vitality due to, 161
Hypoxic cell sensitizers, 104
Hypoxic-specific tracers, 30, 35*f*, 36

**I**

Image fusion, 32, 33–36*f*, 34–36
Image-guided IMRT, 35–36*f*, 36
Immobilization of patient, 12, 34–35*f*

Immune dysfunction, 160
Indium-111, 30
Infection, 122, 160, 162, 163, 165, 166
Innervation
  base of skull, 72*f*
  hypopharynx, 127, 128
  larynx, 139, 141*f*
  nasal cavity, 50, 54*f*
  nasopharynx, 68, 71*f*, 73
  neck, 22*f*, 23*f*
  oropharynx, 101*f*
International Commission on Radiation Units
  and Measurements (ICRU), 38
Ionization chamber, 4–5, 7*f*, 15
Iron filings, intraorbital, 19
Isotopes, creation for PET, 30

**J**

Jaw, muscular dysfunction. *See* Trismus
Jugular lymph nodes
  chains, 21, 25*f*, 68, 149, 155
  upper deep, 78, 95, 121, 136
Jugulodigastric lymph nodes. *See* Subgastric
  lymph nodes
Junction lymph nodes, 78, 95, 121, 136

**L**

Laryngeal ventricle, 18
Laryngectomy, 26*f*, 119, 134, 144, 145,
  147–148, 150
Laryngopharyngectomy, 119, 134
Laryngoscopy, 71, 129, 152
Larynx
  anatomy, 139, 140*f*, 141–142*f*
  general management, 143–145, 147–149,
    148*t*, 149*t*
  imaging, 140, 146*f*
  IMRT, 149–150, 150*t*, 151–153*f*, 152
  incidence of metastasis, 41*t*
  natural history of cancer, 139
  physical examination, 140
  as primary site, 155
  prognostic factors, 143
  sequelae of treatment, 150
  signs and symptoms, 140
  survival results, 149*t*
  TNM staging, 140, 147*t*
Leaf ends, 3
Leukoplakia, 88, 92
Linear accelerator, 2, 10–11
Lip
  anatomy, 85, 86
  general management, 91, 93*t*
  imaging, 88
  as primary site, 155
  survival rate, 93*t*
  symptoms of cancer, 87
  TNM staging, 92*t*
Localization, 12, 13–14*f*, 14
Lymphatic network, 38, 38*f*, 41*t*
Lymph nodes
  base of tongue, 116*f*
  calcifications, 24
  cervical lymph node levels, 21, 26*f*
  clusters, 23, 26*f*
  control results, 47–48
  dissection, incidence of metastasis after, 86,
    91*t*, 143*t*
  hypopharynx, 127–128, 136
  involvement with specific cancer types. *See*
    Metastatic lymph nodes
  larynx, 149
  normal anatomy, 19*f*, 21, 23–25*f*

oral cavity, 85–87, 86f, 95
pathology, 21, 23–24, 24f, 26f
of the tongue, 86f
Lymphoma, 155

## M

Magnetic resonance imaging (MRI)
base of tongue, 116
basics, 18–20
brain, 165
contraindications, 19
floor of the mouth, 89, 91
hypopharynx, 129–131
imaging approach to, 20–28
larynx, 140
lip, 88
nasopharynx, 72–73, 74f, 75f
neck node metastasis of unknown primary, 155
oral tongue, 91
paranasal sinuses and nasal cavity, 56
retromolar trigone, 91
tonsillar fossa, 103f
vs. CT, 18–19, 19f
vs. PET, 31–32, 31t, 32t
Magnetic resonance spectroscopy (MRS), 18
Magnetization transfer imaging (MT), 18
Mandible, 21, 87
Mandibulectomy, 112, 119, 163
Mask, thermoplastic, 12, 12f, 34f
Medications, 152, 162, 163, 164t, 165
Melanoma, 155
Mental state, 165
Metaanalyses
base of tongue cancer, 120
laryngeal cancer, 149
lymph node target volume, 38, 41t
paranasal sinuses and nasal cavity cancer, 58, 60t
Metabolism, 30, 32, 33–35f, 34–35
Metastatic lymph nodes
base of tongue presentation, 114, 116f, 117t, 121
bilateral, 42t, 76, 104t, 155
contralateral, 42t, 86, 88t, 104t, 114
dose prescription and target delineation, 38–48
hypopharynx presentation, 128–129, 129ft, 130ft, 131–132, 131ft
larynx presentation, 140, 143t, 144t, 145t, 147t
micro, 38
nasopharynx presentation, 68, 70t, 76
oral cavity presentation, 85–87, 87t, 88t, 89–91t
paranasal sinus presentation, 56t
and PET, 31, 31t, 33f
target volume, literature review, 38, 41t
tonsillar fossa presentation, 100, 102f, 104t, 112
of unknown primary, 155–158, 156f
[11]C-Methionine (MET), 30, 32
MIMiC, 3
F-18 Misonidazole, 30
Molecular probes, 30, 32
Monitoring, 10, 28, 32, 36, 162
Mortality, surgery-related, 137
MRI. See Magnetic resonance imaging
MRS. See Magnetic resonance spectroscopy
MT. See Magnetization transfer imaging
Mucosa, 28, 28f, 114, 127, 160, 162, 163
Mucositis, 112, 160, 162, 165

Multileaf collimation (MLC), 2, 8, 10
Multiple dose, 1–2
Multiple sclerosis, 165
Musculature
base of tongue, 114, 115f, 118
hypopharynx, 127
jaw, side effects. See Trismus
larynx, 31, 139, 141f, 142f
nasopharynx, 68
neck, 22f, 23f, 40f
tongue, 86f
Musculoskeletal syndromes, 163
Myelopathy, 82–83, 165–166

## N

Nasal cavity
anatomy, 50, 51–52f, 53–55f
general management, 58, 60, 60t
IMRT, 60–61, 61t, 66f
natural history of cancer, 50, 52, 56t
orbital invasion, 52, 55–56f, 58
physical examination, 52, 56
as primary site, 155
prognostic factors, 58
sequelae of IMRT treatment, 61
signs and symptoms, 52, 56
survival rate, 58, 60t
Nasopharynx
anatomy, 68, 69ft, 70ft, 71f
chemotherapy, 77, 78t
general management, 76–77, 76t, 77t
imaging, 18, 21, 72–73, 74f, 75f
IMRT, 77–78, 78t, 79–82f, 81
lymphadenopathy, 25f, 41t, 68, 70t
natural history of cancer, 68, 71, 71f, 72f
as primary site, 155
prognostic factors, 76
sequelae of IMRT treatment, 82–83
signs and symptoms, 71
survival rate, 76, 77, 77t, 81
TNM staging, 71t, 72t, 75t, 76t
Nasoscopes, fiber-optic, 71, 72
National Institute of Standards and Technology (NIST), 4
Natural history of cancer
base of tongue, 114, 115ft, 116t
faucial arch, 100, 102f
hypopharynx, 128–129, 129ft, 130ft, 131ft
larynx, 139
nasal cavity, 50, 52, 56t
nasopharynx, 68, 71, 71f, 72f
oral cavity, 87
paranasal sinuses and nasal cavity, 50, 52, 56t
retromolar trigone, 87, 100
tonsillar fossa, 100, 102f
Neck
anatomy, 20–21, 20f, 22f, 23ft, 40f
asymmetry, 27f
bilateral lymph node involvement, 155
contralateral
data limitations, 38–39
dissection, 95
elective irradiation, 56f, 60
ipsilateral
dissection, 134
radiotherapy, 156, 157t
lower-neck region, 155
of the mandible, 27
with metastasis from unknown primary, 155
mid-neck region, 155
pathology, 19f, 21, 145
posttherapy, 24, 26–28f, 27–28

Neck classification systems
radiologic boundaries, 42, 44t
Robbins' Classification, 38, 38f, 41t, 42
surgical, 38, 38f, 40f, 41t
Neck coil, 18
Neck dissection
axial CT scan, 28f
bilateral, 95
contralateral, 95
ipsilateral, 134
with laryngeal cancer treatment, 148
muscle FDG uptake after, 31
myocutaneous graft, 27f
oral cavity cancer after, 86, 90–91f
with oral cavity cancer treatment, 95
radical, 119
Necrosis
with base of tongue cancer, 114
with irradiation
of the base of tongue, 122
of the larynx, 152
of the nasopharynx, 83
of the oral cavity, 96
overview, 160, 161, 163, 165
of the tonsillar fossa, 112
of the lymph nodes, 23, 26f
osteoradionecrosis, 112, 122, 160, 161, 163
vs. lymph node with hypodense fat, 20f, 23, 26f
Nerve damage
cranial nerves, 76, 82
with irradiation of nasopharynx, 82
optic nerve, 58, 61, 166
NOMOS Peacock system, 3
Normal tissue
avoidance of dermal toxicity, 44, 45–46f, 48, 83
delineation, 65f
protection of specific areas. See Target volume, delineation
target volume dose specification, 47t
tolerance to irradiation, 161t
Nuclear medicine tracers, 30, 32
Nutritional support, 122, 152, 165

## O

Ophthalmalogic side effects
complications from irradiation, 61, 83, 166
sacrifice of the eye, 58
Optical density (OD), 5, 6f
Optic nerve, 58, 61, 166
Oral cavity
anatomy, 85, 85f
contralateral metastasis, 40, 41t, 42f, 88t
IMRT, 95–96, 96t, 97–99f
incidence of metastasis, 41t, 89–91t
lymphatics, 85–87, 87t, 88t
natural history of cancer, 87
as primary site, 155
sequelae of IMRT treatment, 96
TNM staging, 92t
toxic effects of irradiation, 160
Oral disease, stabilization prior to treatment, 160
Oral hygiene, during and after radiation therapy, 160–162, 164t
Oral tongue
anatomy, 85, 86f
general management, 93–94
imaging, 91
incidence of metastasis, 41t, 42f, 86, 88t
natural history of cancer, 87
survival rate, 94t

**172** *Index*

Orbital invasion, 52, 55–56f, 58
Oropharynx
  anatomy, 100, 101f, 117f, 118
  incidence of metastasis, 41t
  lymph nodes, 100, 102f
  as primary site, 21, 155
  TNM staging, 105t
Osteoradionecrosis (ORN), 112, 122, 160,
    161, 163

**P**

Pacemakers, 19
Pain, 160, 162, 163, 164
Palatine arch, 100
Panendoscopy, 31
Paralysis, 129, 134
Paranasal sinuses
  anatomy, 50, 54–55f
  cartilage, 50, 51f
  general management, 58, 60, 60t
  IMRT, 60–61, 61t, 62–66f
  low incidence of metastasis, 40, 42f
  natural history of cancer, 50, 52, 56t
  orbital invasion, 52, 55–56f, 58
  physical examination, 52, 56
  prognostic factors, 58
  sequelae of IMRT treatment, 61
  signs and symptoms, 52, 56
  survival rate, 58, 60t
  TNM staging, 59t
Parapharyngeal lymph nodes. *See* Upper deep
    jugular lymph nodes
Parapharyngeal spaces, 19, 20f, 23ft, 101f, 118,
    130
Parotid glands, 15, 19, 81, 155, 163
Parotid lymph node, 24f, 68
Patient education, 160
Patient immobilization, 12, 34–35f
Patient-specific quality assurance,
    14–15
Phantoms
  anthropomorphic head, to test image fusion,
    34f
  check of single modulated fields, 11
  complete treatment plans, 11
  geometric, 6, 7f, 10
  and positioning of dose distribution, 7
  as source of discrepancy, 10
  types, 6, 7f
Pharyngeal wall, 41t, 42t, 133t
Pharyngectomy, 134, 137
Physical examination
  base of tongue, 114, 116
  hypopharynx, 129
  larynx, 140
  and lymph node micrometastases, 38
  nasopharynx, 71–72, 74t
  oral cavity, 88
  paranasal sinuses and nasal cavity, 52, 56
  tonsillar fossa, 101
Physical modulators, 3–4
Physical therapy, 163
Physics
  IMRT dosimetry, 4–10
  IMRT types, 2–4
  IMRT *vs.* 3DCRT, 1–2
  linear accelerator, 10–11
  patient immobilization and localization,
    12–14
  patient-specific quality assurance,
    14–15
Platinum-based chemotherapy, 104, 120, 149t
Portal attenuators, 3–4

Portal film, 12, 14, 14f
Positron-emitting tomography (PET)
  assessment of treatment response, 32
  brain, 165
  cervical lymph node metastasis, 31
  cost-effectiveness, 32
  CT/PET hybrid machines, 34–35
  detection of recurrence, 31–32, 32t
  FDG, 30, 31
  future developments, 35–36, 35–36f
  image fusion with CT, 32, 33–36f,
    34–36
  impact on treatment planning, 32
  staging head and neck cancer, 31, 31t
  *vs.* CT/MRI, 31–32, 31t, 32t, 33–34f
Posterior cervical lymph nodes, 21, 26f, 68, 78,
    95, 121, 136, 149
Postoperative treatment, laryngeal cancer, 148
Posttherapy, neck, 24, 26–28f, 27–28
Preepiglottic space, 18, 19f, 21, 139, 140f
Prescribed dose. *See* Dose
Pretreatment management, 160, 161
Probes, molecular, 30, 32
Prognostic factors
  hypopharynx, 131–132
  larynx, 143
  nasal cavity, 58
  nasopharynx, 76
  paranasal sinuses and nasal cavity, 58
  tonsillar fossa and faucial arch, 102
Pulmonary nodules, 31
Pulmonary stress, 148
Pyriform sinus, 41t, 42t, 130, 133t

**Q**

Quality-adjusted life-year (QALY), 32
Quality assurance (QA), 4, 10–11, 14–15
Quality of life (QOL), 47, 164

**R**

Radiation therapy
  ispilateral neck, 156, 157t
  laryngeal cancer, 148–149, 148t
  management of acute and late effects,
    160–166
  oral hygiene during and after, 160–162, 164t
  pretreatment management, 160, 161
  3D conformal, 10, 12
Radiographic film, 5, 6, 6f, 10, 15
Reconstructive surgery, 24, 27
Recurrent tumors
  after lymph node dissection, 86, 91f
  after nasopharyngeal cancer, 76t, 77t
  after neck dissection, 86, 90–91f
  after vocal cord carcinoma, 145
  imaging, 18, 31–32, 32t
  indications, 28, 28f
  patterns of failure after definitive IMRT, 48
  patterns of failure without elective neck
    treatment, 56f
Reference distribution, 9f
Retina, 61, 83, 166
Retromolar trigone, 40, 42f, 87, 88, 91,
    100
Retropharyngeal lymph node, 25f, 68, 70t, 78,
    95, 112, 118f, 121, 130, 136, 149
Robbins' Classification, 38, 38f, 41t, 42
Rotation rate, 3

**S**

Saliva, artificial, 164
Salivary glands, 18, 19f, 129, 155, 160, 162.
    *See also* Xerostomia

Scatter dose, 1
Secondary electron transport, 2
Secondary infection, 163
Secondary tumor invasion, 21
Sense of taste, 96, 160, 164
Sequelae of IMRT treatment
  base of tongue, 122
  hypopharynx, 137
  larynx, 150, 152
  nasal cavity and paranasal sinuses, 61
  nasopharynx, 82–83
  neck node metastasis of unknown primary,
    157, 157t
  nerves. *See* Nerve damage
  oral cavity, 96
  skin. *See* Dermal toxicity
  tonsillar fossa, 112
Setup, patient, 2, 10, 15
Sialadenitis, 19f, 27f
Sialogogues, 164, 164t
Signs and symptoms of cancer
  base of tongue, 114
  hypopharynx, 129
  larynx, 140
  nasopharynx, 71
  oral cavity, 87–88
  paranasal sinuses and nasal cavity, 52,
    56
  tongue, 88
  tonsillar fossa and faucial arch, 101
  xerostomia as, 163
Skin cancer, 155
Skull. *See* Base of skull
SMLC. *See* Static multileaf collimation
Smoking, 139, 152, 162
Soft tissue mass, asymmetric, 19f, 20f
Spinal accessory lymph nodes, 21, 155
Spinal cord, 15, 82–83, 161t, 165–166
Spiral computed tomography, 18, 19
Squamous cell carcinoma
  base of tongue, 114, 121, 123–124f
  hypopharynx, 129f, 135
  pyriform sinus, 135
Staging systems
  American Joint Committee on Cancer, 58,
    59t, 75t, 76t
  for PET, 31, 31t
  TNM. *See* TNM staging system
  University of Florida, 58
Standardized uptake value (SUV), 31, 32
Static multileaf collimation (SMLC), 2, 10–11
Stereotactic radiosurgery, 12
Subgastric lymph nodes, 68, 78, 95, 121, 136,
    149, 155
Subglottic larynx, 139, 140f
Sublingual lymph nodes, 19f, 21, 24f
Submandibular lymph nodes, 21, 24f, 78, 95,
    121, 136, 149, 155
Submental lymph nodes, 21, 24f
Supraglottic larynx
  anatomy, 139, 140f, 141f
  carcinoma, 140, 143t, 144ft, 145, 145t,
    147–148, 147t
  incidence of metastasis, 41t, 42t
  as primary site, 155
Suprahyoid neck region, 18
Surgical margin, as prognosis factor, 131
Surgical treatment
  base of tongue cancer, 119
  hypopharyngeal cancer, 134
  with irradiation
    base of tongue cancer, 120, 121t
    hypopharyngeal cancer, 134–135

laryngeal cancer, 148–149, 148*t*, 150
mortality, 137
neck node metastasis of unknown primary, 156
reconstructive, 24, 27
stereotactic radiosurgery, 12
three types, 24
vocal cord cancer, 144–145
Survival results
base of tongue, 121*t*
buccal mucosa, 93*t*
floor of the mouth, 95*t*
hypopharynx, 133*t*
larynx, 149*t*
lip, 93*t*
nasopharynx, 76, 77, 77*t*, 81
neck node metastasis of unknown primary, 156, 157*t*
oral tongue, 94*t*
paranasal sinuses and nasal cavity, 58, 60*t*
tonsillar fossa, 104, 106*t*
SUV. *See* Standardized uptake value
Swallowing, 148, 164
Symptoms. *See* Signs and symptoms of cancer

## T

Target volume
for definitive and postoperative IMRT, 42*t*
delineation
base of tongue, 121, 122–124*f*
and dose prescription, 42–44, 44*t*, 45–46*f*, 47, 47*t*
hypopharynx, 135*f*, 136–137
larynx, 149, 151–152*f*
nasopharynx, 78, 79–80*f*
neck node metastasis of unknown primary, 157, 158*f*
oral cavity, 95, 97–98*f*
paranasal sinuses and nasal cavity, 60–61, 62–64*f*
tonsil, 107–109*f*, 112
determination
base of tongue, 121, 122*t*
and dose prescription, 38, 39–42, 41*t*, 42*t*, 43*t*, 44*t*
hypopharynx, 134*t*, 136
larynx, 149, 150*t*
nasopharynx, 77–78, 78*t*
neck node metastasis of unknown primary, 157, 157*t*
oral cavity, 95, 96*t*
paranasal sinuses and nasal cavity, 60, 60*t*, 61*t*
tonsilar fossa and faucial arch, 104, 106*t*, 112
and management of toxic effects, 160
multiple, 1
phantoms, 11
Taste dysfunction, 96, 160, 164
Taxol, 104, 120
Technetium-99m, 30

Thermoluminescent dosimeters (TLD), 5–6
Thermoplastic mask, 12, 12*f*, 34*f*
3D conformal radiation therapy (3DCRT), 10, 12
[11]C-Thymidine, 30
Thyroid, 24, 155
Time-dose factor, 160
Tissue equivalence, 4
TLD. *See* Thermoluminescent dosimeters
TNM staging system
base of tongue, 116*t*, 119*t*
for cancers of unknown primary, 156*t*
hypopharynx, 132, 132*t*
larynx, 140, 147*t*
lymph node groups in the, 38
nasopharynx, 71*t*, 72*t*, 73, 75*t*, 76*t*
oral cavity and lip, 92*t*
oropharynx, 105*t*
paranasal sinuses, 59*t*
tonsil, 104*t*, 105*t*, 106*t*
Tolerance dose (TD), 160, 161*t*
Tomotherapy, 3
Tomotherapy, Inc., 3
T1-weighted images, 18, 20, 165
Tongue. *See also* Base of tongue; Oral tongue
anatomy, 85, 86*f*
lymph nodes, 86*f*
paralysis, 129
signs and symptoms, 88
Tonsil
carcinoma, 25*f*
incidence of metastasis, 41*t*, 42*t*
lymph nodes, 100, 102*f*
Tonsillar fossa
anatomy, 100, 102*f*
general management, 102, 105–106*t*
IMRT, 104, 106*t*, 107–111, 111*f*, 112
natural history of cancer, 100, 102*f*
prognostic factors, 102
sequelae of IMRT treatment, 112
signs and symptoms, 101
spread of cancer to base of tongue, 114
survival rate, 104, 106*t*
TNM staging, 104*t*, 105*t*, 106*t*
Tonsillectomy, 103
Toxicity
acute and late effects of radiation, 27, 160–166
dermal, 27, 44, 45–46*f*, 48, 83
Tracheoesophageal groove lymph nodes, 21
Tracheotomy, 152
Treatment plan
impact of FDG PET on, 32
modifications to resolve toxic effects, 160
paranasal sinuses and nasal cavity, 58, 60*t*
quality assurance, 15
sources of discrepancies, 8
Tricyclic medications, 163
Trismus
with IMRT, 83, 112, 122

with irradiation, 160
prosthetic aids prior to, 163
as symptom, 88, 101
True vocal cord
anatomy, 139, 140*f*, 142*f*
carcinoma, 140, 143–146, 145*f*
low incidence of metastasis, 40, 42*f*
toxicity effects, 27
T1-weighted images for, 18
T2-weighted images, 18, 20, 165
Tuberculosis, 24
Tumors
classification system. *See* TNM staging system
delineation of margins, 18
dynamics of spread, 21, 38, 68, 70*t*, 71
within fat, 18, 20*f*
location as prognosis factor, 131
within muscle, T2-weighted images for, 18, 19*f*
recurrent. *See* Recurrent tumors

## U

Ulceration, 96, 152, 161, 165, 166
Unknown primary, neck node metastasis of, 155–158, 156*f*
Upper deep jugular lymph nodes, 78, 95, 121, 136
Upper mediastinum lymph nodes, 21
Upper respiratory tract, 160

## V

Vallecula, 139, 140*f*
Vascularization
hypopharynx, 127
larynx, 139
nasopharynx, 73
neck, 22*f*, 23*f*, 40*f*
oropharynx, 101*f*
toxic effects of radiation, 112, 162, 163
Verification and validation
dose distribution, 15
dosimetry of small complex fields, 2
response to discrepancies, 8, 10
serial tomography positioning, 14*f*
using full treatment plan, 11
Vocal cord. *See* False vocal cords; True vocal cord
Voice changes, 129, 139, 140
Voice-sparing surgery, 147

## W

Water equivalence, 4, 11, 15
Weight loss, 12, 122, 129, 140

## X

Xerostomia
with IMRT, 82, 96, 112, 122, 137, 157
overview, 160, 162, 163–164, 164*t*

## Z

Zinc, 164